Special Considerations in Human Airway Management

Edited by Nabil A. Shallik

Published in London, United Kingdom

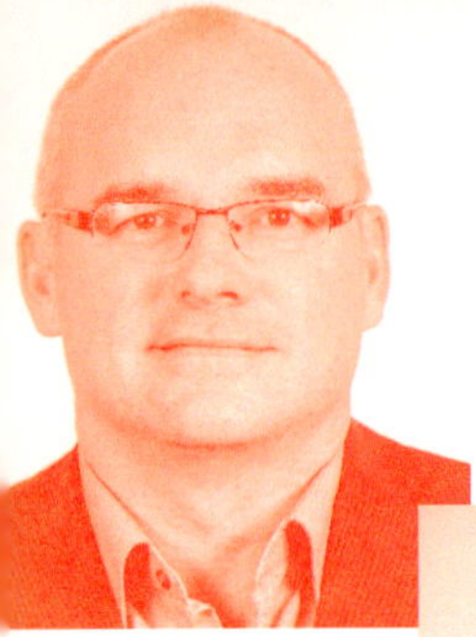
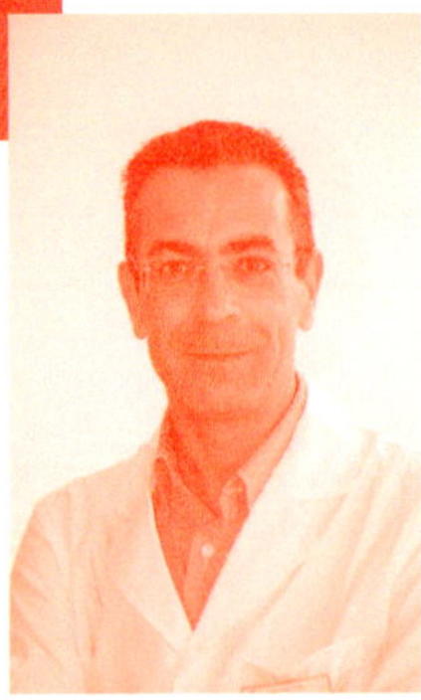
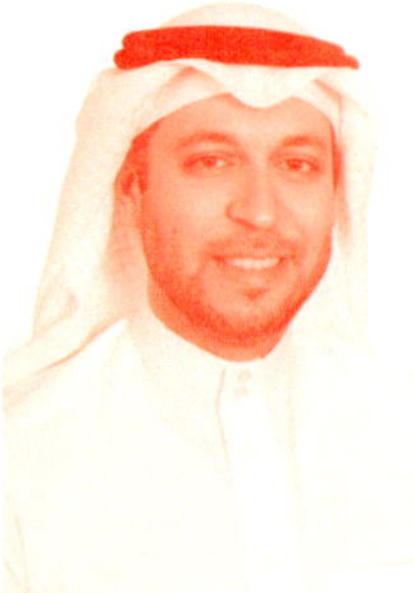
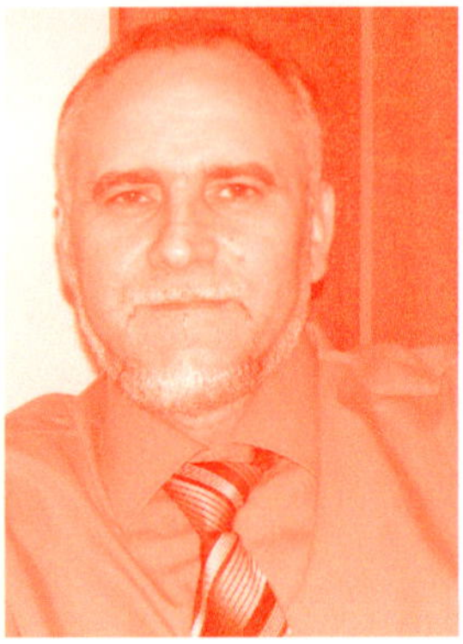
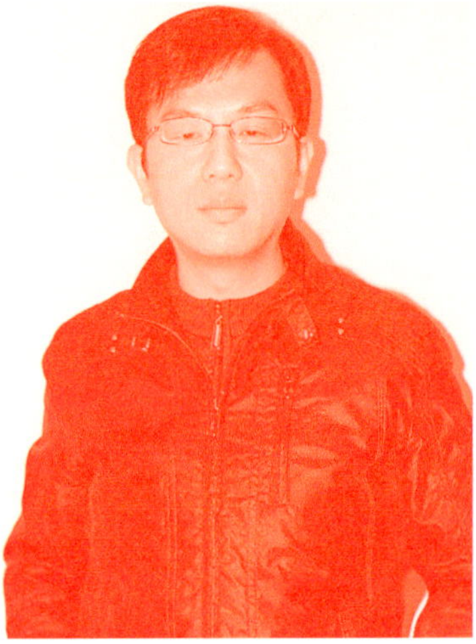
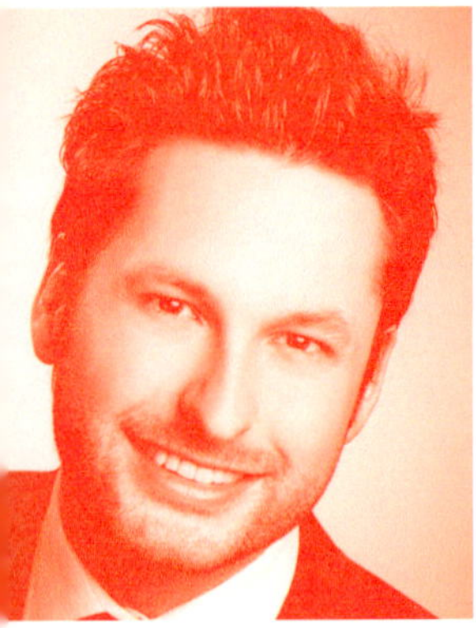
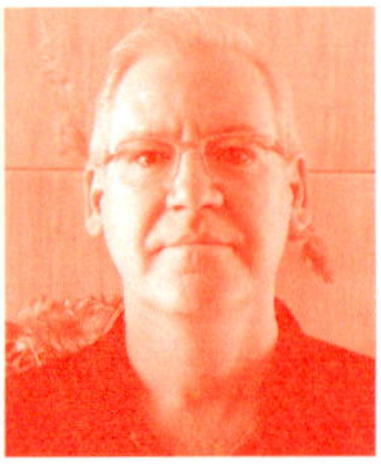

IntechOpen

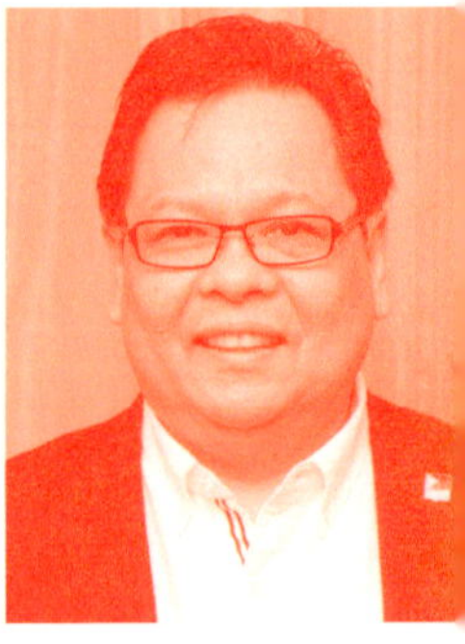
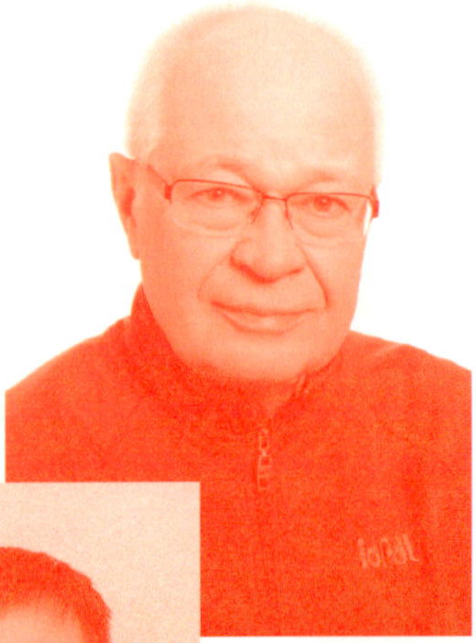
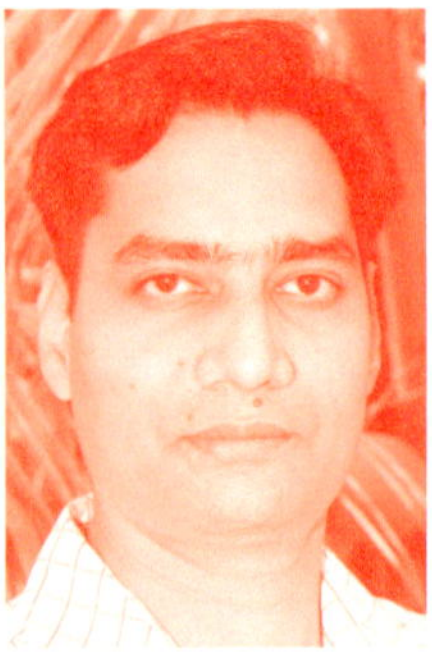
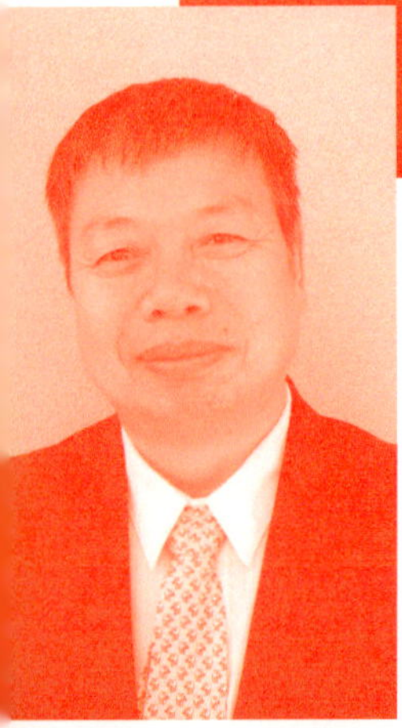
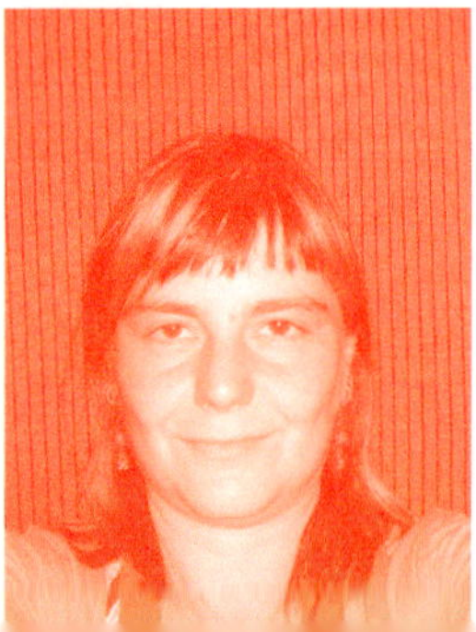
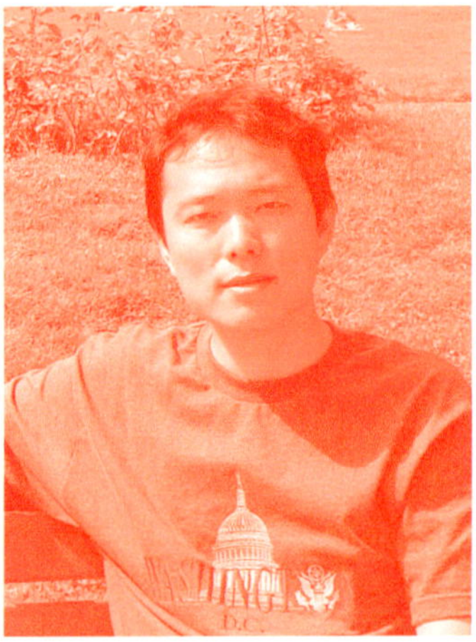

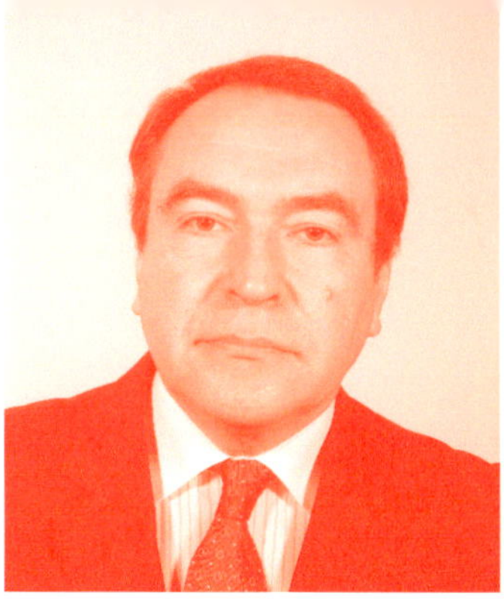
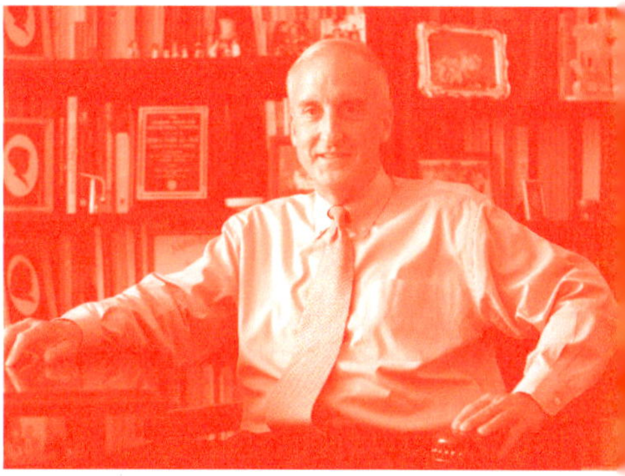
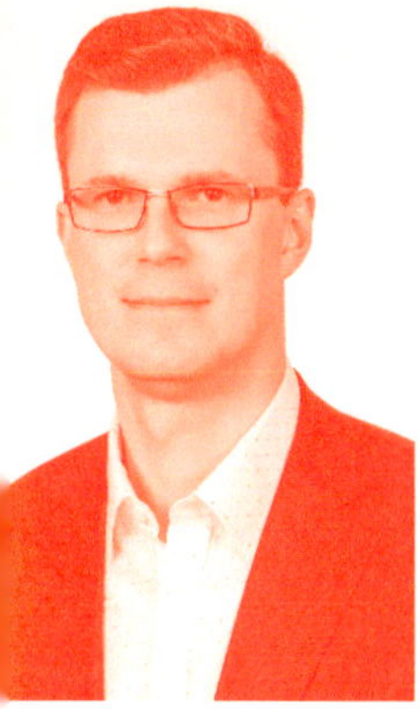
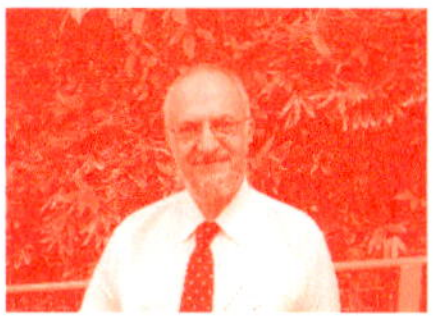
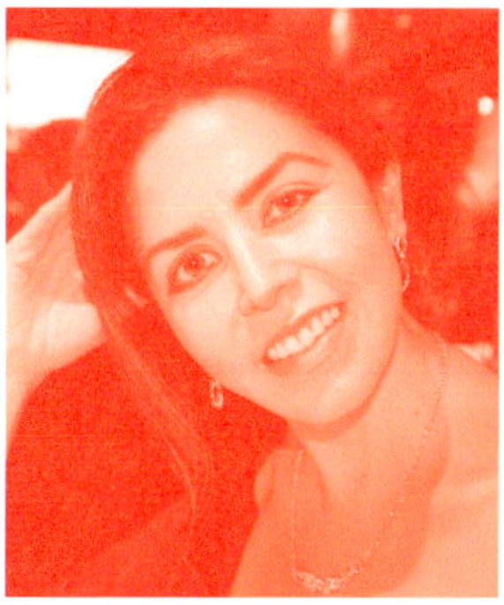

Supporting open minds since 2005

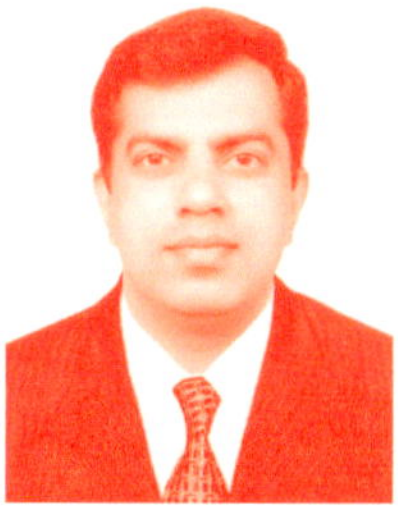
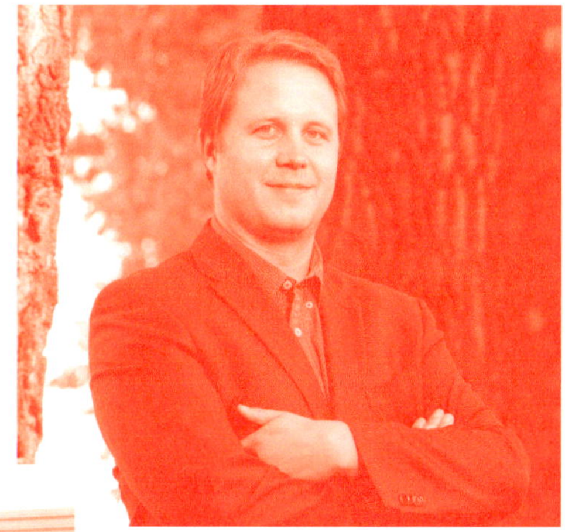
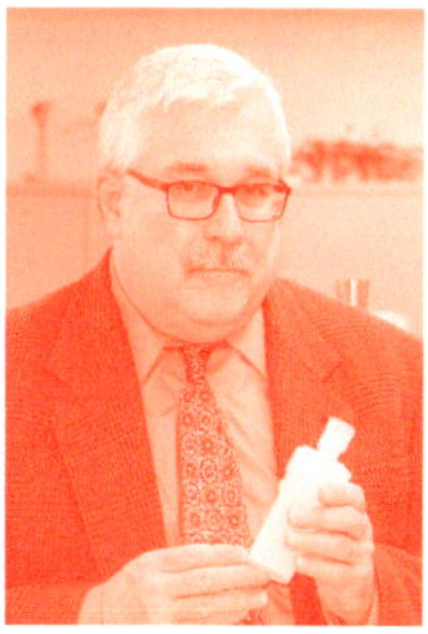
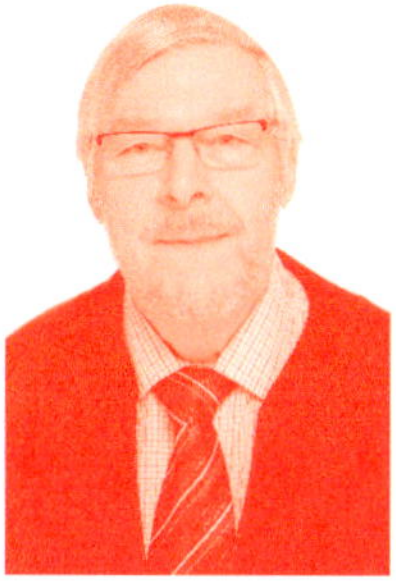
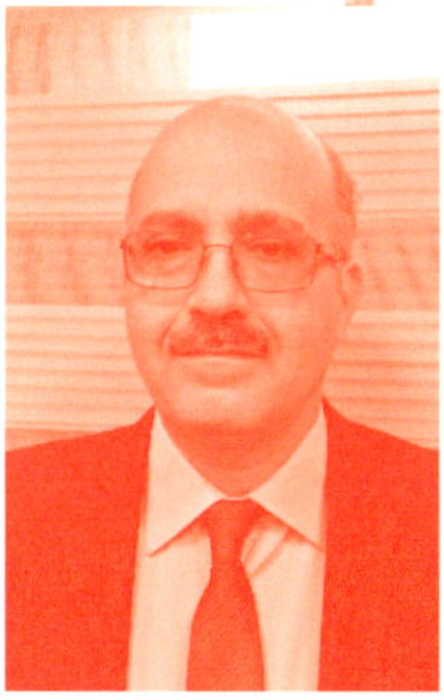
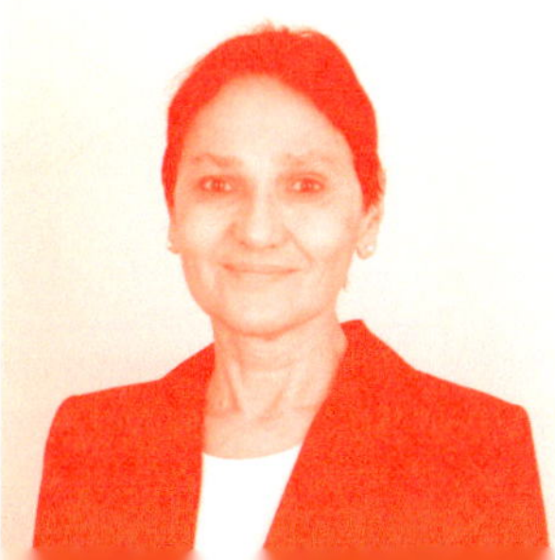
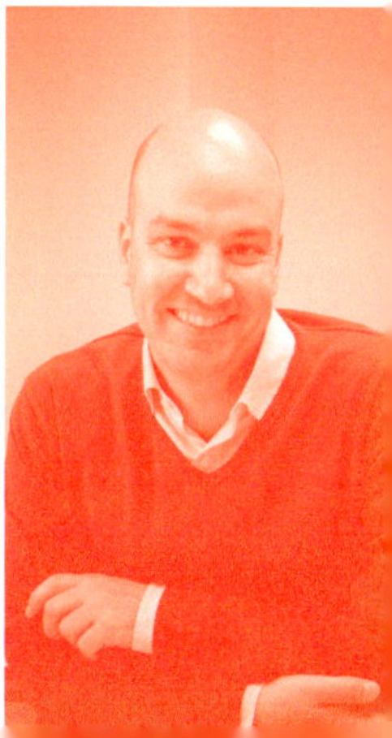

Special Considerations in Human Airway Management
http://dx.doi.org/10.5772/intechopen.91390
Edited by Nabil A. Shallik

Contributors
Nabil A. Shallik, Muhammad Firas Alhammad, Yasser Mahmoud Hammad Ali Hammad, Amr Asem Elfert, Shakeel Moideen, Mashael Al-Khelaifi, Kriti Singh, Saba Al Bassam, Ahmed Zaghw, Arunbha Karmakar, Neethu Arun, Muhammad Jaffar Khan, Mohamed Abdelwahab Elarref, Noran Elarif, Mohamed El-Arref, Mogahed Ismail Hassan Hussein, Muhammad Khan, Muayad M. Radi Al-Khafaji, Abhishek Menon, Furat Abbas, Hossam Makki, Hassan Haider, Lamia Tawfik, Mohammad Al Nobani, Tarek Tageldin, Ayten Saracoglu, Gul Cakmak, Kemal Tolga Saracoglu, Brahim Boudjenah, Surendra M. Chinnapp, Al Moataz Adham, Omed Assaf, Tatjana Goranovic, ELSayed M.E. Elkarta, Magdy Eldegwy, Preethi Reddy, Demetrio Víctor Pérez Civantos, Alicia Muñoz-Cantero, Francisco Fuentes Morillas, Pablo Nieto Sánchez, M Ángeles Santiago Triviño, Natalia Durán Caballero

First published in London, United Kingdom, 2021 by IntechOpen
IntechOpen is the global imprint of INTECHOPEN LIMITED, registered in England and Wales, registration number: 11086078, 5 Princes Gate Court, London, SW7 2QJ, United Kingdom
Printed in Croatia

British Library Cataloguing-in-Publication Data
A catalogue record for this book is available from the British Library

Additional hard and PDF copies can be obtained from orders@intechopen.com

Special Considerations in Human Airway Management
Edited by Nabil A. Shallik
p. cm.
Print ISBN 978-1-83880-387-2
Online ISBN 978-1-83880-388-9
eBook (PDF) ISBN 978-1-83880-547-0

For EU product safety concerns:
IN TECH d.o.o., Prolaz Marije Krucifikse Kozulić 3, 51000 Rijeka, Croatia, info@intechopen.com or visit our website at intechopen.com.

Meet the editor

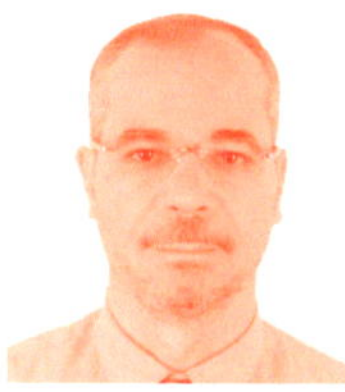

Dr. Nabil A. Shallik, MD, is Assistant Professor of Clinical Anesthesiology at Weill Cornell Medical College, Qatar, Assistant Professor of Clinical Anesthesiology, Qatar University, and Assistant Professor of Anesthesiology and Surgical Intensive Care, Faculty of Medicine, Tanta University, Egypt. He is deputy chair of the anesthesia department and associate head of anesthesia services in Ambulatory Care Center, Hamad Medical Corporation, Qatar. He also works as a senior consultant at Anesthesia, ICU, and Perioperative Medicine at Hamad General Hospital, Qatar. He has published more than fifty articles in national and international peer-reviewed medical journals, including perioperative, pain, and airway publications. He is also a reviewer and editorial board member for many international peer-reviewed medical journals. He is the official reviewer for the Hamad Medical Research Center team. He is the principal author of numerous book chapters and editor of many books. He is a leading researcher in airway management in the Middle East, and his research interests focus on perioperative care and new tools for airway assessment and management. Dr. Nabil is a pioneer in anesthesia education and a dedicated clinical teacher with more than 25 years of anesthesia practice and 20 years of faithful anesthesia teaching. Dr. Nabil is a core faculty member of the Anesthesia Residency Program, and the program's director of head and neck anesthesia & advanced airway management fellowship. He received the Award of Excellence in Medical Education in Qatar and the best teaching material award from the International Sleep Surgery Society. He is a leader of the Anesthesia Department Continuous Professional Development program. As a course director for all airway workshops and courses at Itqan Clinical Simulation and Innovation Center, he is continually testing, inventing, and tailoring basic and advanced educational modules related to airway skills to suit different healthcare providers. Dr. Nabil is an active contributor to international anesthesia societies, including Airway Management Academy, European Airway Management Society, Society of Head and Neck Anesthesia, and Difficult Airway Society. He is the founder of the Difficult Airway Management Training and Innovation Society (DAM Society). He received innovation funding from the Academic Health System in HMC for the development of three projects and is frequently invited as a guest speaker in national and international conferences.

Contents

Preface

Special Considerations in Human Airway Management is an important reference book that is easily navigated and readily available whenever a conceptual gap compromises the reader's airway management knowledge. This book is beneficial for both new trainees and senior staff who are working in the field of airway management.

In combination, knowledge and technology have the immense power to improve healthcare services. This is achieved by excellent use of the best technology for managing medical diseases and the treatment of patients. This book covers both basic and advanced topics and includes an evidence-based scientific background that is designed to help the user apply theoretical knowledge to actual patient situations.

While we did our best to prevent any misinformation and errors, we urge our readers to inform us of any mistakes, including spelling or contextual errors. We also advise that this book is not meant to replace professional or expert guidance and consultation.

Producing an educational resource of this size and complexity would not be possible without the tireless effort of our authors and a broad array of experts. We want to express our gratitude to the staff at IntechOpen who worked tirelessly to produce this book.

We would like to express our sincere gratitude to Mr. Abil Luez, who assisted in capturing most of the book's images. A special thanks to the Department of Anaesthesia, ICU and Perioperative Medicine, Hamad Medical Corporation, and departmental leaders (Drs. Mohamed Hilani, Yasser Hammad, and Mashael Al-Khelaifi) for their tireless support, encouragement, and guidance.

Finally, I would like to dedicate this book to my father and my mother who have taught me over the years and allowed me to succeed, my wife for her support, and my children for their smiles, which keep me going.

Happy reading!

Dr. Nabil A. Shallik
Hamad Medical Corporation,
Tanta Faculty of Medicine,
Weill Cornell Medical College in Qatar,
Qatar University,
Doha, Qatar

Chapter 1

Airway Management in COVID-19 as Aerosol Generating Procedure

Nabil A. Shallik, Muhammad Firas Khader Alhammad, Yasser Mahmoud Hammad Ali Hammad, Elfert Amr, Shakeel Moideen and Mashael Abdulrahman M.S. Al Khelaifi

Abstract

2020 has seen the whole world battling a pandemic. Coronavirus Disease 2019 (COVID-19) is primarily transmitted through respiratory droplets when in close contact with an infected person, by direct contact, or by contact with contaminated objects and surfaces. Aerosol generating procedures (AGPs) like intubation have a high chance of generating large concentrations of infectious aerosols. AGPs potentially put healthcare workers at an increased risk of contracting the infection, and therefore special precautions are necessary during intubation. The procedure has to be performed by an expert operator who uses appropriate personal protective equipment (PPE). Modifications of known techniques have helped to reduce the chances of contracting the infection from patients. The use of checklists has become standard safe practice. This chapter looks at the current knowledge we have regarding this illness and how we should modify our practice to make managing the airway both safer for the patient and the healthcare workers involved. It addresses the preparation, staff protection, technical aspects and aftercare of patients who need airway intervention. It recommends simulation training to familiarize staff with modifications to routine airway management.

Keywords: coronavirus, airway management, intubation, covid 19, novel virus, aerosol generating procedures

1. Introduction

The current outbreak of the novel coronavirus (Severe Acute Respiratory Syndrome Coronavirus 2 – SARS CoV-2) (COVID-19) was first reported as a cluster of pneumonia cases on Dec 31st, 2019 from Wuhan, Hubei province, China. The World Health Organization (WHO) declared COVID-19 as a public health emergency of international concern (PHEIC) on Jan 30th, 2020, and on March 11th, 2020 WHO characterized the spread of coronavirus as a pandemic.

We know that COVID-19 is primarily spread through respiratory droplets when in close contact with an infected person, or by contact with contaminated objects and surfaces. This puts healthcare workers attending to an infective patient at risk of contracting the illness, and airway management, being an AGP, would be the riskiest of all interventions. AGPs like intubation have a high chance of generating large concentrations of infectious aerosols. Therefore, special precautions are necessary during intubation. The procedure has to be performed by an expert operator who uses personal protective equipment (PPE) such as FFP3 or N95 masks, protective goggles, disposable long sleeved gowns, disposable double gloves and leg coverings. It is important to recognize mask ventilation and open suctioning of airways as AGPs. If possible, thorough preoxygenation and a rapid sequence induction and intubation (RSII) should be performed. Heat and moisture exchanger (HME) must be positioned between the mask and the breathing circuit or between the mask and the ventilation balloon. Personnel involved in the room should be kept to a minimum and this should be decided beforehand. Small changes to what we know as conventional airway management has been studied and improved upon to keep both COVID 19 patients and staff looking after them safe. This chapter looks at the details inside operating theater and kindly note that the airway management of COVID 19 patient in Intensive care settings are discussed in much details in other chapter in this book.

2. Epidemiology

Corona virus pandemic has evolved since December 2019 in Wuhan, China. Starting from Wuhan the novel virus named Severe Acute Respiratory Syndrome Coronavirus 2 (SARS-CoV-2) invaded all the over the globe [1], causing corona virus disease 2019 (COVID 19) [2]. As of July 2020, infected cases are increasing incredibly around the world. Based on current real-time reports, the estimated infected cases is fifteen million cases reported and more than 610.000 deaths worldwide [3]. The number of infected cases is expected to increase as the second peak is rising in most countries.

3. Transmission

COVID19 pandemic started as an outbreak in Wuhan with mainly transmission from animal to human. This theory was raised after most primarily infected people had visited or worked in seafood the market at Wuhan [4], and later on person to person transmission has been identified [5].

It is well known today that corona virus transmission is established by droplet. This is simply droplets with size 5–10 micron that can carry the virus. However till there is now no clear evidence to support airborne transmission (droplets size less than 5 micron which can carry the virus and able to remain in air for a period of time) but considering that this is still possible, the recommendation is to manage aerosols generating procedures as highly contaminating [6]. Experimental studies have revealed that the virus can be detected on different surfaces after these surfaces are exposed to the virus between 4 hours to 3 days depending on the surface type, the virus is more stable on plastic and stainless-steel surfaces [7].

4. Airway assessment

Airway assessment is recommended whenever there is airway management. Generally speaking the evidence behind airway assessment does not show high specificity nor sensitivity except for previous difficult intubation history, COVID 19 patients mostly need urgent or emergent interventions i.e. intubation. In these circumstances' airway evaluation is not always practical It is worth mentioning that most of these patients are critically ill. COVID 19 is known to cause laryngitis and upper airway oedema is not uncommon in this population which could make intubation challenging [8]. In COVID 19 patient's general recommendation for airway assessment will apply when it is possible and unanticipated difficult airway should be kept in mind.

COVID 19 patients are critically ill which preclude standard airway assessment.

The difficult airway is defined as:

The difficult airway is "*the clinical situation in which a conventionally trained anaesthesiologist experiences difficulty with facemask ventilation, difficulty in supraglottic device ventilation, difficulty in tracheal intubation or all three*" [9].

4.1 Steps for airway assessment

History: previous difficult intubation history, last meal, previous critical events, smoking, drooling, dysphagia, recent burn in face or upper respiratory system, head or neck trauma, OSA, snoring hoarse voice stridor.

Physical examination: mouth, face, neck, teeth, Mallampati score.

Investigations: X-Ray, USG (ultrasonography), CT, MRI, nasal endoscopy, 3D & Virtual Endoscopy (VE), can be used for airway assessment.

Many score systems and tools have been developed to predict difficult airway; useful tools might be used like:

The 6 D methods (**Table 1**): [10], **LEMON** score system (**Table 2**) [11] **MMMMASK** mnemonics (**Table 3**), or **OBESE** mnemonics (**Table 4**). (**please refer to other book's chapters for more details).**

The most important recommendation for health care provider who will take a history or will do examination of the airway of suspected or infected COVID 19, is to wear full PPE to protect himself or herself from the infection.

5. Personal protection and optimal environment

Health care workers (HCW) are at a high risk to be infected with SARS-COV-2 (COVID 19) in particular during any aerosol generating procedures. As discussed before the main transmission route appears to be by respiratory droplets and contact transmission. Not surprisingly these droplets have very high virus load [13]. In view of this protecting personnel who are managing airways in COVID 19 patients must be at the most priority. Aerosol generating procedures vary in their ability to infect HCW but intubation tracheostomy, non-invasive ventilation (NIV) and bag mask ventilation (BMV) appear to carry the highest risk [14].

All efforts should be made to protect HCW providing airway management this will include many aspects to keep in mind. We can summarize them as following:

- Full PPE (personal protective equipment)
- Surface decontamination
- Equipment decontamination
- Negative pressure room
- Minimizing health care workers during active procedure
- Waste management

Sign of difficulty	Description	Quantitative or qualitative findings reported to be associated with difficulty	Acceptable findings not usually associated with difficulty
1. Disproportion	• Increased size of tongue in relation to pharyngeal size	• Mallampati class III or IV	• Mallampati class I or II
	• Airway swelling	• Possibly difficult to assess	
	• Airway trauma (blunt or penetrating)	• Blunt or penetrating airway trauma	• Midline trachea
	• Tissue consolidation (e.g., secondary to radiation)	• Tracheal deviation	• No contractures of the neck
		• Neck asymmetry	• No surgical airway scar
2. Distortion	• Neck mass	• Voice changes	• Mobile laryngeal anatomy
	• Neck hematoma	• Subcutaneous emphysema	• Easily palpated thyroid cartilage
	• Neck abscess	• Laryngeal immobility	• Easily palpated cricoid cartilage
	• Arthritic changes in the neck joints	• Nonpalpable thyroid cartilage	
	Previous surgical airway	• Nonpalpable cricoid cartilage	
3.Decreased thyromental distance	• Anterior larynx and decreased mandibular space	• Thyromental distance >7 cm (˜3 finger breadths) measured from the superior aspect of the thyroid cartilage to the tip of the chin	• Thyromental distance ≥7 cm (–3 finger breadths)
		• Receding chin	• No receding chin
4.Decreased Inter-incisor gap	• Reduced mouth opening	• Distance between upper and lower incisors (i.e., inter-incisor gap) <4 cm (<2 finger breadths) • Mandibular condyle fracture • Rigid cervical spine collar	• Inter-incisor gap <4 cm (–2 finger breadths)
5. Decreased range of motion in any or all of the joints of the airway (i.e., atlanto-occipital joint, temporomandibular joints, cervical spine); atlantooccipital range of motion is critical for assuming the sniffing position	• Limited head extension secondary to arthritis, diabetes, or other diseases	• Head extension <35°	• Head extension ≥35° of atlanto-occipital extension
	• Previous neck radiation and/or radical surgery	• Neck flexion <35°	• Cervical spine flexion ≥35°

Sign of difficulty	Description	Quantitative or qualitative findings reported to be associated with difficulty	Acceptable findings not usually associated with difficulty
	Neck contractures secondary to burns or trauma	• Short, thick neck	• Long, thin neck
		Cervical spine collar or cervical spine immobilization	• No cervical spine collar or cervical spine
6. Dental overbite	• Large angled teeth disrupting the alignment of the airway axes and possibly decreasing the inte-rincisor gap	• Dental overbite	• No dental overbite

Table 1.
Shows 6 D methods for airway assessment: [11].

LEMON	Criterion	Score
L	**Look externally:** • facial trauma • large incisors • beard or mustache • large tongue	(1–4) 1 1 1 1
E	**Evaluate:** • incisor distance • hyoid-mental distance • thyroid-to-mouth distance	(1–3) 1 1 1
M	**Mallampati**	1
O	**Obstruction**	1
N	**Neck mobility**	1

Table 2.
Shows LEMON score for airway assessment [12].

MMMMASK	Description
M	Male gender
M	Mask seal which is affected by bread or being edentulous
M	Mallampati grade 3or4
M	Mandibular
A	Age
S	Snoring and OSA
K	Kilograms (weight)

Table 3.
Shows MMMMASK mnemonics difficult airway.

OBESE	Description
O	Obese (BMI >26 kg/m2)
B	Bearded
E	Edentulous
S	Snoring
E	Elderly (>55 years)

Table 4.
Shows OBESE mnemonics for difficult mask ventilation.

It is well known today that use of full PPE reduces the risk of infection in corona virus family [15], Based on retrospective study published on March 2020, hospital acquired infection was 41.3% from those 29% were health care workers from different specialties [16].

Level 3 (enhanced) is recommended in COVID 19 suspected or confirmed cases airway management for better understanding it is worth to mention here in summary what are the level of PERSONAL protection for healthcare workers [17] **(Table 5).**

The person who is performing the intubation should wear a third pair of gloves and remove them immediately after intubation [18].

Minimizing number of people during intubation is preferred in order to reduce risk of exposure. The interval time after intubation should be taken into consideration. The required waiting period will vary between 15 and 30 minutes [19].

Level 1 SICPs	**Standard Infection Control Precaution** • Disposable apron • Disposable gloves
Level 2 CONTACT	**DIRECT/INDIRECT CONTACT PRECAUTIONS** • Fluid-resistant disposable gown • Disposable gloves
Level 2 DROPLET	**DROPLET (RESPIRATORY) PRECAUTIONS** • Fluid-resistant disposable gown • Disposable gloves • Fluid-resistant Type IIR surgical face mask and goggle or visor
Level 2 AIRBORNE	**AIRBORNE (RESPIRATORY) PRECAUTIONS** • Fluid resistant disposable gown • disposable gloves • Filtering face piece 3 (FFP3) respirator and eye protection or a powered hood respirator
Level 3 ENHANCED	**ENHANCED PRECAUTIONS** • Reinforced fluid-resistant long-sleeved surgical gown • Disposable fluid-resistant hood (if wearing a gown without an attached hood) • Full length disposable plastic apron • FFP3 respirator or powered hood respirator • Disposable full-face visor • 2 sets of long or extended cuff non-sterile, non-latex disposable gloves • Surgical wellington boots or closed shoes • Disposable boot covers

Table 5.
Levels of personal protective equipment (PPE) for healthcare workers when providing patient care. (copied from health protection Scotland, "levels of personal protective equipment (PPE) for ward patient care").

Negative pressure rooms with good rates of air exchange (> 12 exchanges per hour) is recommended to minimize risk of airborne exposure, in case not available portable HEPA filters or negative air flow, can be considered to reduce risk.

It is very important to have a clear plan for the airway management team. The plan should be discussed in detail with clarifying the rescue one in case unanticipated difficult airway management appear.

Staff who should avoid involvement in airway management: Immunocompromised or pregnant health care workers are advised not enroll in airway management for COVID 19 patients. Also, HCW above age of 60 years old mortality curve will increase remarkably in COVID 19 and patients with cardiac disease chronic respiratory disease; diabetes; recent cancer; and perhaps hypertension that is why it is recommended to exclude HCW who have any of these co-morbidities [20].

6. Non-invasive methods of ventilation in aerosol generating procedure

6.1 Nasal cannula

Low-flow nasal oxygen (nasal cannula) may provide some oxygenation during apnoea (apnoeic oxygenation) and might therefore delay or reduce the extent of hypoxemia during tracheal intubation [21] however, literature suggests this beneficial effect might be worthless in patients with primary respiratory failure like in COVID 19 patients [22]. Till now, there is no evidence that low flow nasal canula can generate aerosols, in COVID 19 patients so, it is not recommended to use it routinely during intubation [23].

6.1.1 High flow nasal cannula

Using high flow nasal cannula (HFNC) 30–70 L/min significantly increases the risk of spreading exhaled gas [24], debate around using HFNC in COVID 19 considering it prolong apnoea time remarkably however there is few predisposed disadvantage: when used in deteriorating patients it is delaying intubation in severely ill patients who really need intubation, exhausting hospital oxygen reserves as a results in very high demand [25], when used during intubation risk of generating aerosol that carrying the virus [26].

Important note: after a few hours of ventilation by high flow nasal cannula (HFNC), the oropharyngeal airway and trachea become extremely dry, due to a high oxygen flow reaching 60 L/min. Which leads to difficulty in passing the endotracheal tube (ETT). So, make sure that the tube and the intubation equipment are very well lubricated to allow the tube to go easily through the vocal cords. Our personal experience is to soak the pharyngeal cavity with 10 ml 0.9% saline and some gel to allow a sufficient lubrication for this purpose.

6.1.2 Non-invasive ventilation

Data regarding use of non-invasive ventilation (NIV) in COVID 19 patients is limited but based on recent systematic review published recently the evidence for using NIV in COVID 19 patient is currently low in quality however it might reduce mortality and increase risk of healthcare worker transmission [27]. Many centres recommend to use NIV in view of limited resources in pandemic regions or using hyperbaric oxygen therapy in preventing mechanical ventilation in COVID-19 in other centers [28–30].

7. Intubation

7.1 Introduction

Endotracheal intubation is considered a very high-risk procedure in COVID 19 patients. For many reasons usually COVID 19 patients who need intubation urgently are critically ill patients with severe hypoxemia and respiratory failure. Desaturation is very quick because of depleted oxygen reserve and high consumption with regards to severe inflammatory status also involvement of other organ failure makes airway management of these cases are challenging. Special attention to the previous mentioned points may provide avoidance of major complications and avoidable deaths ensuring the safety of healthcare workers involved. Sever hypoxemia during ICU intubation has been reported in 25% [31]. In general, physiologically and anatomically airway management in critically ill patients consider challenging.

7.2 Before intubation

All equipment should be prepared with tracheal intubation checklist (see - **Figure 1**) [33] and preferably COVID 19 airway intubation trolley to be prepared figure [34], medications should be prepared in advance, crash trolley should be handy before progress to intubation.

7.2.1 Communication

In operating theater or in ICU setting delegated person, an outside-room "runner" to provide additional outside-room equipment and medications.

The runner can communicate with the inside personnel using special pager or phone kept inside water seal cover.

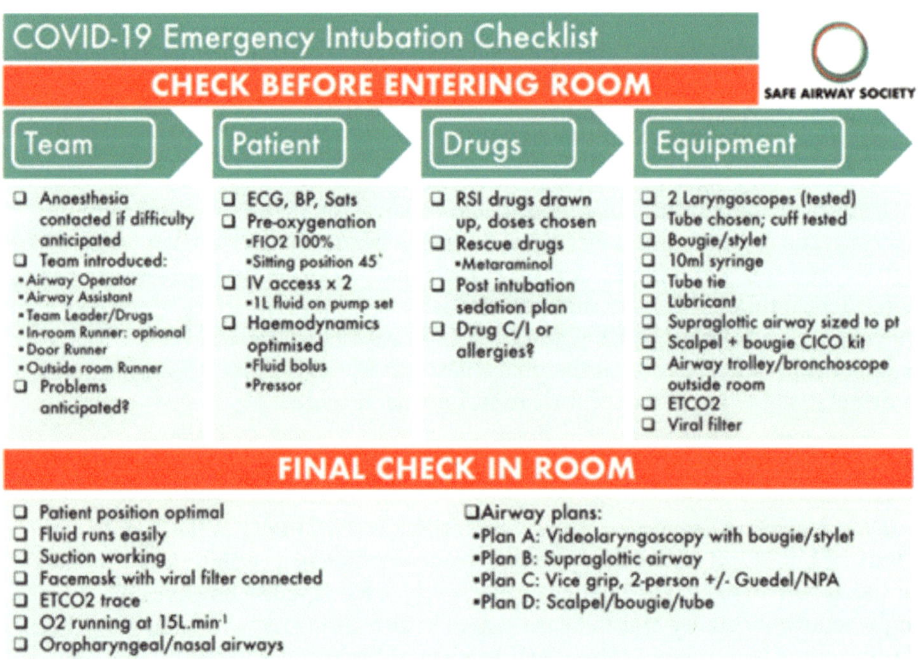

Figure 1.
Checking list an example of emergency intubation checklist from safe airway society [32].

Optimizing communication: wearing full PPE make communication is really difficult so it is very important to use clear language with loud voice repeating the order to make sure communication is efficient. As recognizing a person with full PPE is somewhat difficult so, it is recommended to put sticker with individual name on top of visor [35].

7.2.2 Virus filters

Using of heat moisture exchanger (HME filter) has been advised by many centers which can filter the viruses including Corona virus by 99 percent. HME filter should be attached most proximal to patient i.e. directly to ETT or between the mask and bag of Ambu, another alternative to HME filter that can be used is high efficiency particulate air filter (HEPA filter). Another HME filter is kept between expiratory limb of anesthesia circuit and anesthesia machine (**Figure 2**).

7.2.3 Video laryngoscope

In covid 19 pandamic Video laryngoscopy is recommended as first line option for airway management the rational be [44]:

Higher chance for ETT pass first attempt, reducing chance of infection for the intubator by increasing the distance between the patient airway and the incubators face also use of special drapes is possible and might increase the level of protection, better intubation view can be achieved especially in full PPE situation where the face shield and googles (with fog) are obstructing clear view.

Two pieces of video laryngoscope (display, single use probe) are better to be used to make sure the intubator's face is far away from the patient's mouth during the procedure [36] in addition, first pass success rate is much higher in experienced manager with video laryngoscope than direct laryngoscope.

7.2.4 Pre-oxygenation

Preoxygenation is crucial part before intubating covid 19 patients as these patients are ill and prone to very rapid desaturation due to the nature of the disease. When it is possible 3–5 minutes of preoxygenation is recommended using non rebreathing mask with 10–15 liter/O2 which provide 100% Fio2, if NRM is not enough modified non invasive ventilation might needed with close circuit and HEPA filter. If bagging the patient is inventible for preoxygenation this should be done with two hand technique with HEPA filter however avoiding bagging the patient is always recommended when it is possible [38].

Ideally pre-oxygenation could avoid necessity of bag mask ventilation but there is no guarantee especially in critical COVID 19 patients.

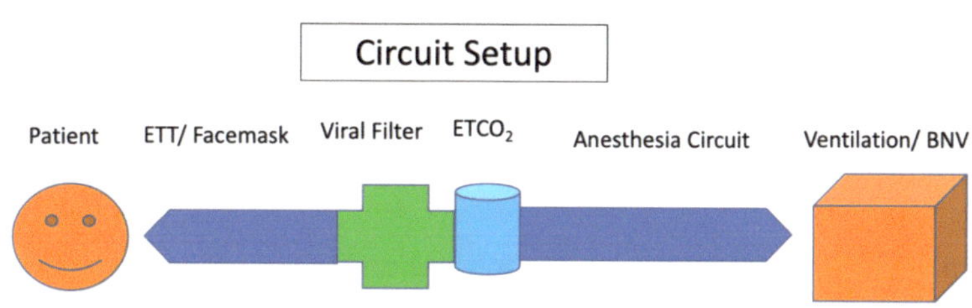

Figure 2.
Ventilation circuits setup (image courtesy Dr. Nabil Shallik).

Keeping the patient in 45 degree (reverse Trendelenburg positioning)may help in increasing apnea time improving the preoxygenation .

7.2.5 Fibroscopic intubation

Flexible bronchoscope can be used in anticipated difficult airway however, it is not advised to be used routinely. But if you in real need in difficult case, better to shift to single use fibro scope [37].

7.3 During intubation

Endotracheal Tube (ETT) confirmation site should be confirmed by $ETCO_2$ because full PPE will make auscultation much difficult and using stethoscope impractical. Clinically observing chest rising may help in precluding unilateral intubation. Also seeing the ETT passing through vocal cord and recording using video laryngoscopic screen is the best way of confirmation of endotracheal intubation.

As most of COVID 19 patients who need mechanical ventilation will have ARDS so, lung protective mechanical ventilation strategies should be used (target tidal volume less than 6 mL·kg − 1 predicted body weight, plateau pressure $\leq$ 30 cm H20, target SaO2 88–95% and pH $\geq$ 7.25 [38].

The most experience intubator should perform the intubation in order to achieve high first pass success [39] and reduce the contamination and the intubator should use a technique which he is familiar and comfortable with.

Many of novel devices have been introduced trying to achieve high level of protection during the intubation procedure itself, like novel intubation plastic box and plastic cover. Yet there is no definite evidence that such these devices could really protect the intubator from the aerosols [40], few articles suggested that and current studies are ongoing to prove it.

One of the common novel devices recently introduced is intubation novel box. First time had been described by Dr. Lai Hsien-yung [41], The device composed of a transparent plastic cube covering a patient's head and shoulders, with access holes for the intubating procedure and additional hole for an assistance. These device have been discussed in medical literature [42]but more commonly on social media and medical education websites, often being praised for their ingenuity (**Figure 3**).

Brown et al., has created "Barrier System for Airway Management of COVID-19 Patients" it is simply a plastic drape attached to a plastic bag as a protective measure during end tracheal intubation and extubation [43].

7.4 Some tips and tricks during intubation

- Modified Rapid Sequence Induction and Intubation (RSII) is advised as it reduces the time to intubation as securing the airway, with or without cricoid pressure. Drugs of choice are discussed later [44]

- Bag mask ventilation should be minimized unless there it is indicated 3–5 minutes of pre-oxygenation with 100% will help.

- Optimizing the patient position for intubation is recommended as any other intubation tool as video-laryngoscope will be used straight line head which suppose make the intubation more convenient, in obese patient ramping position is recommended.

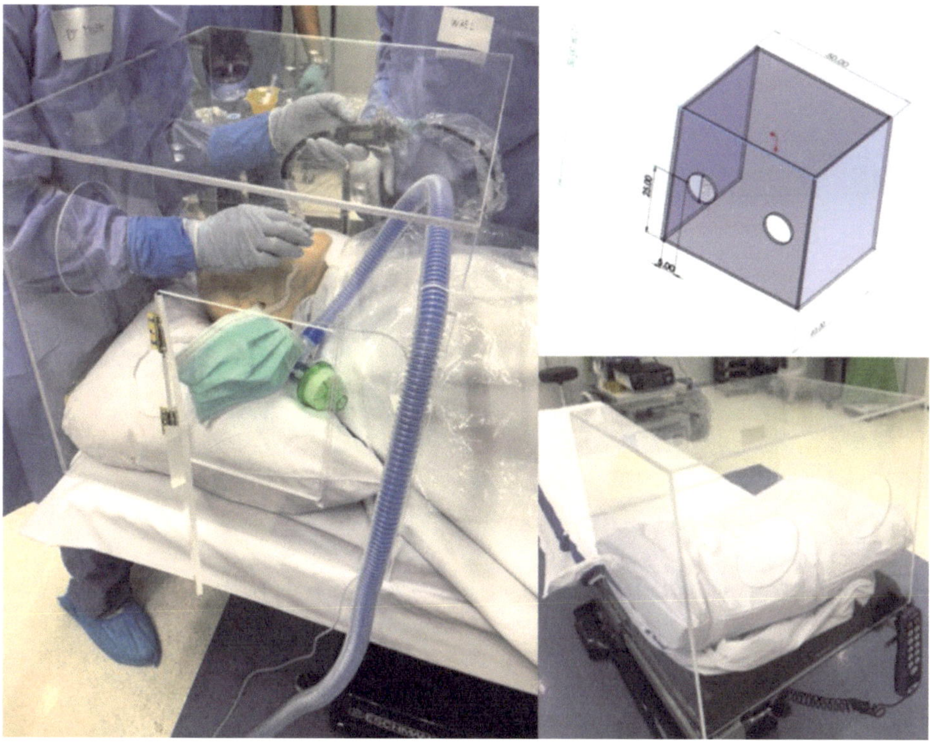

Figure 3.
Plastic intubation box (image courtesy Dr. Nabil Shallik).

- In cardiovascular instability induction agents should be chosen carefully for the best hemodynamic stability i.e. (Ketamine, Etomidate).

- Regardless of the choice of induction agents, ensure that the patient is deep enough before starting intubation to prevent coughing and straining during intubation and this will lead to aerosolization of organisms.

- As RSII is recommended, the rapid acting muscle relaxant should be used in a good dose to ensure complete relaxation that the patient will not cough for example (Succinylcholine 1.5 mg/kg, Rocuronium1.2 mg/kg).

- As many patients could have severe hypotension, loaded vasopressors should be immediately available for bolus or infusion. Phenylephrine, Ephedrine can be used as a first line.

- Some experts recommended Continuous Positive Airway Pressure (CPAP) with good sealing as this might help to delay desaturation with apneic oxygenation, using proper size oral airway after induction will help in maintaining the airway patency. If CPAP is not enough to prevent desaturation, then bag-mask ventilation should start with two hand technique and minimal oxygen flow and minimal airway pressure (**Figure 4**).

- While video-laryngoscope is the best option to start yet using adjunctive is pretty helpful for C-MAC Macintosh blade and C-MAC D-blade (Karle Storz, Germany); it is a good idea to use Gum Elastic Bougie (GEB) in case needed. Also, stylet can be used to ease intubation with GlideScope (Verathon, Burnby, BC, Canada). If video

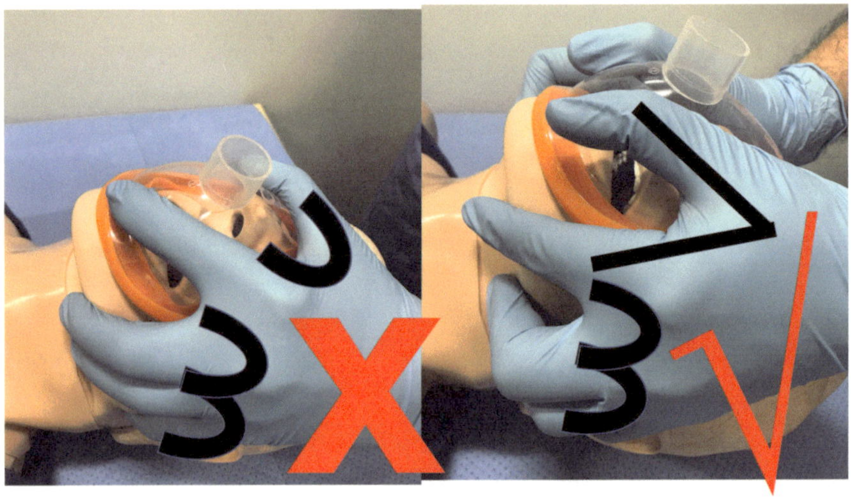

Figure 4.
(√): Two-handed two-person bag-mask technique with the VE hand position; the second person squeezes the bag. (X): The CE hand position, which should be avoided. (image courtesy Dr. Nabil Shallik).

laryngoscope is not available for any reason direct laryngoscopy could be other option using Macintosh blade with Gum Elastic Bougie (GEB) help.

- Tube size should be reliable with patient condition and should be the biggest diameter size that fit the patient preferably supplied with subglottic suction port.

- After tube insertion under direct vision, inflate the ETT cuff between 20–30 cmH_2O then connect the circuit provided by HME/HEPA filter, anesthesia machine or mechanical ventilator should be in standby mode at this point, after making sure the ETT cuff is inflated well, we can start mechanical ventilation. Waiting for capnography waveform to confirm correct tube site and observing chest movement as mentioned before.

- Please note that auscultation is not practical with full PPE and difficult to perform so, we have to rely on other parameters. Airway pressure can help the intubator or heath care provider to figure out a bronchial intubation as well as circuit leak. The reason of not using auscultation is not the impractibal procedure, the reason is not to increase the contamination risk)

- During intubation if suction needed it is advised to use close loop suction, in line catheter suction.

- Some procedure will increase the risk of circuit disconnection or ETT displacement so, attention during these procedures must be taken to avoid any complication and contamination: examples of these procedures are patient proning, nasogastric tube insertion, Trans Esophageal Echocardiography (TEE) procedure, or oral suctioning.

- For ultimate reducing possible contamination during ventilation It is recommended by safe airway society to arrange the circuit in this order, i.e. keep the $ETCO_2$ sample line always distal

- to the patient.

- **Difficult airway management:**

Difficulty can happen in many aspects:

1. Facemask ventilation is not adequate,

2. Placement of a supraglottic airway (SGA) is difficult,

3. Laryngoscopy and tracheal intubation: inability to intubate the patient.

4. Same consideration for non- COVID patients will be applied in COVID19 patients, nevertheless the reason of difficulty, the crucial part is to have a pre-prepared plan and being well ready in order to avoid any serious complications.

5. COVID 19 intubation trolley should be ready.

6. The cause of difficult airway actually is multifactorial including the effect of patient factors, the clinical setting, and the skills of the practitioner.

7. There are many local institutional policies and algorithm to manage anticipated and unanticipated difficult airway (**Figure 5**).

Declare the status clearly to team members is very important, in case FONA needed the recommended technique is the one to minimize aerosol generating i.e. The scalpel bougie-tube technique as using high flow oxygen could generate

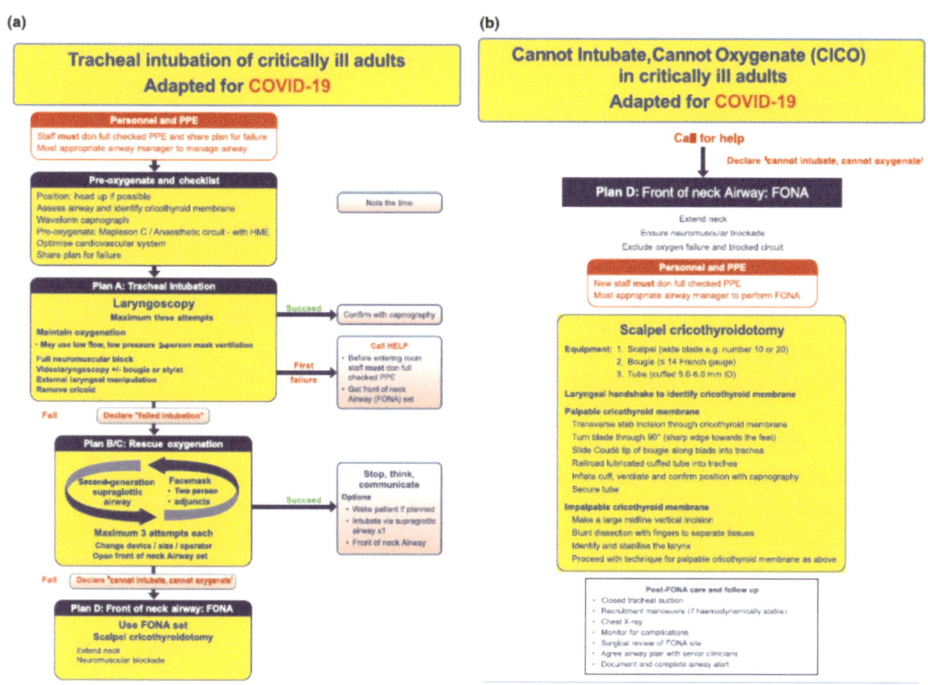

Figure 5.
(a) Tracheal intubation adapted for COVID 19 patient & (b) CICO adapted for COVID 19 patients. Taken with permission from Difficult Airway Society (DAS) 2015 guidelines [45].

aerosols and contamination [46], Front neck kit should be available immediately in case needed however it is better keep nearby the room not inside to avoid contaminate it.

8. Tracheostomy

A lot of COVID 19 patients need long time ventilation that many cases will undergo tracheostomy, currently there is debate about the proper time case selection tracheostomy technique. The major indication for tracheostomy is to facilitate mechanical ventilation for a long period, while reducing complications from a trans-laryngeal endotracheal tube and weaning from ventilation. Airway obstruction, laryngeal oedema might be an emerging feature of COVID-19 which indicate urgent tracheostomy [47, 48].

When elective tracheostomy is done, an inflated tracheostomy tube cuff via which pressure support ventilation can be delivered affords a closed system for controlled weaning of respiratory support.

Tracheostomy in COVID 19 patients is like intubation a high risk for aerosol generating same consideration will apply for intuatbion however based on recent reports for tracheostomised COVID 19 patients it is recommended to use of enhanced PPE, with PAPRs(powered air-purifying respirators), eye protection, fluid-repellent disposable surgical gown, and gloves If a PAPR is not available, we advise the use of a fit-tested filtering face piece 3 (FFP3) or N95 mask with an additional fluid shield, minimizing number of people during the procedure is necessary.

Surgical tracheostomies were generally favored over percutaneous tracheostomies during the SARS outbreak, however, percutaneous techniques have subsequently advanced and no data are available to establish superiority of one approach over the other from the standpoint of infectious transmission or safety. Single-use bronchoscopes with a sealed ventilator circuit are preferable when doing percutaneous tracheostomies.

Good sedation should ensure during the procedure to avoid cough and muscle relaxant might be used.

9. Extubation

Like intubation, extubation is an aerosol generating procedure (AGPs) and need special attention in COVID 19 patients.

Specific considerations during extubation include [49]:

i. Strategies for supporting respiration after extubation, such as noninvasive ventilation (NIV) and high-flow nasal oxygen (HFNC), are relatively contraindicated because of their ability to aerosolize SARS-CoV-2

ii. Extubation should ideally take place in a negative pressure room, if available.

iii. All non-essential staff should exit the room before extubation.

iv. Personal protective equipment (PPE) with airborne precautions is required during extubation and for personnel entering the room for a variable period of time after extubation, dependent on room ventilation.

v. Limit the need for subsequent staff interactions with:

- Prophylactic and anti-emetics.
- Adequate analgesia; consider regional anesthesia. (What kind of regional anesthesia for extubation? If it is an advice for surgery it should take place above???)

vi. Perform oropharyngeal suction with vigilance, as this may generate aerosols.

vii. Antitussive drugs, such as Remifentanil, Lidocaine, and Dexmedetomidine, reduce the risk of coughing and minimize agitation on extubation.

Ensure good sedation before extubation. Efforts to prevent cough during extubation should be implanted including possible use of medications like Dexmedetomidine, Lidocaine, and/or opioids if there is no contraindication.

10. Extubation technique

Many techniques have been described to minimize exposure to aerosols during extubation although no clear evidence behind them [50].

- Extubation under plastic cover
- Mask over tube technique with attached filter
- Extubation with LMA as alternative to ETT (contraindicated; as it can generate aerosol and contact contamination,
- Extubation with lightweight barrier hood device [51]

10.1 Endotracheal tube exchange

On the ICU there are times the ETT may need to be changed, either due to blockage or damage to the cuff. This is usually done with a tube exchanger, with the new ETT railroaded over the bougie. The lungs of a COVID-19 patient are diseased and more prone to trauma. It is advised to avoid blindly introducing a bougie into the trachea with the possibility of advancing it too deep, and thus damaging the airways, with a potential to cause a pneumothorax. If the airway is not predicted to be difficult, paralyzing the patient, preoxygenation, extubation and then reintubation with a fresh ETT using a video-laryngoscope would be the gentler way to do it.

11. Single vs. reusable equipment during COVID19 outbreak

- Ideally single use equipment is the best option in such a huge pandemic like COVID 19 pandemic, however because of the high transmission rate, applying this does not look practical especially with enormous number of infected people. It is really advised to avoid reusable equipment that will guarantee patient and health care provider safety as well. Actually, this fact utmost true when invasive equipment is used [52, 53].

- As a general rule any non-invasive equipment contaminated with patient secretions (blood, urine, vomit, or faces) or has been used with contact in suspected or confirmed COVID 19 patients must decontaminated with,1,000 parts per million available chlorine (ppm av. cl) [54]
- The real concern in single use equipment is shortage of these devices, and in highly demand situation replacement will be quite difficult.
- If re-usable equipment has been used special consideration should be taken in decontamination process following local and manufacture recommendation is a must.

12. Conclusion

Managing the airway in a patient who is potentially infective with a droplet infection needs thorough understanding of the disease process and the modifications to airway management technique, that have been seen to reduce harm to the patients and reduce spread to the airway operators. The COVID 19 pandemic has taught us better ways to manage the airway, which can be used in all aerosol generating procedures. Formulating a plan early with good preparation and using checklists, meticulous patient assessment, personal protection for staff, modification of technique and good after care are the cornerstones to achieving safe airway management in COVID19 patients and all AGPs in general.

(Best Practice Recommendations) Airway Management in Patient with Suspected Novel Coronavirus (COVID19): Permission from Qatar Difficult Airway Society (QMAD) (Figure 6)

Keep in your mind YOUR personal protection is the priority.

1. Please review the material and use droplet/contact isolation precautions (PPE – face mask, long-sleeved gown, gloves, overhead, overshoes with eye protection and fit-tested particulate respirators (N95 or equivalent, or higher level of protection) when interacting with patients' blood, body fluids, secretions (including respiratory secretions) and non-intact skin.

2. Standard precautions should always be routinely applied in all areas of health care facilities. Standard precautions include: hand hygiene; prevention of needle-stick or sharps injury; safe waste management; cleaning and disinfection of equipment; and cleaning of the environment.

3. Before intubation, review and practice wearing and removing the protective barrier mask, gloves and clothing of the infected patient. Pay close attention to avoid self-contamination.

4. Most skilled anesthetists available to perform suitable airway management technique, if possible. Avoid junior intubation for sick patients.

5. Check carefully the followings; standard ASA monitoring, I.V. access, equipment, drugs, ventilator and suction.

NAS Ver/03/20

Airway Management in Patient with Suspected Novel Coronavirus (nCoV) (Best Practice Recommendations)

1. Keep in mind YOUR personal protection is the priority.
2. Please review the material and use droplet/contact isolation precautions (PPE – face mask, long-sleeved gown, double gloves, overhead, overshoes with eye protection and fit-tested particulate respirators (N95 or equivalent, or higher level of protection) when interacting with patients' blood, body fluids, secretions (including respiratory secretions) and non-intact skin.
3. Standard precautions should always be routinely applied in all areas of health care facilities. Standard precautions include hand hygiene; prevention of needle-stick or sharps injury; safe waste management; cleaning and disinfection of equipment; and cleaning of the environment.
4. Before intubation, review and practice wearing and removing the protective barrier mask, gloves and clothing of the infected patient. Pay close attention to avoid self-contamination.
5. Most skilled anesthetists available to perform suitable airway management techniques, if possible. Avoid junior intubation for sick patients.
6. Check carefully the followings; standard ASA monitoring, I.V. access, equipment, drugs, ventilator, and closed suction unit.
7. Avoid awake fiberoptic intubation unless highly indicated. An atomized local anesthetic will aerosolize the virus.
8. Consider disposable Videolaryngoscopes to protect your face or single use Fiberscope.
9. Avoid mask ventilation, unless absolutely essential. If unable to intubate, place the SGA as a bridge. Avoid using SGA as a primary airway. Avoid/minimize the leak during Positive Pressure Ventilation.
10. Plan for rapid sequence intubation (RSI) and ensure skilled assistants able to perform cricoid pressure if needed. RSI may need to be modified if the patient has a very high alveolar-arterial gradient and is unable to tolerate a short period of apnea or has a contraindication to succinylcholine. If manual ventilation is predicted, small tidal volumes should be applied.
11. Three to five minutes of preoxygenation with oxygen 100% and RSI in order to avoid manual ventilation of the patient's lungs and potential aerosolization of virus from airways.
12. Avoid THRIVE/HFNC because it will aerosolize the virus and spread the infection inside and outside the patient's airway.
13. Ensure high-efficiency Heat & Moisture Exchange (HME) filters interposed between facemask and breathing circuit or between the facemask and self-inflating (Ambo) bag. These HME filters should be antibacterial and antiviral characters.
14. Ensure using two HME filters, one beside Endotracheal Tube (ETT) before right angle connection and a second filter at the expiratory limb of the anesthesia circuit.
15. $ETCO_2$ sample line is connected to sideway of the HME filter.
16. After intubation, confirm the correct position of the tracheal tube.
17. Start mechanical ventilation only after cuff inflation and stabilize your patient.
18. Avoid patient coughing during extubation and put a wide plastic cover around the face mask.
19. All airway equipment must be sealed in a double zip-locked plastic bag and removed for decontamination and disinfection.
20. Assigned personnel should then wipe down surfaces with appropriate disinfectant (as directed by our hospital infection control policy) after exiting the negative-pressure atmosphere.
21. After removing your PPE, avoid touching your hair or face before washing hands.
22. The HMC infection control department will provide additional updates regarding the management of patients at the various hospital facilities.

References:

Figure 6.
Qatar difficult airway society (QMAD)airway management in COVOD 19 patients.

6. Avoid awake fiberoptic intubation unless highly indicated. Atomized local anesthetic will aerosolize the virus. Consider disposable videolaryngoscopes.

7. Plan for rapid sequence intubation and intubation (RSII) and ensure skilled assistant able to perform cricoid pressure if needed. RSI may need to be modified, if patient has very high alveolar-arterial gradient and is unable to tolerate short period of apnea or has a contraindication to succinylcholine. If manual ventilation is predicted, small tidal volumes should be applied.

8. Three to five minutes of preoxygenation with oxygen 100% and RSI in order to avoid manual ventilation of patient's lungs and potential aerosolization of virus from airways.

9. Avoid THRIVE/HFNC because will aerosolize the virus and spread the infection inside and outside patient's airway.

10. Ensure high efficiency hydrophobic filter interposed between facemask and breathing circuit or between facemask and self-inflating (Ambo) bag.

11. After intubation; confirm correct position of tracheal tube.

12. Start mechanical ventilation and stabilize your patient.

13. All airway equipment must be sealed in double zip-locked plastic bag and removed for decontamination and disinfection.

14. Assigned personnel should then wipe down surfaces with appropriate disinfectant (as directed by our hospital infection control policy) after exiting the negative-pressure atmosphere.

15. After removing your PPE, avoid touching your hair or face before washing hands.

16. Hospital infection control department will provide additional updates regarding the management of patients at the various hospital facilities.

Author details

Nabil A. Shallik[1,2,3,4*], Muhammad Firas Khader Alhammad[1], Yasser Mahmoud Hammad Ali Hammad[1,2], Elfert Amr[5], Shakeel Moideen[1] and Mashael Abdulrahman M.S. Al Khelaifi[1,2]

1 Department of Anaesthesia, ICU and Perioperative Medicine, HMC, Doha, Qatar

2 Weill Cornell Medical College in Qatar, Doha, Qatar

3 Qatar University, Doha, Qatar

4 Tanta Faculty of Medicine, Tanta, Egypt

5 UIC College of Medicine, Chicago, USA

*Address all correspondence to: nshallik@hamad.qa

References

[1] 'Naming the Coronavirus Disease (COVID-19) and the Virus That Causes It' <https://www.who.int/emergencies/diseases/novel-coronavirus-2019/technical-guidance/naming-the-coronavirus-disease-(covid-2019)-and-the-virus-that-causes-it> [accessed 17 June 2020].

[2] Harapan Harapan and others, 'Coronavirus Disease 2019 (COVID-19): A Literature Review', *Journal of Infection and Public Health*, 13.5 (2020), 667–73 <https://doi.org/https://doi.org/10.1016/j.jiph.2020.03.019>.

[3] 'COVID-19 Map - Johns Hopkins Coronavirus Resource Center' <https://coronavirus.jhu.edu/map.html> [accessed 17 June 2020].

[4] WHO, 'Novel Coronavirus (2019-NCoV) 22 January 2020', *WHO Bulletin*, JANUARY, 2020, 1–7 <https://www.who.int/docs/default-source/coronaviruse/situation-reports/20200122-sitrep-2-2019-ncov.pdf>.

[5] Jasper Fuk Woo Chan and others, 'A Familial Cluster of Pneumonia Associated with the 2019 Novel Coronavirus Indicating Person-to-Person Transmission: A Study of a Family Cluster', *The Lancet*, 2020, 514–23 <https://doi.org/10.1016/S0140-6736(20)30154-9>.

[6] 'Modes of Transmission of Virus Causing COVID-19: Implications for IPC Precaution Recommendations' <https://www.who.int/news-room/commentaries/detail/modes-of-transmission-of-virus-causing-covid-19-implications-for-ipc-precaution-recommendations> [accessed 17 June 2020].

[7] Neeltje Van Doremalen and others, 'Aerosol and Surface Stability of SARS-CoV-2 as Compared with SARS-CoV-1', *New England Journal of Medicine* (Massachussetts Medical Society, 2020), 1564–67 <https://doi.org/10.1056/NEJMc2004973>.

[8] B. A. McGrath, S. Wallace, and J. Goswamy, 'Laryngeal Oedema Associated with <scp>COVID</Scp> –19 Complicating Airway Management', *Anaesthesia*, 75.7 (2020), 972–972 <https://doi.org/10.1111/anae.15092>.

[9] Jeffrey L. Apfelbaum and others, 'Practice Guidelines for Management of the Difficult Airway: An Updated Report by the American Society of Anesthesiologists Task Force on Management of the Difficult Airway', *Anesthesiology* (The American Society of Anesthesiologists, 2013), 251–70 <https://doi.org/10.1097/ALN.0b013e31827773b2>.

[10] James M. Rich, 'Recognition and Management of the Difficult Airway with Special Emphasis on the Intubating Lma-Fastrach/Whistle Technique: A Brief Review with Case Reports', *Baylor University Medical Center Proceedings*, 18.3 (2005), 220–27 <https://doi.org/10.1080/08998280.2005.11928072>.

[11] Rich, James M., 'Recognition and Management of the Difficult Airway with Special Emphasis on the Intubating Lma-Fastrach/Whistle Technique: A Brief Review with Case Reports', Baylor University Medical Center Proceedings, 18.3 (2005), 220–27 <https://doi.org/10.1080/08998280.2005.11928072>

[12] Sunanda Gupta, Rajesh Sharma, and Dimpel Jain, 'Airway Assessment: Predictors of Difficult Airway', *Indian J Anaesth*, 49.4 (2005), 257–62.

[13] Dawei Wang and others, 'Clinical Characteristics of 138 Hospitalized Patients with 2019 Novel Coronavirus-Infected Pneumonia in Wuhan, China', *JAMA - Journal of the American Medical Association*, 323.11 (2020), 1061–69 <https://doi.org/10.1001/jama.2020.1585>.

[14] Khai Tran and others, 'Aerosol Generating Procedures and Risk of Transmission of Acute Respiratory Infections to Healthcare Workers: A Systematic Review', *PLoS ONE* (Public Library of Science, 2012) <https://doi.org/10.1371/journal.pone.0035797>.

[15] Mark Loeb and others, 'SARS among Critical Care Nurses, Toronto', *Emerging Infectious Diseases*, 10.2 (2004), 251–55 <https://doi.org/10.3201/eid1002.030838>.

[16] Wang, Dawei, Bo Hu, Chang Hu, Fangfang Zhu, Xing Liu, Jing Zhang, and others, 'Clinical Characteristics of 138 Hospitalized Patients with 2019 Novel Coronavirus-Infected Pneumonia in Wuhan, China', *JAMA - Journal of the American Medical Association*, 323.11 (2020), 1061–69 <https://doi.org/10.1001/jama.2020.1585>.

[17] health protection Scotland, 'Levels of Personal Protective Equipment (PPE) for Ward Patient Care' <http://webcache.googleusercontent.com/search?q=cache:z2Ta_6e3Ch4J:www.nipcm.hps.scot.nhs.uk/media/1437/2019-02-11-aide-memoire-for-levels-of-personal-protective-equipment-ppe-for-healthcare-workers-for-patient-care.pdf+&cd=1&hl=en&ct=clnk&gl=qa&client=fir> [accessed 22 June 2020].

[18] Mengqiang Luo and others, 'Precautions for Intubating Patients with COVID-19', *Anesthesiology* (Lippincott Williams and Wilkins, 2020), 1616–18 <https://doi.org/10.1097/ALN.0000000000003288>.

[19] 'COVID-19 and Anesthesia FAQ - Anesthesia Patient Safety Foundation' < https://www.apsf.org/covid-19-and-anesthesia-faq/#clinicalcare.> [accessed 22 June 2020].

[20] Zunyou Wu and Jennifer M. McGoogan, 'Characteristics of and Important Lessons from the Coronavirus Disease 2019 (COVID-19) Outbreak in China: Summary of a Report of 72314 Cases from the Chinese Center for Disease Control and Prevention', *JAMA - Journal of the American Medical Association* (American Medical Association, 2020), 1239–42 <https://doi.org/10.1001/jama.2020.2648>.

[21] A. Higgs and others, 'Guidelines for the Management of Tracheal Intubation in Critically Ill Adults', *British Journal of Anaesthesia*, 120.2 (2018), 323–52 <https://doi.org/10.1016/j.bja.2017.10.021>.

[22] Joshua M. Gleason, Bill R. Christian, and Erik D. Barton, 'Nasal Cannula Apneic Oxygenation Prevents Desaturation during Endotracheal Intubation: An Integrative Literature Review', *Western Journal of Emergency Medicine*, 19.2 (2018), 403–11 <https://doi.org/10.5811/westjem.2017.12.34699>.

[23] 'COVID-19 Transmission Assessment Report | Vapotherm - Mask-Free NIV' <https://vapotherm.com/blog/transmission-assessment-report/> [accessed 23 July 2020] Chinese Medical Association Respiratory Branch Respiratory Therapy Group, 'Expert Consensus on Respiratory Therapy Related to New Coronavirus Infection in Severe and Critical Patients', *Chinese Journal of Tuberculosis and Respiratory Medicine*, 2020.

[24] Agarwal, Arnav, John Basmaji, Fiona Muttalib, David Granton, Dipayan Chaudhuri, Devin Chetan, and others, 'High-Flow Nasal Cannula for Acute Hypoxemic Respiratory Failure in Patients with COVID-19: Systematic Reviews of Effectiveness and Its Risks of Aerosolization, Dispersion, and Infection TransmissionLes Canules Nasales à Haut Débit Pour Le Traitement de l'insuffisance Respiratoire Hypoxémique Aiguë Chez Les Patients Atteints de La COVID-19: Comptes Rendus Systématiques de

l'efficacité et Des Risques d'aérosolisation, de Dispersion et de Transmission de l'infection', Canadian Journal of Anesthesia/Journal Canadien d'anesthésie, 2020, 1 <https://doi.org/10.1007/s12630-020-01740-2>

[25] *Will Loh NH,Tan Y,Taculod J, et al.* The impact of high-flow nasal cannula (HFNC) on coughing distance: implications on its use during the novel coronavirus disease outbreak. Can J Anesth 2020; DOI: https://doi.org/10.1007/s12630-020-01634-3

[26] Respiratory Therapy Group, Chinese Medical Association Respiratory Branch, 'Expert Consensus on Respiratory Therapy Related to New Coronavirus Infection in Severe and Critical Patients', *Chinese Journal of Tuberculosis and Respiratory Medicine*, 2020

[27] Holger J. Schünemann and others, 'Ventilation Techniques and Risk for Transmission of Coronavirus Disease, Including COVID-19', *Annals of Internal Medicine*, 2020 <https://doi.org/10.7326/m20-2306>.

[28] M. A. Baugh, 'HIV: Reactive Oxygen Species, Enveloped Viruses and Hyperbaric Oxygen', *Medical Hypotheses*, 55.3 (2000), 232–38 <https://doi.org/10.1054/mehy.2000.1048>.

[29] Stephen R. Thom, 'Hyperbaric Oxygen: Its Mechanisms and Efficacy', *Plastic and Reconstructive Surgery*, 127. SUPPL. 1 S (2011), 131S <https://doi.org/10.1097/PRS.0b013e3181fbe2bf>.

[30] Kerry Thibodeaux and others, 'Hyperbaric Oxygen Therapy in Preventing Mechanical Ventilation in COVID-19 Patients: A Retrospective Case Series', *Journal of Wound Care*, 29. Sup5a (2020), S4–8 <https://doi.org/10.12968/jowc.2020.29.Sup5a.S4>.

[31] A. Higgs and others, 'Guidelines for the Management of Tracheal Intubation in Critically Ill Adults', *British Journal of Anaesthesia*, 120.2 (2018), 323–52 <https://doi.org/10.1016/j.bja.2017.10.021>.

[32] Brewster, David J, Nicholas Chrimes, Thy B T Do, Kirstin Fraser, Christopher J Groombridge, Andy Higgs, and others, 'Consensus Statement: Safe Airway Society Principles of Airway Management and Tracheal Intubation Specific to the <scp>COVID</Scp>−19 Adult Patient Group', *Medical Journal of Australia*, 212.10 (2020), 472–81 https://doi.org/10.5694/mja2.50598

[33] safe airway society, 'Safe Airway Society', Infographic <https://www.safeairwaysociety.org/covid19/> [accessed 23 July 2020]

[34] David J Brewster and others, 'Consensus Statement: Safe Airway Society Principles of Airway Management and Tracheal Intubation Specific to the <scp>COVID</Scp> −19 Adult Patient Group', *Medical Journal of Australia*, 212.10 (2020), 472–81 <https://doi.org/10.5694/mja2.50598>.

[35] Saito, Tomoyuki, Asuka Taguchi, and Takashi Asai, 'Videolaryngoscopy for Tracheal Intubation in Patients with COVID-19', British Journal of Anaesthesia (Elsevier Ltd, 2020) <https://doi.org/10.1016/j.bja.2020.06.002>

[36] D Hall and others, 'Videolaryngoscopy Increases 'Mouth-to-mouth'Distance Compared with Direct Laryngoscopy', *Anaesthesia*, 75.6 (2020), 822–23.

[37] Mengqiang Luo and others, 'Precautions for Intubating Patients with COVID-19', Anesthesiology (Lippincott Williams and Wilkins, 2020), 1616–18 <https://doi.org/10.1097/ALN.0000000000003288>.

[38] Randy S. Wax and Michael D. Christian, 'Practical Recommendations for Critical Care and Anesthesiology Teams Caring for Novel Coronavirus (2019-NCoV) Patients', *Canadian Journal of Anesthesia* (Springer, 2020), 568–76 <https://doi.org/10.1007/s12630-020-01591-x>.

[39] Louise Park, Irene Zeng, and Andrew Brainard, 'Systematic Review and Meta-analysis of First-pass Success Rates in Emergency Department Intubation: Creating a Benchmark for Emergency Airway Care', *Emergency Medicine Australasia*, 29.1 (2017), 40–47.

[40] Clyde T. Matava, Julie Yu, and Simon Denning, 'Clear Plastic Drapes May Be Effective at Limiting Aerosolization and Droplet Spray during Extubation: Implications for COVID-19', *Canadian Journal of Anesthesia* (Springer, 2020), 902–4 <https://doi.org/10.1007/s12630-020-01649-w>.

[41] 'Taiwanese Doctor Invents Device to Protect US Doctors against Coronavirus | Taiwan News' <https://www.taiwannews.com.tw/en/news/3902435> [accessed 11 July 2020].

[42] Robert Canelli and others, 'Barrier Enclosure during Endotracheal Intubation', *The New England Journal of Medicine* (NLM (Medline), 2020), 1957–58 <https://doi.org/10.1056/NEJMc2007589>.

[43] Sarah Brown and others, 'Barrier System for Airway Management of COVID-19 Patients', *Anesthesia & Analgesia*, 131.1 (2020), e34–35 <https://doi.org/10.1213/ane.0000000000004876>.

[44] T M Cook and others, 'Consensus Guidelines for Managing the Airway in Patients with COVID-19: Guidelines from the Difficult Airway Society, the Association of Anaesthetists the Intensive Care Society, the Faculty of Intensive Care Medicine and the Royal College of Anaesthetist', *Anaesthesia*, 75.6 (2020), 785–99.

[45] Jeffrey L. Apfelbaum and others, 'Practice Guidelines for Management of the Difficult Airway: An Updated Report by the American Society of Anesthesiologists Task Force on Management of the Difficult Airway', *Anesthesiology* (The American Society of Anesthesiologists, 2013), 251–70 <https://doi.org/10.1097/ALN.0b013e31827773b2>.

[46] 'Anesthesia in Patients with Positive COVID Status & Difficult Airway | Department of Anesthesiology and Pain Medicine' <https://www.anesthesia.utoronto.ca/anesthesia-patients-positive-covid-status-difficult-airway> [accessed 23 July 2020]

[47] Brendan A. McGrath and others, 'Tracheostomy in the COVID-19 Era: Global and Multidisciplinary Guidance', The Lancet Respiratory Medicine (Lancet Publishing Group, 2020) <https://doi.org/10.1016/S2213-2600(20)30230-7>.

[48] B. A. McGrath, S. Wallace, and J. Goswamy, 'Laryngeal Oedema Associated with <scp>COVID</Scp>–19 Complicating Airway Management', *Anaesthesia*, 75.7 (2020), 972–972 <https://doi.org/10.1111/anae.15092>.

[49] David F. D'Silva and others, 'Extubation of Patients with COVID-19', British Journal of Anaesthesia (Elsevier Ltd, 2020), e192 <https://doi.org/10.1016/j.bja.2020.03.016>.

[50] Aaron W. Kangas-Dick and others, 'Safe Extubation during the COVID-19 Pandemic', Respiratory Medicine (W.B. Saunders Ltd, 2020), 106038 <https://doi.org/10.1016/j.rmed.2020.106038>.

[51] Choi, G.Y., Wan, W.T., Chan, A.K., Tong, S.K., Poon, S.T. and Joynt, G.M.,

2020. Preparedness for COVID-19: in situ simulation to enhance infection control systems in the intensive care unit. British Journal of Anaesthesia.

[52] Choi, G.Y., Wan, W.T., Chan, A.K., Tong, S.K., Poon, S.T. and Joynt, G.M., 2020. Preparedness for COVID-19: in situ simulation to enhance infection control systems in the intensive care unit. *British Journal of Anaesthesia*.

[53] Wong, J., Goh, Q.Y., Tan, Z. *et al.* Preparing for a COVID-19 pandemic: a review of operating room outbreak response measures in a large tertiary hospital in Singapore. *Can J Anesth/J Can Anesth* **67**, 732–745 (2020). https://doi.org/10.1007/s12630-020-01620-9

[54] https://assets.publishing.service.gov.uk/government/uploads/system/uploads/attachment_data/file/877533/Routine_decontamination_of_reusable_noninvasive_equipment.pdf

Chapter 2

Airway Management in the Pre-Hospital Setting

Lamia Tawfik, Mohammad Al Nobani and Tarek Tageldin

Abstract

This chapter explores the different techniques and challenges faced by emergency medical providers during pre-hospital airway management of critically ill patients. It is a crucial topic that has a major impact on patient's safety. Improper airway management in this category of patients can lead to catastrophic results in terms of morbidity and mortality, this fact stimulates the ongoing improvement and evolution in this area of practice. We explore some of the debatable topics in pre-hospital airway management like airway management in the pediatric group, the use of medication assisted intubation and rapid sequence intubation in the field as well as the role of video assisted intubation and it's challenges in the field. The up-to-date practices and research findings in the most recent related articles are discussed here in this chapter.

Keywords: airway management, pre-hospital, paramedics, endotracheal intubation, advanced airway management techniques, basic airway management techniques

1. Introduction

Prehospital airway management is a core component of emergency services, it is a vital and challenging skill of emergency service responders around the globe. The advancement of pre-hospital airway control procedures and equipment represents the evolution of pre-hospital triage and emergency care.

The spectrum of airway management outside of the hospital involves a wide array of skills and techniques, starting with basic airway skills that are included in basic life support training (BLS) such as mouth to mouth or mouth to nose ventilation and use of the simple oxygen face masks, moving to intermediate airway management techniques like bag mask ventilation or use of oral and nasal airway devices, ending with advanced airway management techniques like use of supraglottic devices, endotracheal intubation or surgical airway techniques.

Prehospital airway management services are provided by a spectrum of providers who have different levels of training and skills. For example, basic airway skills can be provided by a lay person since it has been taught to the public for decades now. Intermediate and advanced skills are performed by emergency medical service responders, who also have a variable level of training. The majority of the Emergency Medical Service (EMS) systems around the world utilize non-physician providers, while in other countries they do operate with a physician staffed EMS.

2. Challenges in airway management

Airway management in the prehospital setting has major challenges. Achieving a successful airway management requires a collection of adjustments that involve equipment, personnel and medication in a simultaneous fashion. In addition to the logistic challenges an effort in identifying the patient who need urgent advanced airway management techniques from those whom basic airway maneuvers are adequate. Over the years prehospital airway management has become progressively formalized, local and international associations in different countries has put in place guidelines to improve patient safety and standardize the process. Although there are noticeable differences in EMS infrastructure in different countries which are reflected in those different guidelines, needless to say the purpose of those guidelines is the same, with the main focus being the patient safety.

In general, most of the protocols suggest that advanced airway management techniques should only be carried out by appropriately skilled personnel, at the same time attention should focus on performing high quality basic airway maneuvers when personnel with advanced airway skills aren't immediately available.

3. Airway management equipment and techniques in the prehospital setting

3.1 Mouth to mouth ventilation

In certain circumstances, when other airway equipment's aren't available this technique can be used initially to maintain oxygenation and ventilation. A barrier should be used to avoid infection transmission [1].

3.1.1 Techniques

Adults:

Head-tilt/chin-lift to open the airway while pinching the person's nose closed and the hand over his head. The lips have to surround the mouth to create a seal. Start to blow into the person's mouth for one second and watch the chest rise. This maneuver is contraindicated when cervical spine injuries are suspected.

Pediatrics:

Head-tilt/chin-lift to open the airway. The lips have to surround the mouth and nose of the child to create a seal. Blow gently the child's nose mouth for one second. Note that the infant's lungs need a smaller volume of air than an adult., Watch the chest rise while blowing.

3.2 Spontaneous breathing

It is performed when the rescuer is dealing with a spontaneously breathing patient assisting him to maintain adequate oxygenation and ventilation, with the aid of simple of equipment such as oral or nasal airway devices that can maintain upper airway patency.

Oxygenation can be maintained via simple face mask, nasal cannula or non-rebreathing face mask. Continuous positive pressure ventilation (CPAP) by applying a fitting mask to allow CPAP with spontaneous ventilation can also be implemented in special circumstances when deemed appropriate. This method is found to decrease rates of intubation and mortality [2].

3.3 Bag-mask-ventilation (BMV)

It is a standard maneuver for initial airway management, the mask applied to the patient's mouth and nose with a properly tight seal being formed between the patient's mouth and the mask to improve oxygenation and ventilation.

It can also be used if endotracheal intubation is planned to avoid oxygen desaturation during the process of intubation.

BMV can be applied by one person using one hand bag mask ventilation technique or by two providers using two hand bag mask ventilation technique in cases were mainting proper seal and proper ventilation becomes difficult.

3.4 Oropharyngeal and nasopharyngeal airways

They are used frequently by prehospital rescuers for spontaneous and assisted breathing to improve both oxygenation and ventilation. They should be avoided in patients suffering from facial and head injuries.

The oropharyngeal airway device is ideal for use in unresponsive or unconscious patients who have depressed airway reflexes. Keeping in mind that patient with intact gag reflex might not be able to tolerate the device. On the other hand, The nasopharyngeal airway is usually better tolerated by conscious patients, it is useful also in patients having trauma to oral structures. The proper size should be carefully selected.

3.5 Supra-glottic airway devices (SGA)

SGA is a broad term for devices which sits above the glottic opening, examples includes laryngeal masks, Proseal LMA, Intubating LMA (ILMA, Fastrach), LMA Supreme, LMA Protector, i-gel (with non-inflatable cuff).

The ease of use for non-experienced personnel, makes those devices an appealing option for the use in the out of hospital environment or remote setup. SGA insertion does not require sophisticated skills, it provides proper means of ventilation and oxygenation in unconscious patients. Those features helped the adoption of such devices and increased their use worldwide. Moreover, SGA has become a backup tool in failed intubation in accordance with the difficult airway algorithm by the American Society of Anesthesia (ASA) [3]. Unfortunately, these devices do not protect from aspiration and may induce soft tissue trauma.

3.6 Extra-glottic airway devices

These devices have an extra advantage over the other SGA by having large pharyngeal tubes to seal the oropharynx or esophageal balloons to seal the esophagus so they can provide oxygenation and ventilation with reasonable protection from aspiration. They are easy to use and do not require advanced training.

A group of airways includes Laryngeal tube [4], Esophageal tracheal airway (Combitube) which be either inserted in the trachea or esophagus, King laryngeal tube (LT), Rusch EasyTube unlike the Combitube, Intubating Laryngeal Tube Suction Disposable (iLTS-D).

3.7 Endotracheal intubation (ETI)

Endotracheal intubation is considered the gold standard method of airway management, which allows proper oxygenation, positive pressure ventilation, positive end-expiratory pressure (PEEP), and protection from gastric content aspiration.

The performance of ETI requires advanced training and highly skilled personnel, keeping in mind that out of hospital ETI is carried out in suboptimal environment and unusual positions. First attempt ETI among EMS providers in an Australian cohort study was found to be around 80%, non the less, the paramedic experience was not associated with improved patient survival [5]. But in other studies the first-pass intubation was correlated with improved return of spontaneous circulation rate and survival [6]. Those conflicting result highlights the importance of the approach to airway management, experience in performing one specific procedure like ETI does not warrant a better outcome, moreover literature suggest that out of hospital ETI is not achieving the goals it intended for and that in some cases it might even cause harm [7].

The fundamental role of performing ETI in the Field is to improve patient outcome. There are multiple studies that have looked into the morbidity and mortality of field ETI compared to other airway management maneuvers like the use of supraglottic/extra-glottic devices or bag mask ventilation, most of the studies had an inconclusive results on survival or outcome. In a recent study of the national database of Thailand registry that looked into the return of spontaneous circulation (ROSC) in out of hospital cardiac arrest patients who received ETI vs. bag mask ventilation, both groups had comparable ROSC rate although the bag mask ventilation group had less severe condition and received faster treatment [8]. In a meta-analysis by Benoit and his colleagues that investigated the outcome of out of hospital ETI vs. SGA insertion in patients with cardiac arrest among more than 75,000 patients, they concluded that patients who arrested outside of the hospital had better outcome when they received ETI rather than SGA device by EMS providers, specifically speaking ROSC, survival to hospital admission and neurological outcome were all better in the ETI group [9]. Similar conclusion was demonstrated by a study of the Korean nationwide registry that studied the survival of out of hospital cardiac arrest in approximately 100,000 patients who received bag mask ventilation vs. ETI vs. SGA, ETI group had favorable outcomes compared to both other groups [10].

Out of hospital endotracheal intubation brings a lot of challenges to the provider, other than just performing the procedure itself, other complication can occur, like misplacement of the endotracheal tube, hemodynamic changes associated with the intervention and their pathophysiological impact on the disease process itself, intervention with the resuscitation efforts, airway trauma and others.

In an observational study at level trauma center the rate of endotracheal misplacement without the use of continuous end-tidal carbon dioxide (ETCO2) monitoring was around 23%, using ETCO2 continuous monitor reduced it to around zero [11].

3.8 Rapid sequence intubation versus no-medication intubation

Rapid Sequence Intubation (RSI) is an airway management technique that aims toward controlling the airway in the emergency setting in the fastest and safest means possible, that might require the use of anesthetic induction agents and neuromuscular blocking agents in order to minimize the possibility of gastric content aspiration during endotracheal intubation. Rapid sequence induction technique is further discussed in another chapter.

The debate over whether to use RSI vs. intubation without the use of medications to facilitate the process of intubation in the prehospital setting is still ongoing. Despite that the use of medications in RSI provides optimum conditions for successful endotracheal intubation but it does not goes without risks, mainly because of the significant hemodynamic changes associated with the use of anesthetic induction agents and the possibility of development of difficult airway scenario and loss of spontaneous ventilation after the use of muscle relaxants.

The use of medications to assist endotracheal intubation provides conditions that properly optimize the procedure. Factors that might be associated with failure to intubate like inability to pass the tube through the vocal cords, inability to visualize the cords, trismus and presence of gag reflex, can all be resolved with the use of medications to assist the endotracheal tube insertion [12]. Bernard et al. in a randomized clinical trial concluded that the neurological outcome of patients with severe traumatic brain injury was better when out of hospital RSI is performed by paramedics compared with intubation in the hospital setting [13].

In a study that evaluated the outcome in patients with severe traumatic brain injury who received RSI by paramedics compared to matched non intubated historical controls, concluded that RSI group had increase in mortality [14]. Moreover RSI led to prolonged on scene time and thus delayed transfer to the hospital.

Therefor the decision whether to incorporate RSI vs. non medication intubation should be individualized based on the level of training of EMS providers as well as the level of resources provided by the health care system.

4. Special considerations

4.1 Trauma

Management of hypoxia thus management of the airway is of a paramount importance for trauma victims, trauma is one of the leading causes of death among the young adult population, and number of potentially preventable prehospital death is high, reaching up to 43% according to a recent review [15], the majority are due to the missed opportunity of performing a proper basic airway management technique.

Airway management of trauma cases is challenging due to many factors, some are directly related to the type of trauma like trauma to the face or the respiratory tract, while others are related to the hypovolemia as a result of the trauma insult. Cervical spine injuries present a specific set of challenges that would render managing the airway in such population quite difficult and might need special equipment and techniques to maintain patient safety.

Since upper airway obstruction is one of most important factors of morbidity and mortality in trauma victims, identifying the factors that would lead to airway mismanagement is very important. Factor that would contribute to airway mismanagement include [16]:

Inability to recognize an inadequate airway
Inability to establish a clear airway with or without airway device
Inability to recognize a misplaced airway device
Failure of maintenance of a previously established airway due to displacement of the airway device
Inability to recognize the need for ventilation
Aspiration of gastric content

Special attention to patients who might have potential inadequate respiration such as patient with decreased level of consciousness due to head injury or intoxication, patients with direct trauma to the airway, facial and maxillary region, neck, larynx or throat, patient with significant blood loss and patients who might develop respiratory failure due to a blast, inhalational injury or exposure to chemical agent.

In most of the cases of trauma victims, simple maneuvers are usually sufficient to overcome upper airway obstruction, but in cases were simple techniques were ineffective the aim should be toward establishing a definitive airway technique. In an prospective observation study Lockery and his colleagues investigated the effectiveness prehospital advanced airway management in trauma patient, among the patient whom had received advanced airway management technique around 57% of them had airway compromise upon there arrival to the trauma centers, the success rate of ETI for non-physician paramedic was 64% and 11% reached a health care facility with unrecognized esophageal intubation. While physician-paramedic teams achieved definitive airway management for all patients [17]. Therefore, level of training, and availability of expertise are important in situations when advanced airway technique is warranted in trauma patient population group.

Advanced airway management techniques include ETI or a surgical airway. Below is a list of the most common indications for advanced airway technique in trauma victims.

Apneic patient
Protect from aspiration of vomitous content or airway bleeding
Reduced level of consciousness (Glasgow Coma Scale <8)
Significant faciomaxillary fractures
Patient who is at risk of upper airway obstruction: neck hematoma, laryngeal and tracheal injury
Inhalational injury with impending or potential airway compromise
Failure to maintain oxygenation using facemask or BiPAP/CPAP

It is recommended to assume that patients with major trauma, head and facial injuries, decreased level of consciousness or with neck pain as having cervical spine injury thus warranting cervical immobilization techniques to prevent further damage. Cervical immobilization has been known to attribute to difficulties with laryngoscopic view and hence difficult airway management. In a prospective study by Heath, that investigated the effect of different cervical spine immobilization techniques on the ease of laryngoscopy, poor view on laryngoscopy (grade 3 or 4) was more encountered when the cervical spine immobilized using rigid collar, tapes and sandbags compared to in-line manual immobilization. Therefore, manual in-line stabilization of cervical spine is the method of choice during tracheal intubation [18].

5. Pediatrics

Airway management in pediatrics is relatively difficult and requires highly skilled and professional personnel, this difficulty is based on the physiological, anatomical differences between infant, pediatric, and adult airways [19]. These differences included in the following table:

Large occiput
Relatively larger tongue and small mouth
High and anterior larynx
Large and floppy epiglottis
Subglottic narrowing at the cricoid cartilage

Foreign body aspiration is a common problem in the pediatric population, it may cause severe airway obstruction and might mandates immediate intervention. Other causes that might mandate airway intervention in the pediatric group include epiglottitis, viral croup, trauma, seizures, hypoxia, and cardiac arrest.

The use of prehospital advanced airway management techniques in the pediatric population have shown to have a conflicting result, in a recent nationwide cohort study, that looked into the outcome of out of hospital cardiac arrest in the pediatric population of japan, the use of advanced airway management technique including ETI and supraglottic devices did not demonstrate any improvement in 1-month survival or functional status when compared to the use of basic airway techniques [20].

Despite the conflicting results of the use of advanced airway management techniques, the use of supraglottic airway devices has been shown to easy, simple and with minimal complications in simulated pediatric cardiac arrest scenarios [21].

A useful tool to help guiding the sizes and dosages of the equipment and medications in the pediatric group is the Broselow Pediatric Emergency Tape, also known as the Broselow Tape, a color-coded tape that matches the measured height to the child's expected weight and other needed information.

6. Inhalation injury

Inhalational injury is a broad non-specific term that encompasses damage inflicted by heat, smoke, or chemical irritants to the respiratory tract or lung tissue.

Inhalational injury is commonly associated with burn injuries, around 10–20% of burn victims also suffered from inhalational injury complications that increased morbidity and mortality [22], moreover inhalation injury is considered an independent predictor of mortality in burn victims.

All burn patients should receive humidified 100% oxygen though a facemask to displace carbon monoxide [23], Advanced Life support of the American burn association recommends early endotracheal intubation, if there is any of the following indicators:

- Signs of Airway obstruction
- Total burn surface area more than 40%
- Extensive facial burns or involvement of the oral cavity
- Significant facial edema.
- Difficult swallowing
- Signs of respiratory distress
- Disturbed level of consciousness
- In patient with large burns, absence of qualified personnel to perform intubation during transfer.

7. Prehospital airway management during COVID 19 pandemic

Current recommendations for the airway management of patient with respiratory failure due to novel Corona virus II infection are focusing on in-hospital health care providers. While neglecting to provide guidance for EMS providers in the pre-hospital setting.

The in-hospital airway management recommendations of COVID-19 patients can be summarized in the following points:

1. Always use proper personal protective equipment (PPE) during the contact with the patient.

2. A surgical mask should be placed over the patient face to reduce the risk of spreading the infection, it can be placed over a nasal canula as well.

3. Bag-mask-ventilation should be restricted to minimum if any to minimize aerosol generation.

4. Rapid sequence intubation technique with video laryngoscopy is highly recommended.

Regarding the pre-hospital airway management, EMS providers should be able to identify suspected COVID 19 patients. To screen the patients EMS providers should inquire about the following: Recent history of travel, close contact with a known COVID 19 case, or with a person with flu like symptoms, worsening dyspnea, myalgia, sore throat, dry cough and/or GI symptoms. All precautions should be taken when dealing with patients reporting difficulty in breathing, or flu like sickness.

When handling COVID 19 patients appropriate PPE should be worn. That includes N95 mask, gown, gloves, and eye protection. To prevent further contamination a surgical mask should be provided to the suspected patient as soon as possible.

Similar to the in-hospital airway management protocols, rapid sequence intubation with video laryngoscopy is highly recommended when endotracheal intubation is warranted in the prehospital setting. Providers should not attempt more than one endotracheal intubation trial, if it wasn't successful the provider should proceed to SGA insertion. HEPA filter should be applied to avoid equipment contamination. Bag-mask ventilation should be restricted to minimum, but in scenarios where the bag-mask ventilation is inevitable two-person mask ventilation technique, and the use of airway adjuncts are recommended to improve the mask seal [24].

8. Future developments

The use of video assisted devices for endotracheal intubation has been gaining solid ground over the past recent years, especially as the cost of the technology has become lower.

Several recent studies have concluded that the use of video assisted devices has significantly increased the first-pass success rate as well as the overall success rate compared to the use of direct laryngoscopy [25–27]. Moreover, the use of video assisted devices for intubation has shown a faster learning curve compared to direct laryngoscopy [28], such feature might increase the use of advanced airway techniques by the paramedics in the field over time.

One of the downsides of using video assisted devices in the field is the potential difficulty of visualizing the vocal cords in the presence of blood and vomitus specially in trauma patients, another downside is that direct sun light might interfere with the visualization of video monitor [29].

Author details

Lamia Tawfik*, Mohammad Al Nobani and Tarek Tageldin
Hamad Medical Corporation, Qatar

*Address all correspondence to: lamia_tawfik@hotmail.com

References

[1] Berg MD, Schexnayder SM, Chameides L, et al. Part 13: Pediatric basic life support: 2010 American Heart Association guidelines for cardiopulmonary resuscitation and emergency cardiovascular care. Circulation. 2010;**122**(SUPPL. 3). DOI: 10.1161/CIRCULATIONAHA.110.971085

[2] Hubble MW, Richards ME, Jarvis R, Millikan T, Young D. Effectiveness of prehospital continuous positive airway pressure in the management of acute pulmonary edema. Prehospital Emerg Care. 2006;**10**(4):430-439. DOI: 10.1080/10903120600884848

[3] Caplan RA, Benumof JL, Berry FA, et al. Practice guidelines for management of the difficult airway: An updated report by the American Society of Anesthesiologists Task Force on Management of the Difficult Airway. Anesthesiology. 2003;**98**(5):1269-1277. DOI: 10.1097/00000542-200305000-00032

[4] Gaitini L, Madrid V, Capdevila M, Ariño JJ. The laryngeal tube. Revista Española de Anestesiología y Reanimación. 2008;**55**(4):232-241. DOI: 10.1016/S0034-9356(08)70554-1

[5] Dyson K, Bray JE, Smith K, et al. Paramedic intubation experience is associated with successful tube placement but not cardiac arrest survival. Annals of Emergency Medicine. 2017;**70**(3):382-390.e1. DOI: 10.1016/j.annemergmed.2017.02.002

[6] Carlson JN, Wang HE. Paramedic intubation: Does practice make perfect? Annals of Emergency Medicine. 2017;**70**(3):391-393. DOI: 10.1016/j.annemergmed.2017.03.024

[7] Wang HE, Yealy DM. Out-of-hospital endotracheal intubation: Where are we? Annals of Emergency Medicine. 2006;**47**(6):532-541. DOI: 10.1016/j.annemergmed.2006.01.016

[8] Yuksen C, Phattharapornjaroen P, Kreethep W, et al. Bag-valve mask versus endotracheal intubation in out-of-hospital cardiac arrest on return of spontaneous circulation: A national database study. Open Access Emerg Med. 2020;**12**:43-46. DOI: 10.2147/OAEM.S229356

[9] Benoit JL, Gerecht RB, Steuerwald MT, McMullan JT. Endotracheal intubation versus supraglottic airway placement in out-of-hospital cardiac arrest: A meta-analysis. Resuscitation. 2015;**93**:20-26. DOI: 10.1016/j.resuscitation.2015.05.007

[10] Kang K, Kim T, Ro YS, Kim YJ, Song KJ, Do SS. Prehospital endotracheal intubation and survival after out-of-hospital cardiac arrest: Results from the Korean nationwide registry. The American Journal of Emergency Medicine. 2016;**34**(2):128-132. DOI: 10.1016/j.ajem.2015.09.036

[11] Silvestri S, Ralls GA, Krauss B, et al. The effectiveness of out-of-hospital use of continuous end-tidal carbon dioxide monitoring on the rate of unrecognized misplaced intubation within a regional emergency medical services system. Annals of Emergency Medicine. 2005;**45**(5):497-503. DOI: 10.1016/j.annemergmed.2004.09.014

[12] Wang HE, Lave JR, Sirio CA, Yealy DM, Wang H. Paramedic Intubation Errors: Isolated Events or Symptoms of Larger Problems?2020. DOI: 10.1377/hlthaff.25.2.501

[13] Bernard SA, Nguyen V, Cameron P, et al. Prehospital rapid sequence intubation improves functional outcome for patients with severe traumatic brain injury: A randomized controlled trial. Annals of Surgery. 2010;**252**(6):959-965. DOI: 10.1097/SLA.0b013e3181efc15f

[14] Davis DP, Hoyt DB, Ochs M, et al. The Effect of Paramedic Rapid Sequence

Intubation on Outcome in Patients with Severe Traumatic Brain Injury. 2003. doi:10.1097/01.TA.0000053396.02126.CD

[15] Oliver GJ, Walter DP, Redmond AD. Are prehospital deaths from trauma and accidental injury preventable? A direct historical comparison to assess what has changed in two decades. Injury. 2017;**48**(5):978-984. DOI: 10.1016/j.injury.2017.01.039

[16] Khan RM, Sharma PK, Kaul N. Airway management in trauma. Indian Journal of Anaesthesia. 2011;**55**(5):463-469. DOI: 10.4103/0019-5049.89870

[17] Lockey DJ, Healey B, Crewdson K, Chalk G, Weaver AE, Davies GE. Advanced airway management is necessary in prehospital trauma patients. British Journal of Anaesthesia. 2015;**114**(4):657-662. DOI: 10.1093/bja/aeu412

[18] HEATH KJ. The effect on laryngoscopy of different cervical spine immobilization techniques. Anaesthesia. 1994;**49**(10):843-845. DOI: 10.1111/j.1365-2044.1994.tb04254.x

[19] Apfelbaum JL, Hagberg CA, Caplan RA, et al. Practice guidelines for management of the difficult airway: An updated report by the American Society of Anesthesiologists Task Force on Management of the Difficult Airway. Anesthesiology. 2013;**118**(2):251-270. DOI: 10.1097/ALN.0b013e31827773b2

[20] Okubo M, Komukai S, Izawa J, et al. Prehospital advanced airway management for paediatric patients with out-of-hospital cardiac arrest: A nationwide cohort study. Resuscitation. 2019;**145**:175-184. DOI: 10.1016/j.resuscitation.2019.09.007

[21] Chen L, Hsiao AL. Randomized trial of endotracheal tube versus laryngeal mask airway in simulated prehospital pediatric arrest. Pediatrics. 2008;**122**(2). DOI: 10.1542/peds.2008-0103

[22] Walker PF, Buehner MF, Wood LA, et al. Diagnosis and management of inhalation injury: An updated review. Critical Care. 2015;**19**(1). DOI: 10.1186/s13054-015-1077-4

[23] Weiss SM, Lakshminarayan S. Acute inhalation injury. Clinics in Chest Medicine. 1994;**15**(1):103-116

[24] Hart J, Tracy R, Johnston M, et al. Recommendations for prehospital airway management in patients with suspected COVID-19 infection. The Western Journal of Emergency Medicine. 2020;**21**(4):809-812. DOI: 10.5811/westjem.2020.5.47540

[25] Boehringer B, Choate M, Hurwitz S, Tilney PVR, Judge T. Impact of video laryngoscopy on advanced airway management by critical care transport paramedics and nurses using the CMAC pocket monitor. BioMed Research International. 2015;**2015**:821302. DOI: 10.1155/2015/821302

[26] Jarvis JL, McClure SF, Johns D. EMS Intubation Improves with King Vision Video Laryngoscopy. In: *Prehospital Emergency Care*. Vol 19. Taylor and Francis Ltd; 2015:482-489. doi:10.3109/10903127.2015.1005259

[27] Wayne MA, McDonnell M. Comparison of traditional versus video laryngoscopy in out-of-hospital tracheal intubation. Prehospital Emerg Care. 2010;**14**(2):278-282. DOI: 10.3109/10903120903537189

[28] Kaplan MB, Ward DS, Berci G. A new video laryngoscope - an aid in intubation and teaching. J Educ Perioper Med JEPM. 2003;**5**(1):E025 http://www.ncbi.nlm.nih.gov/pubmed/27175418. Accessed July 29, 2020

[29] Trimmel H, Kreutziger J, Fitzka R, et al. Use of the glidescope ranger video laryngoscope for emergency intubation in the prehospital setting: A randomized control trial. Critical Care Medicine. 2016;**44**(7):e470-e476. DOI: 10.1097/CCM.0000000000001669

Chapter 3

Airway Management Outside the Operating Room

Shakeel Moideen

Abstract

An anesthesiologist is an expert at airway management in the clinical environment. He or she has mastered knowledge of the anatomy and physiology of the normal and potentially abnormal airway. The environment of the operating room (OR) has been considered to be their most familiar area of work, where they feel most confident. Airway management outside this area is known to put patients at an increased risk of complications. This chapter addresses the important facets of this indispensable skill when used outside the operating room, taking into consideration both anesthesiologists and non-anesthesiologists as operators. Since the intensive care unit (ICU) is a similar environment to the OR, a separate chapter has been written for airway management in the ICU. Therefore, this chapter will concentrate on other areas outside the OR. It will not address resuscitation scenarios.

Keywords: outside OR, remote locations, airway complications, sedation, standalone anesthesia

1. Introduction

> *The most compelling educational effort for the anaesthesia community should be to reduce the frequency and severity of complications related to managing the airway—Benumof 1995.*

Airway management outside the operating theater is associated with increased risks when compared with the management of the airway done in the operating theater setting [1]. Except for the resuscitation scenario, airway management is always associated with the administration of sedative medication to facilitate a procedure being performed. This could be diagnostic or therapeutic in nature. It is understood that the responsibility of managing the airway lies on the physician who prescribes the sedative drug, unless there is the presence of an assigned anesthesiologist to that area. The anesthesiologist is considered the expert for airway management in the clinical environment, who has mastered knowledge of the anatomy and physiology of the airway, usually with years of experience in dealing with the normal airway. They are also trained to handle the potentially abnormal airway and are most familiar with the newer equipment available for the management of the airway. The operating room has always been associated with terms such as being the anesthesiologist's home or backyard. It is their most familiar area of work, where they feel most confident. The reason for this is that this area is most prepared to handle problems with the airway, not only in terms of equipment and available expert help, but also in terms of ergonomics. Airway management outside this area is known to put patients at an increased risk of airway complications. This chapter addresses the important facets of this invaluable skill when used outside the operating room, taking into consideration both anesthesiologists and non-anesthesiologists as operators. Since the intensive care unit is a highly specialized area, similar to the OR, a separate chapter has been written for airway management in the ICU. Therefore, this chapter will concentrate on other areas outside the OR. It will not address resuscitation scenarios where immediate airway management is unplanned and is a life-saving procedure, and may be needed in any area of the hospital and beyond.

2. Anticipating difficulty is key

As with any skill, preparation is fundamental and is the secret to avoiding harm to patients. Ideally, all patients needing airway manipulation outside the OR should be assessed for potential difficulty, and prepared just as they would be for an elective procedure in the OR. One of the reasons airway management is more difficult outside the OR than inside is due to the fact that there may not be enough time to learn about the patient's physical condition and to predict risk of difficult airway or aspiration. Whenever possible patients should be assessed for comorbidities, drug allergies and fasting status. An airway assessment should be completed. There are many aides-memoires to help with a quick but relatively thorough assessment of the airway to predict difficulty with mask ventilation and intubation. These should be available in all areas for the physician to refer to, ideally attached to the difficult airway trolley. Risk factors for difficult mask ventilation include an increased body mass index (BMI), history of obstructive sleep apnea (OSA), presence of a beard that may disrupt the seal of the face mask, being edentulous and having limited mandibular protrusion. A difficult laryngoscopy is anticipated when a patient has limited mouth opening, a Mallampati score of III or IV, limited head and neck movements, is obese and has an increased neck circumference.

Patient preparation is also important. A patient who is not fasting adequately is at a higher risk of aspiration of gastric contents during induction of anesthesia and intubation. Standard airway equipment and monitoring that conforms to international safety standards should be readily available. These are discussed below. For intubating patients, it is sometimes difficult to get optimal positioning of the patient outside the OR. The OR tables allow all kinds of position changes, but the trolleys and ward beds are not as versatile. In obese patients, one has to try to achieve the ramp position to aid intubation. Outside the OR, one may need to improvise to achieve this. The Oxford HELP® (Head Elevating Laryngoscopy

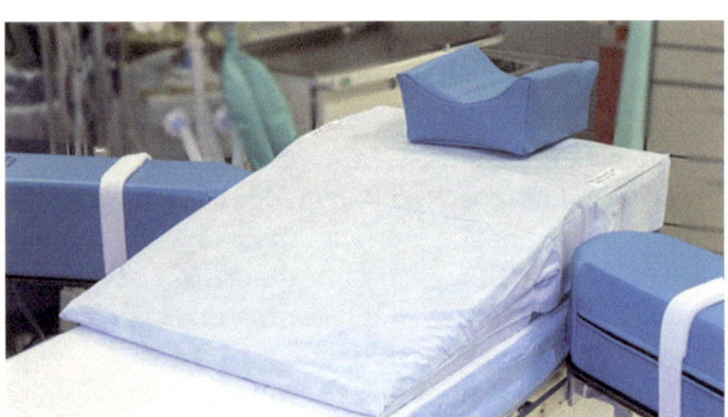

Figure 1.
Troop Elevation Pillow® System.

Pillow) and the Troop Elevation Pillow® System (**Figure 1**) are examples of adjuncts used to achieve optimal laryngoscopy position in obese patients.

3. Areas outside the OR

There are many areas in hospitals outside of operation theaters and ICUs where sedation or general anesthesia is given for various reasons. This could be to aid uncomfortable diagnostic or therapeutic procedures or for patients who do not have the capacity to understand the need for such essential procedures. The medication that a patient receives defines where on the continuum of sedation (**Table 1**) they lie, which in turn decides the airway support needed.

Every hospital facility will have different areas where airway management will be required or needed to be on standby. Airway management in some areas such as the ICU and prehospital setting will be discussed in other chapters. These are some of the other areas:

3.1 The radiology suite

Most hospitals have a very large radiology suite. It can consist of MRI scanners, CT scanners and interventional radiology suites. Patients requiring both diagnostic and therapeutic procedures in these areas may need some form of sedation or analgesia to tide over the procedure. They may even need a general anesthetic. These areas need to be equipped from the start with all the airway kit that is required in an operating room setting. It is important to have MRI compatible airway equipment, as airway difficulties can arise when the patient is in the scanner tunnel. Laryngoscopes need to be non-ferromagnetic and MR compatible anesthetic machines, ventilators and vaporizers are available. Having long breathing circuits is the alternative to having MR compatible machines.

Another problem faced in scanner suites is the inability to prop-up the head-end of the patient. This can sometimes lead to partial airway obstruction in the deeply sedated patient who is spontaneously breathing. Partial obstruction to breathing causes movement artifacts on the head and neck scans. Nasal or oral airways can be carefully used in these deeply sedated patients (**Figure 2**).

The coils used in MR magnets need to be kept cold in order to maintain superconductivity. This is often achieved by immersing them in liquid helium. If the machine gets quenched (usually an emergency process involving the rapid boil-off

	Depth			
Signs	**Minimal**	**Moderate**	**Deep**	**General anesthesia**
Responsiveness	Alert/awake	Responds to verbal stimuli	Responds to painful stimuli	Unresponsive
Ventilation	Unaffected	Adequate	Maybe inadequate	Frequently inadequate
Airway	Unaffected	No intervention	Intervention maybe needed	Intervention often required
Cardiovascular	Unaffected	Maintained	Usually maintained	Maybe impaired

Table 1.
Sedation continuum.

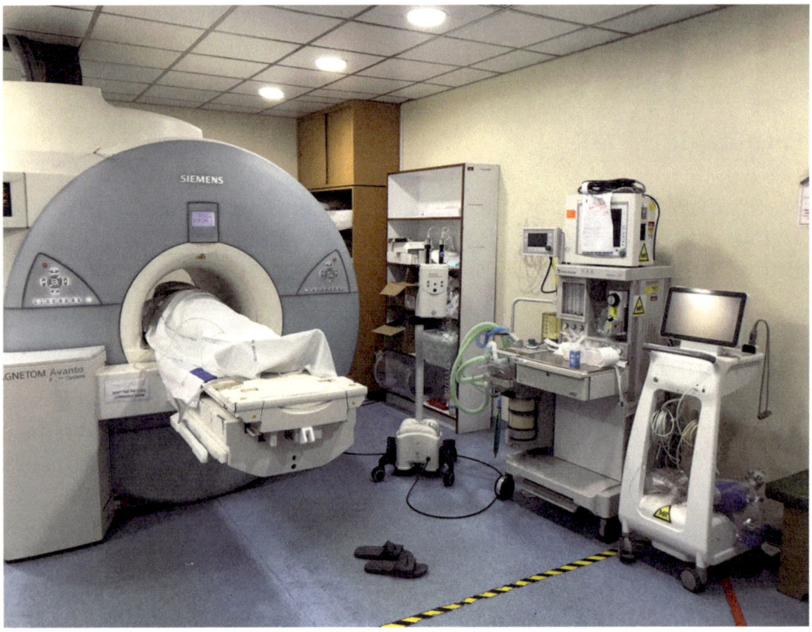

Figure 2.
The MRI room with the patient's airway in the tunnel and not easily accessible to the operator.

of the cryogen that causes an immediate loss of superconductivity, to shut down the magnetic field) and if there is damage to the quench pipe, the build-up of helium within the scanning room could potentially lead to asphyxiation. The use of oxygen sensors is vital to the safe conduct of anesthesia.

3.2 The neuroradiology suite

The neuroradiology suite would require a special mention, as they may be standalone from the rest of the radiology suite. These are very similar to the interventional radiology suites used by radiologists for other procedures, but the incidence of the patient needing intubation and a general anesthesia over just deep sedation is more here. Apart from the general risks of working in a dark environment with high radiation as is mentioned in the general risks below, these areas should be set up to mirror an OR as far as possible. It is comparable to the hybrid CT/MRI ORs that exists in many hospitals these days.

3.3 The gastroenterology suite

The gastroenterology suites conduct many procedures that can warrant the patient to be either sedated or anesthetized. These include edoscopic retrograde cholangiopancreatography (ERCP) and papillotomy, esophageal or colonic dilatation and stenting, enteroscopies, and endoscopic sleeve gastroplasties. ERCP procedures need to be done with the patient in the prone position and in a fluoroscopy room. These rooms are usually small and crowded with equipment other than airway equipment. Apart from doing these under GA, these procedures have also been done under deep sedation with no adjunct airway device except supplemental oxygen via nasal prongs. One has to bear in mind the difficulty of airway access in these cases and plan airway management at the outset based on the expected duration of the procedure and expertise of the operator. Frequent suctioning of the oral cavity may be required in the unprotected airway.

The gastroenterology suites have started doing more bariatric work than in the past. These include simple procedures like intra-gastric balloon insertions and removals, and also complicated longer procedures like the sleeve gastroplasties. Obesity is by itself a pointer of airway risk and this should be taken into consideration when planning to intubate these patients. This includes having trained staff familiar with the bariatric airway, proper preparation of the patient, positioning the patient well using a ramp, good pre-oxygenation, and having a skilled person for post procedure monitoring.

3.4 Electroconvulsive therapy (ECT) suite

ECT is still being used in patients who have severe major depression or bipolar disorders who have not responded to maximal medical management strategies. Small electrical currents are passed through the brain, intentionally triggering a brief seizure, which has been known to alter brain chemistry, reversing symptoms. This procedure requires a GA, with the patient given an induction agent and a small dose of muscle relaxant to prevent trauma during seizures. It is vital to establish that the patient is fasting (some patients do not have mental capacity and are not able to give proper history) to avoid aspiration of gastric contents. These are very brief procedures and do not usually require an extensive airway armamentarium, but backup airway equipment should be standard. Since suxamethonium, a depolarizing muscle relaxant is used to achieve safety during the brief period of seizure (and therefore a short period of apnea), it is vital to pre-oxygenate the patient well to increase the safe apneic time.

3.5 The in-vitro fertilization (IVF) suite

The IVF suite usually requires sedation and analgesia for egg retrieval. Mild to moderate sedation is usually sufficient, but some patients slip into deep sedation and airway support may be warranted. These areas need to be equipped with a dedicated airway trolley as airway problems are not uncommon.

3.6 Oncology

Stand-alone oncology units do procedures that usually require general or spinal anesthesia, or at times deep sedation. These include brachytherapy and bone marrow aspirations, among other procedures. In spite of being a stand-alone facility for the immunocompromised, these areas usually have OR setups with the usual airway kit.

3.7 Cardiology

The cardiac catheter lab provides an area for interventional procedures and has similarities to the neuro-interventional suite although deep sedation or general anesthesia is not usually necessary in adult patients. Apart from interventional cardiology, sedation is also given for Transesophageal Echocardiograms (TEE). This is similar to having an esophagogastroscopy and the airway needs are that of the gastroenterology suite. Cardioversions may be done in this area or as an emergency in the ED. These patients usually get a dose of sedative medication, but muscle relaxants are not necessary.

Ventilation in some patients needs the use of room air to study the blood gases physiology in certain critical congenital heart lesions.

3.8 ENT procedure room

The Ear, Nose and Throat clinic usually has a procedure room to carry out minor procedures. Local anesthesia of the airway is usually used to access the laryngeal inlet for vocal cord injections. The clinic also performs tracheostomy tube changes and tracheostomy wound management. Routine tracheostomy changes must be done only during the daytime and during working hours except in an emergency. At least two trained practitioners are required during the tracheostomy tube change procedure. No drugs are usually given to hamper the patient's respiratory efforts, but the difficult airway trolley should always be available along with a good functioning suction machine.

3.9 Emergency department

The resuscitation areas in the ED are usually equipped to intubate and ventilate patients. In the other acute areas of the ED, procedures may be done for non-fasted patients (such as cardioversions, TEEs and fracture reductions). These areas should be well equipped with anesthetic machines and airway trolleys. One needs to keep in mind the need for a fiberoptic scope in case of airway swelling in severe allergies or burns.

3.10 Wards and other areas

The resuscitation team may need to intubate a patient in any area of the hospital. Basic airway kit and intubation equipment are available in all ward areas (**Figure 3**).

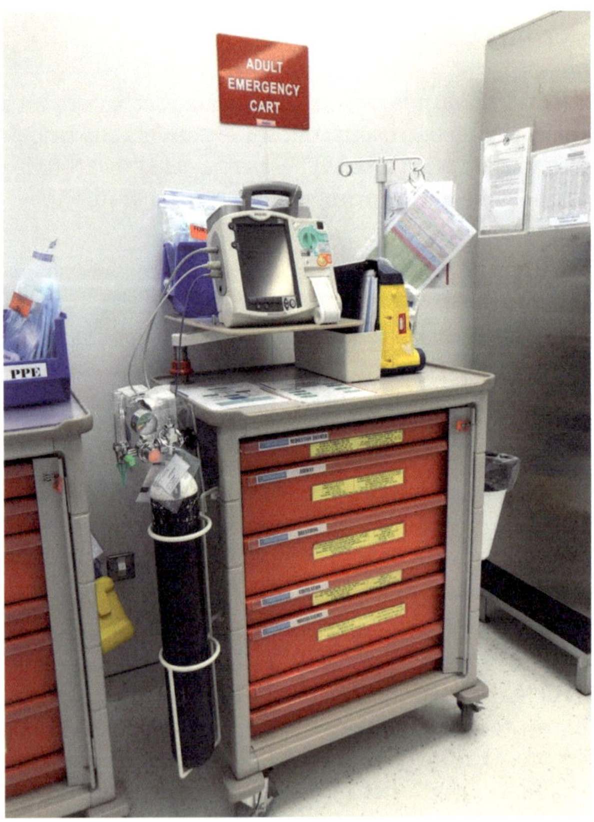

Figure 3.
A resuscitation trolley with airway equipment on the ward.

Ventilation is usually achieved with the use of a bag-valve-mask device until a definite portable ventilator is made available for transfer of the patient to the ICU.

4. Challenges in these areas

Working in different areas outside the OR comes with its own difficulties. These may be specific to the area like the radiology suite or can be general differences to the OR.

Dark rooms: Rooms where fluoroscopy or ultrasound is used tend to have low lighting to enable visual clarity of the images for the operator (**Figure 4**). This makes it difficult to observe the patient and to monitor notes. An alternate source of light should always be available [2]. The monitor should be clearly visible in this environment (**Figure 5**).

Remote location: When airway management is undertaken away from other trained personnel and specialist equipment, it is important to formulate a plan to getting help quickly in case of a crisis.

Unfamiliar equipment: Different areas are equipped with different airway kit. The anesthetic machines may be basic models with minimal monitors. It is important to familiarize oneself with the equipment available prior to use, as they may be very different to those available in the OR.

Lack of skilled staff: As mentioned above, skilled support staff may be at a distance, and having a plan to inform and seek help needs to be in place before starting.

Limited patient access during procedures: Whether the patient is in the MRI tunnel or fully draped on the interventional radiology table, it is difficult to manipulate the patient's airway once the procedure has begun. The decision to maintain the patient's airway using a particular technique should be taken keeping this in mind.

Crowded rooms: The rooms mentioned above can be very crowded with equipment essential to the procedure being performed (**Figure 4**). In the

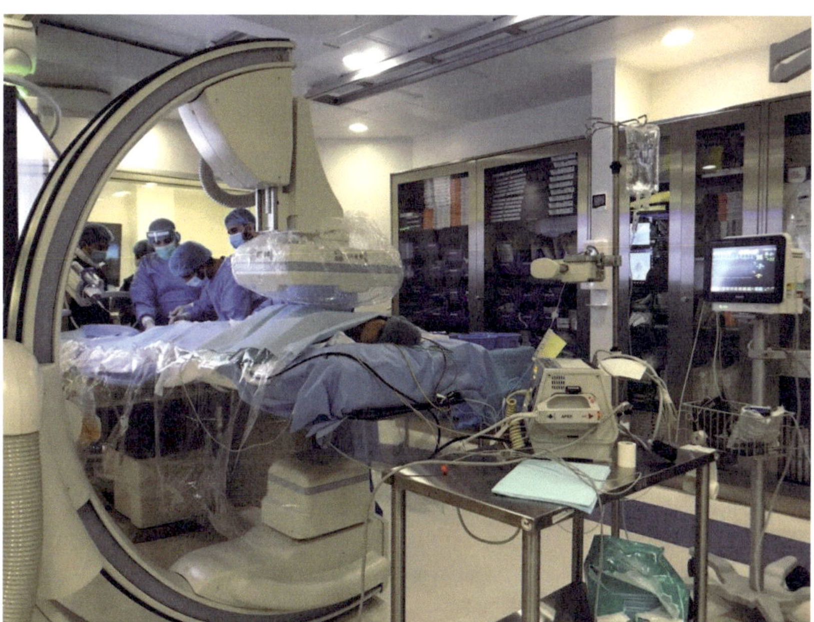

Figure 4.
A dimly-lit crowded interventional radiology room.

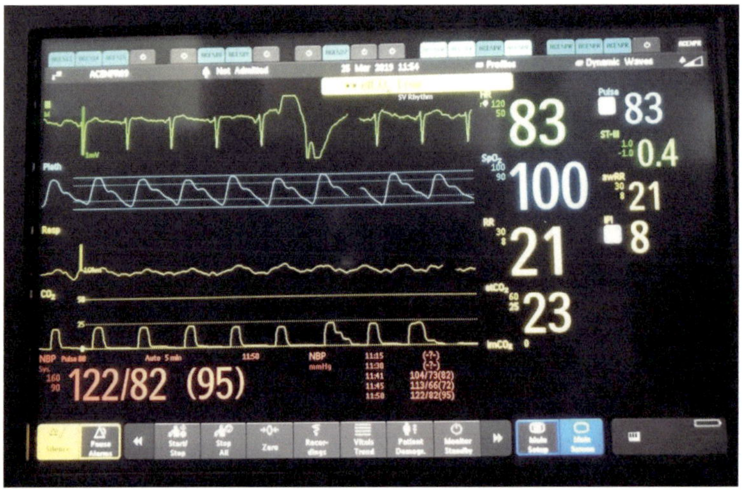

Figure 5.
Basic monitoring.

fluoroscopy rooms, the C-arms of the fluoroscope will move in multiple axes and can come in the way of airway or monitoring equipment intra-procedure. Very little consideration is given to airway equipment placement in these areas as not all procedures require patient sedation or airway manipulation. It is therefore important to reshuffle equipment, in discussion with the operator, to make sure airway maintenance and management is kept safe throughout the procedure.

Radiation exposure: Patients and staff are exposed to high doses of ionizing radiation in the radiology suite. Radiation exposure poses a significant health risk. Measures taken to minimize exposure and risk during the procedure include wearing protective lead aprons, thyroid shields, eye protection, radiation exposure badges (to log exposure) and distancing oneself as far as possible from the radiation source.

5. Sedation outside OR

With respect to administrating sedation outside the OR environment two aspects need to be emphasized:

Oxygen therapy modalities: These could be either low-flow administration or high-flow administration [3]. Low-flow methods are usually employed for the majority of sedation that happens outside the OR. These may be via nasal cannulae with flow rates between 2 and 6 L/min or face masks, including simple masks, venturi masks, or non-rebreathing masks, with flow rates up to 15 L/min. High-flow nasal cannula (HFNC) is a nasal cannula with the capability of delivery humidified oxygen at flow rates that exceed the inspiratory pressure of the patient (60–70 L/min). It allows delivery of 100% oxygen, and can be given to achieve transient apneic oxygenation.

Medication for sedation: Choosing sedative agents that cause minimal depression of the ventilatory drive is safer when dealing with patients away from the OR. Fentanyl and Midazolam are the most commonly used sedative agents, with an added advantage of having antagonists available. Ketamine and Ketamine-Propofol mixtures are also used. Dexmedetomidine is known to preserve upper airway reflexes and the ventilatory drive. Propofol should be used only with the option

Drug	IV dose in Adults	Onset	Duration	Comments
Midazolam	1–2 mg titrated boluses (×3)	1–5 min	30–90 min	Usually used along with Fentanyl
Fentanyl	0.5–2 mcg/kg	2–3 min	20–30 min	Can cause hypoventilation
Propofol	1 mg/kg then 0.5 mg/kg q5 min	<1 min	3–10 min	Causes drop in BP, reduced inotropy (caution in hypovolemic patients and HF patients) Can cause hypoventilation or apnea
Ketamine	0.25–1 mg/kg	30 sec	5–10 min	Does not depress ventilatory drive Has bronchodilatory effects Can cause hypersalivation (may need anticholinergic) Can cause increase in HR, BP, ICP and emergence delirium
Dexmedetomidine	0.5–1 mcg/kg over 10 min	5–30 min	1–2 h	Minimal respiratory depression Can decrease SVR and HR

Table 2.
Commonly used drugs for sedation (BP-blood pressure, HF-heart failure, HR-heart rate, ICP-intracranial pressure, SVR-systemic vascular resistance).

of airway rescue available, as the patient may move from deep sedation to general anesthesia (**Table 2**).

6. Monitoring

Maintaining standards of monitoring is the most important modality used to ensure the safety of the patient and to avoid airway complications. Adherence to the current best practice guidelines [4] is essential when planning and equipping areas outside the OR. This should include the pulse oximeter and capnograph. Failure of capnography contributed to 74% of cases of death or persistent neurological injury [5]. **Figure 5** shows a snapshot of a monitor used in a patient who is deeply sedated with a Target Controlled Infusion (TCI) of Propofol, spontaneously breathing with supplemental oxygen delivered via a nasal cannula. No other airway adjuncts were necessary. The nasal cannula is incorporated with a sampling port for expired gases (**Figure 6**) and a clear $EtCO_2$ (end tidal carbon dioxide) trace and value is displayed on the monitor. In a fully open circuit as is with nasal prongs, the value displayed is dependent on the flow of oxygen delivered and the depth of breathing. Although the exact value displayed is not of true significance always, the characteristics of the trace and the trend of the number displayed warns clinicians of impending airway compromise and the need to intervene.

Capnography use has the highest potential to prevent deaths from airway complications outside of the operating theater complex [6, 7].

Monitoring depth of sedation has been looked at using a bispectral index (BIS) monitor. The depth of sedation is calculated by measuring cerebral electric activity via an electroencephalogram (EEG). The BIS algorithm processes the frontal EEG and converts the signal to a waveform on the BIS monitor, and displays a number between

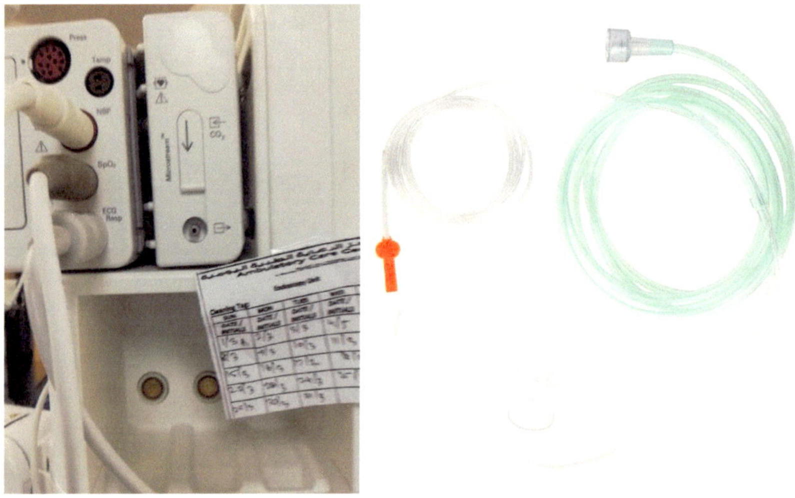

Figure 6.
A capnography module for the monitor and a nasal cannula with an oxygen tubing and an integrated CO_2 sampling line that fits into the module.

100 (fully awake) and 0 (no brain activity). This has proved very useful during general anesthesia in avoiding awareness due to inadequate hypnosis, by keeping values between 40 and 60, but its use to achieve a particular level of sedation on the continuum of sedation has proved difficult to interpret. Levels of 60–70 have been postulated and the aim should be to avoid letting the patient slip into general anesthesia from deep sedation, risking apnea and hypoxia. This has not always correlated to an adequate level of sedation and most operators adjust the level of sedation based on response to any stimulus the patient experiences during the procedure.

7. Improving airway management outside the OR

At least 25% of major airway events are from outside of the OR environment [8]. Complications are associated with hypoxia, aspiration, unrecognized esophageal intubation, airway trauma and obesity.

As we have seen above, areas outside the OR need to be prepared with equipment to manage the airway in a patient who may need it. We should plan and equip every area where this is anticipated, usually due to the fact that we as clinicians give patients drugs to aid procedures to happen, putting them in harm's way. Apart from eternal vigilance and monitoring, we should be prepared to step up the management of the airway that can become compromised.

Capnography is a tool that has become part of the basic standards of monitoring the world over, in patients having sedation or general anesthesia. It is a very important tool to detect a deterioration in ventilation in a spontaneously breathing patient due to increasing levels of sedation. All staff involved with sedating patients need to be trained in its use.

Checklists have improved patient care [9]. In areas where intubations are not routinely carried out, an intubation checklist has proved invaluable. Checklists have also helped in pre-assessment of patients and has helped recognize potential difficulties. For example, obesity is recognized as an increased risk factor for airway complications. These allow for thorough back-up strategy planning, both for intubation and extubation, as it may not be routine in areas outside the OR.

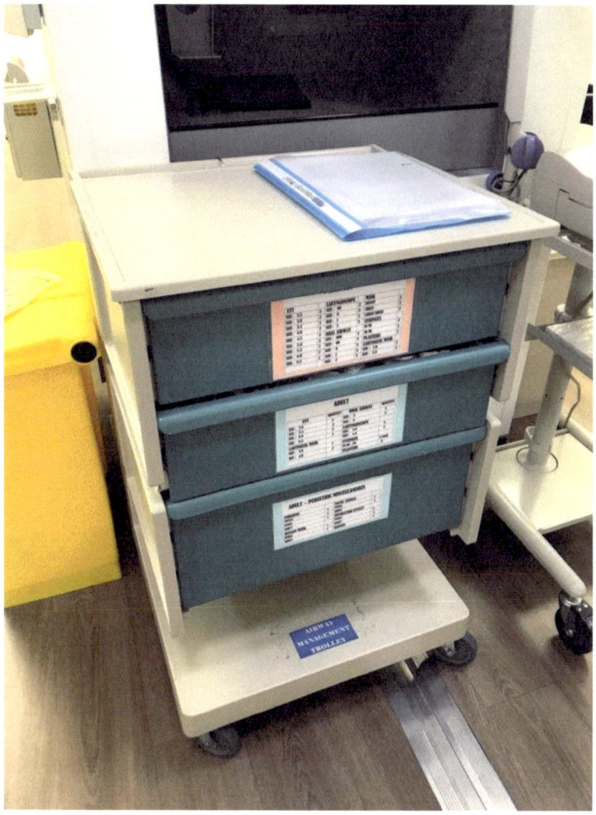

Figure 7.
An airway trolley in a patient recovery area.

The availability of the difficult airway trolley (**Figure 7** and **Table 3**) is paramount in areas where airway maneuvers are planned. These require regular checking and maintenance with replacement and stocking done every day. Since many areas exist outside the OR for airway procedures and since not every area is used on a daily basis unlike the OR, a designated person should be responsible to oversee this task. Every area should also have a plan to access video-laryngoscopes and fiberoptic bronchoscopes without much delay. Front of neck access equipment should always be available on the difficult airway trolley, and regular training should happen among the staff who look after the airway of patients.

Apart from airway equipment that is routinely used in the OR, certain newer developments in airway management have potential roles in areas outside the OR [11]. These include Laryngeal Mask Airways (LMA) modified with a separate channel to allow endoscope access into the esophagus, and high flow nasal oxygen delivery devices. Examples of the separate channel devices include the LMA® Gastro™ Airway from Teleflex, and the Gastro-Laryngeal Tube from VBM Medizintechnik GmbH (**Figure 8**). These modified airway devices have made it easier to anesthetize patients for ERCPs and upper endoscopy procedures.

The use of heated and humidified high flow nasal cannula (HFNC) with flows of 60–70 L/min has also become increasingly popular in deeply sedated patients outside the OR [12]. This can be used in various areas and addresses the concerns of transient apneas and hypoventilation and hypercarbia. It is recommended to use transcutaneous carbon dioxide ($TcCO_2$) monitoring during prolonged use of HFNC in patients who may go apneic.

Level	Contents
On top of trolley	• Difficult airway algorithm flowchart • Direct access phone numbers to anesthesia/ICU/ENT • Portable monitor for videolaryngoscope
On the side of trolley	• Introducers/bougies • Airway exchange catheter • Suction catheters
Drawer 1	• Laryngoscope handles • Laryngoscope blades: Macintosh sizes 3 and 4 • Videolaryngoscope blades depending on make • Endotracheal tubes: sizes 5–8 • Stylet • Lubrication gel • Cuff inflation syringe 10 ml • Magill forceps • Adhesive tape or tie
Drawer 2	• Second-generation supraglottic airway devices (SADs) sizes 3, 4, 5 • Lubrication gel • Inflation syringe 20 ml • Orogastric tube sizes 12, 14
Drawer 3	• Facemask sizes 3, 4 • Oropharyngeal airways sizes 7–11 • Nasopharyngeal airways sizes 6–8 • Syringe 10 ml
Drawer 4	• Emergency front of neck access—scalpel blade 10, bougie, endotracheal tube size 6.0

Table 3.
An example of an adult difficult airway trolley [10].

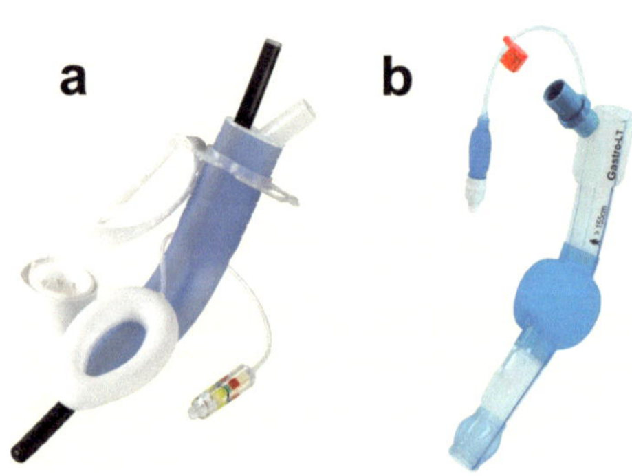

Figure 8.
(a) LMA® gastro™ airway; (b) gastro-LT.

8. Human factors and team working

Human factors such as poor team working, poor communication and failure to call for help all contribute to airway critical events. Human factors extend to institutional organization and structure, equipment availability and use of standard operating protocols (SOP) [13].

Junior staff should always have senior help readily available, and non-anesthesiologists should have a system in place to get anesthetic help in case of problems. All staff involved in airway management outside the OR should undergo airway training, both basic and advanced, and have annual refresher practice sessions of the less used skills, preferably in a dedicated simulation lab. They should also be familiar with the interpretation and use of capnography along with other monitoring equipment.

Communication channels and links should be established between various departments and senior clinicians in the Emergency Department, Anesthesia, Intensive Care Unit and ENT (Ear Nose and Throat surgery department). Regular audits should take place of airway management problems or events, in all areas.

High-fidelity simulator training provides anesthesiologists and other doctors involved in sedating patients outside the OR with the opportunity to develop their technical and non-technical skills for managing rare and dangerous scenarios related to airway management. It provides a safe multidisciplinary learning environment, and simulators can replicate a specific aspect of airway management, or the entire outside OR working environment.

9. Post-procedure care

Post-procedure care should be the same as that required after an anesthetic in the operating room. This should be the rule, irrespective of the procedure done. If the patient has had sedative drugs or a general anesthetic, they are prone to having airway complications in the recovery phase. The risk is dependent on the drugs used, airway technique applied intra-procedure, and the duration of the procedure.

Ideally a designated area of the corresponding suite should be available for patient recovery. This should be adequately equipped with facilities and trained personnel like a theater recovery room. This is an area that needs to cater to the monitored recovery of different kinds of patients, from those who may have had only moderate sedation, all the way to the patient who has had a full general anesthetic (with an indwelling endotracheal tube) for a few hours.

For most, such a facility may not be available, and depending on the area, may not be possible. This would require patients to be transported to the main theater recovery room (the post-anesthetic care unit-PACU). For safe transfer one must ensure that adequate equipment and personnel are available in advance, and organized with the PACU team. It is vital to have the location of recovery and logistics of transfer if required, planned in advance, before embarking on anesthetizing in a remote location.

Safe post procedure discharge from the intervention unit to the ward or home should be done following local discharge criteria. At the least patients should have vital parameters (Heart rate, blood pressure, oxygen saturation on room air and respiratory rate) within 20% of pre-procedure baseline levels, not be too sedated (either alert or responding to verbal stimulation), have a core temperature of more than 36°C, have no nausea or vomiting, and be pain free. The patient should be able to sip fluids orally without features of aspiration or coughing.

10. Conclusion

Airway management outside the OR can be a challenging task, not just due to the situationally difficult airway that can arise, but also due the different environments having different SOPs, differences in equipment availability and expertise of personnel present. It is crucial to standardize equipment availability in all areas where sedation will be given. This has to be drawn up and agreed upon with the anesthetic department. The need for the availability of special equipment like the video-laryngoscope or the fiberoptic bronchoscope will be decided depending on local protocols. Having capnography in all these areas is of utmost importance for patient safety in this day and age. Staff involved in monitoring these patients need to be educated in its use. The importance of eternal vigilance cannot be emphasized enough. Airway management can be more of a challenge in these areas and in an attempt to prevent a deterioration in the airway of a patient, constant monitoring by a dedicated member of staff is paramount throughout the procedure and into the recovery phase. The ability to manage airway emergencies must be a skill mastered by all staff involved in sedating patients outside the OR and this can only be made possible through regular training. Airway management outside the operating room is challenging. Difficult airway management guidelines from the Difficult Airway Society (DAS), UK, or the American Society of Anesthesiologists (ASA) remain the standard reference guide [14].

Author details

Shakeel Moideen
Hamad Medical Corporation, Doha, Qatar

*Address all correspondence to: smoideen@hamad.qa

References

[1] Brindley PG, Beed M, Law JA, et al. Airway management outside the operating room: How to better prepare. Canadian Journal of Anesthesia. 2017;**64**:530-539

[2] Royal College of Anaesthetists. Guidelines for the provision of anaesthesia services (GPAS), Chapter 7: Guidelines for the Provision of Anaesthesia Services in the Non-Theatre Environment. UK: Royal College of Anaesthetists; 2020. Available from: https://www.rcoa.ac.uk/gpas/chapter-7 [Accessed: 13 August 2020]

[3] Weekley MS. Oxygen administration. StatPearls Publishing; 2020. Available from: https://www.ncbi.nlm.nih.gov/books/NBK430685/

[4] CSPP. Standards for Basic Anesthetic Monitoring [Internet]. 2015. Available from: https://www.asahq.org/-/media/sites/asahq/files/public/resources/standards-guidelines/standards-for-basic-anesthetic-monitoring.pdf?la=en&hash=C4F2C7F3F5FBC209A7D43190DF3FD958E78FBAC9 [Accessed: 10 May 2020]

[5] Cook T, Woodall N, Harper J, Benger J. Major complications of airway management in the UK: Results of the Fourth National Audit Project of the Royal College of Anaesthetists and the Difficult Airway Society. Part 2: Intensive Care and Emergency Departments. British journal of anaesthesia. 2011;**106**:632-42. DOI: 10.1093/bja/aer059

[6] Cook TM, MacDougall-Davis SR. Complications and failure of airway management. BJA: British Journal of Anaesthesia. 2012;**109**(suppl_1):i68-i85. DOI: 10.1093/bja/aes393

[7] AAGBI Safety Statement. The Use of Capnography Outside the Operating Theatre Updated Statement from the Association of Anaesthetists of Great Britain & Ireland (AAGBI). May 2011. Available from: https://anaesthetists.org/Portals/0/PDFs/Archive%20guidelines%20PDFs/Archived_guidelines_Standards_monitoring_capnography_outside_operating_theatre_2011.pdf?ver=2018-06-28-154808-040 [Accessed: 13 August 2020]

[8] Cook T, Behringer EC, Benger J. Airway management outside the operating room: Hazardous and incompletely studied. Current Opinion in Anaesthesiology. 2012;**25**:461-469

[9] Russ S, Rout S, Sevdalis N. Do safety checklists improve teamwork and communication in the operating room? A systematic review. Annals of Surgery. 2013;**258**:856-871

[10] Bjurstrom M. The difficult airway trolley: A narrative review and practical guide. Anesthesiology Research and Practice. 2019. DOI: 10.1155/2019/6780254

[11] Mort T. The supraglottic airway device in the emergent setting. Its changing role outside the operating room. Anesthesiology news guide to airway management, Anesthesiology News. 2011;**37**:59-71

[12] Kuzhively J, Pandit JJ. Anesthesia and airway management for gastrointestinal endoscopic procedures outside the operating room. Current Opinion in Anaesthesiology. 2019;**32**(4):517-522

[13] Sevdalis N, Hull L, Birnbach DJ. Improving patient safety in the operating theatre and perioperative care: Obstacles, interventions and priorities for accelerating progress. British Journal of Anaesthesia. 2012;**109**(Suppl 1):i3-i16

[14] Neyrinck A. Management of the anticipated and unanticipated difficult airway in anesthesia outside the operating room. Current Opinion in Anaesthesiology. 2013;**26**(4):481-488

Chapter 4

Airway Trauma: Assessment and Management

Yasser Mahmoud Hammad Ali Hammad and Nabil A. Shallik

Abstract

Recognizing airway trauma and safety management is challenging for any anaesthesiologist. Many types of airway injuries require identifying airway anatomy correctly; early assessment and proper management are crucial for saving many lives. Proper management involves the classification of those patients into three categories. Each one has a unique and different control. Knowing your capabilities and skills are very important for safe airway management. It does not matter where you are but skills, knowledge of airway management algorithms and tools you have. After reading this book chapter, the participant will be able to define airway trauma, proper airway risk assessment and safety management.

Keywords: airway obstruction, facial injuries, intubation, mandibular fractures, maxillary fractures, maxillofacial injuries, surgical airway

1. Introduction

Many head and neck procedures have special and challenging requirements for anaesthesia care beyond airway management; however, securing the airway in patients with maxillofacial and neck trauma is crucial and lifesaving. Direct traumatic airway injury is rare (incidence <1%); hence, the airway assessment and management are not well structured because physicians rarely treat such cases [1, 2].

Trauma to the airway carries a life threatening situation because it can cause by itself airway obstruction or obstruction by blood, secretions, tissue oedema, debris and vomitus. It may be associated with cervical spine injury which will worsen intubating conditions. Finally, the risk of airway obstruction continues to postoperative period and the decision to extubate in part is based on the prevention of reintubation and/or to prevent postoperative airway obstruction by tissue oedema in certain types of trauma and facial bone fixation.

There are specific situations in patients with facial and neck trauma, as described by Hutchison et al. [3] to adversely affect the airway:

1. The displacement of posterior-inferior-fractured maxilla parallel to the inclined plane of the base of the skull can block the nasopharyngeal airway.

2. In the supine patient, a bilateral fracture of the anterior mandible may cause the tongue and the fractured symphysis to slide posteriorly and block the oropharynx.

3. Exfoliated and/or fractured teeth, bone fragments, vomitus, blood and secretions as well as foreign bodies, such as dentures, debris and shrapnel, may block the airway anywhere along the oropharynx and larynx.

4. Haemorrhage from open wounds or severe nasal bleeding may contribute to airway obstruction.

5. Trauma-induced soft tissue oedema and swelling can cause delayed airway compromise.

6. Trauma to the larynx and the trachea can cause displacement of the epiglottis, arytenoid cartilages and vocal cords, thereby increasing the risk of cervical airway obstruction.

2. Airway trauma and findings, modified from Jain et al. and De Angelis studies

2.1 Maxillofacial trauma

- Dento-alveolar: Exfoliated and/or fractured teeth, soft tissue lacerations, swelling and oropharyngeal bleeding [4, 5]. Gastric distension from swallowing of the blood can cause regurgitation and aspiration while securing the airway.

- Bilateral or comminuted parasymphyseal mandibular fractures: It can lead to posterior tongue displacement in supine position and airway obstruction. Movement to sitting position can relieve the obstruction, however those injuries may be associated with cervical spine injury.

- Temporo-mandibular fractures: A condylar fracture and displacement can prevent mouth opening. The mouth may be locked open or closed. Trismus which is secondary to the spasm of the masseter muscle due to irritation may be the cause of mouth lock.

- Mid-face fractures: Unilateral or bilateral Le Fort fractures (I-II&III) may cause airway compromise via maxillary prolapse, oedema or hemorrhage. Le Fort fractures II&III may be associated with fracture base of the skull with CSF leakage from the nose, epistaxis and oedema. Ng and colleagues reported establishing an emergency airway in 22 (34%) of 64 patients presenting with Le Fort fractures; the severity of the Le Fort fracture also correlated with an increased need for intubation [6].

- Zygomatic and orbital fractures: It can cause retro-bulbar hemorrhage and vision loss, traumatic mydriasis and increased intraocular pressure.

- Fracture base of the skull (temporal, occipital, sphenoid and ethmoid bones): It can cause peri-orbital ecchymosis (Raccoon eyes), Battle's sign, CSF rhinorrhea and cranial nerves palsy.

2.2 Neck and laryngeal trauma

- Penetrating trauma to the neck can cause arterial injury in 12–13% of the cases, and venous injury in 18–20% of the patients as reported by Britt et al. [7].

- Blunt trauma can cause airway obstruction by tissue disruption, oedema and hematoma. It can be associated with cervical spine (C-spine) injury. C-spine injury at or above C4 and C5 can cause airway obstruction by laryngeal oedema and apnea by diaphragmatic paralysis and neurogenic shock [8].

- Laryngeal trauma: The clinical presentation may not reflect the severity of the injury; some patients may present with delayed airway obstruction after blunt trauma to the neck. Others are associated with fracture base of the skull, C-spine injury, pharyngeal, oesophageal and vascular injury [9].

Patients with neck trauma including the trachea can be presented with one or combination of the following symptoms and signs: subcutaneous emphysema, crepitus, external bleeding, ecchymosis, hematoma, dyspnea, hypopnea, stridor, wheezing, cough, dysphonia, hoarseness, pain with phonation, dysphagia, drooling, haemoptysis, tracheal deviation and nerve injury [4].

3. Airway assessment and management

Despite the incidence of airway traumatic injury being low, it is associated to injuries, or to the airway obstruction and severe hypoxemia [1, 2].

According to a retrospective review of 12,187 civilian patients treated at a regional trauma Canadian centre, mortality was 36% in blunt airway trauma and 16% in penetrating airway trauma [1].

The definitive airway assessment and instantaneous management may be performed as soon as indicated, whether outside the hospital in case of profuse bleeding with airway compromise or inside the hospital, as it may cause early death in trauma. Securing the airway should be done with cervical spine stabilization to avoid spinal cord injury and based on the advanced trauma life support (ATLS) concept for managing patients who have sustained life-threatening injuries [3, 10].

The airway should be reevaluated frequently at least for several hours. The symptoms and signs of airway obstruction described before should be carefully examined, for example, inspiratory stridor suggests impending loss of airway. Ability to speak and answer simple questions indicates a patent airway, enough respiratory effort to generate voice and enough blood pressure to perfuse the brain [11].

A thorough history and physical examination should be made for every patient before the initiation of anaesthetic care and airway management. However, this should not delay the immediate securing of the airway in case of its compromise; as indicated in the Advanced Trauma Life Support Manual, there are three underlying concepts:

1. Treat the greatest threat to life first.

2. The lack of a definitive diagnosis should never impede the application of an indicated treatment.

3. A detailed history is not essential to begin the evaluation of a patient with acute injuries [12].

Gruen et al. found 16% of inpatients' deaths among 2594 trauma patients due to failure to establish and/or secure the airway and oxygenation [13].

This is followed by the standard preoperative airway assessment, which attempts to identify risk factors for difficult bag mask ventilation combined with difficult direct laryngoscopy [14].

The next step is to evaluate the traumatized airway and the adjoining structures using direct or video laryngoscopy, fiberoptic bronchoscopy (FOB) or ultrasonic imaging, with or without sedation and topical anaesthesia.

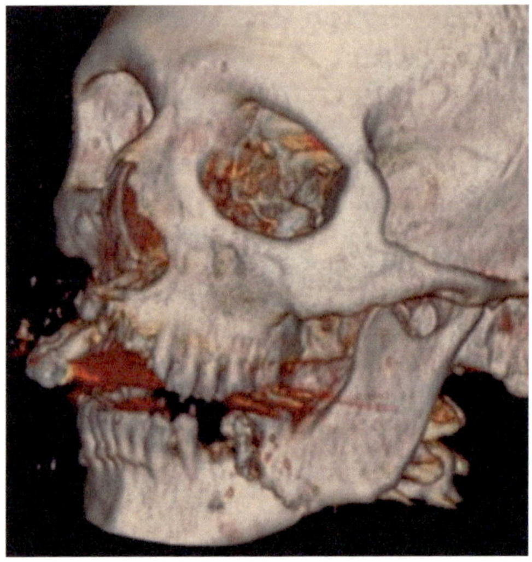

Figure 1.
3-D CT reconstruction showing loose teeth and bone that can cause airway obstruction.

If airway is maintained and there is no need for intubation, then computerized Tomography (CT) and Magnetic Resonance Imaging (MRI) can be performed. Imaging provides comprehensive information about airway and surrounding.

Virtual endoscopy and 3-D reconstruction of upper airway could be done, and all the injuries are identified, and the risk of airway compression is evaluated (**Figure 1**).

Once the airway risk assessment is done, the choice of airway management and possible interventions should be planned before the induction of anaesthesia.

4. Preintubation check list

1. Oxygen mask and nasal cannula oxygen running
2. Suction working
3. Bag Mask Value (BMV) ready
4. Different sizes of Guedel's oral airway
5. Laryngoscope functioning
6. Endotracheal tube (ETT)
7. Supraglottis airway (SGA) device ready
8. Intravenous line functioning (and blood pressure cuff on opposite arm)
9. Assistant designated to provide manual in-line stabilization (MILS)
10. Medications drawn up (including paralytic, even if not planning to use it)
11. Patient position optimized (if possible)
12. Airway plan verbalized with all personnel involved

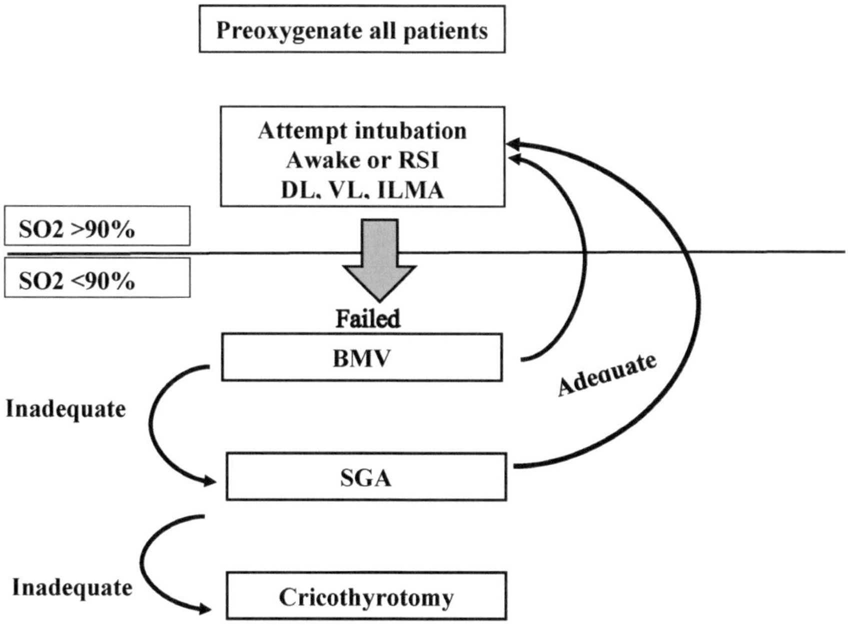

Figure 2.
Airway management algorithm (SO_2 = oxygen saturation, RSI = rapid sequence induction, DL = direct laryngoscopy, VL = video laryngoscopy, ILMA = intubating laryngeal mask airway, BMV=bag mask ventilation, SGA = Supraglottis airway.

The optimal airway management depends on the availability of expertise and equipment, not the location of the care. Communication should be clear between team members, concerning the airway plan and the role of each of them. Regardless of who oversees airway management, it should be clear who will make the decision to proceed and who will perform the procedure if a cricothyrotomy or surgical airway is required. Reardon et al. suggested airway management algorithm (**Figure 2**) [15].

5. Suggested airway management technique

5.1 Preoxygenation

Preoxygenation is critical to success and safety of emergency intubation, especially when rapid sequence induction and intubation (RSI) is used. The best way to provide high fraction of inspired oxygen (FiO_2; 100) for preoxygenation is by using a standard reservoir facemask with the oxygen flow rate set as high as possible. Patients should be preoxygenated for 3 min or 8 maximal capacity breaths if time is short. It is best to preoxygenate patients in a head-elevated position or in reverse Trendelenburg, especially if the patient is obese. Apneic oxygenation is a relatively new concept that can help prevent oxygen desaturation during RSI. This is best accomplished by placing a nasal cannula (with an oxygen flow rate more than 15 L/min) under the facemask during preoxygenation and leaving it in place during intubation [16].

Patients may be classified into the following three groups when deciding how to intubate:

- Group 1 (G1): Those at low risk of difficulty.

- Group 2 (G2): Those at higher risk of difficulty (as the real difficulty is uncertain).
- Group 3 (G3): Those with known airway difficulty or are highly likely to be difficult.

Patients with low risk of difficulty G1: Needs direct laryngoscopy and standard equipment with usual backup.

Patients with a higher risk of difficulty and uncertainty G2: Different plans should be ready, including video laryngoscopy (VL), suitable laryngeal masks (LMA) and emergent surgical airway.

Patients who are known difficult G3: Awake technique and spontaneous ventilation are maintained; fiberoptic intubation or elective surgical airway (tracheostomy).

5.2 Awake fiberoptic intubation

The technique has the advantage that patient is breathing throughout, however it has many disadvantages and limitations when used for management of patients with airway trauma.

The airway visualization is challenging with ongoing haemorrhage, the use of local anaesthetic is difficult due to trauma and hemorrhage and the procedure itself needs cooperative patient and expert anaesthesiologist.

When airway management is beyond emergency situations, the patient is stable with $SpO_2 > 90\%$ and in operating theater, the following situations should be considered:

5.3 Patients with full stomach

In general, all patients with trauma should be managed as with full stomach until proved otherwise. The risk of regurgitation and aspiration of food or swallowed and ingested blood is high.

Evacuating the contents of the stomach may be tried by the insertion of nasogastric tube before starting airway management in cooperative patients and in the absence of contraindications as mid face fractures. Applying cricoid pressure in not indicated any more with induction of anaesthesia in patients with trauma [17, 18] as it may itself hamper endotracheal tube insertion, may cause rupture oesophagus and its efficiency is suspected [19, 20].

5.4 Patients with C-spine injury

Any patient with trauma to the head and neck is considered to have C-spine injury till proved otherwise [21, 22].

Those patients are kept in neck collar and cervical spine inline stabilization during insertion of endotracheal tube to prevent neck movement, which may worsen intubating conditions [8].

Indirect video laryngoscopy (**Figure 3**) is proved to be useful compared to conventional direct laryngoscopy in some studies, when used for patients who need to be immobilized during intubation [23–25].

5.5 Nature of injury and decision making

According to the nature of maxillofacial trauma and the previous classification to six criteria either single or mixed, the decision of endotracheal intubation and

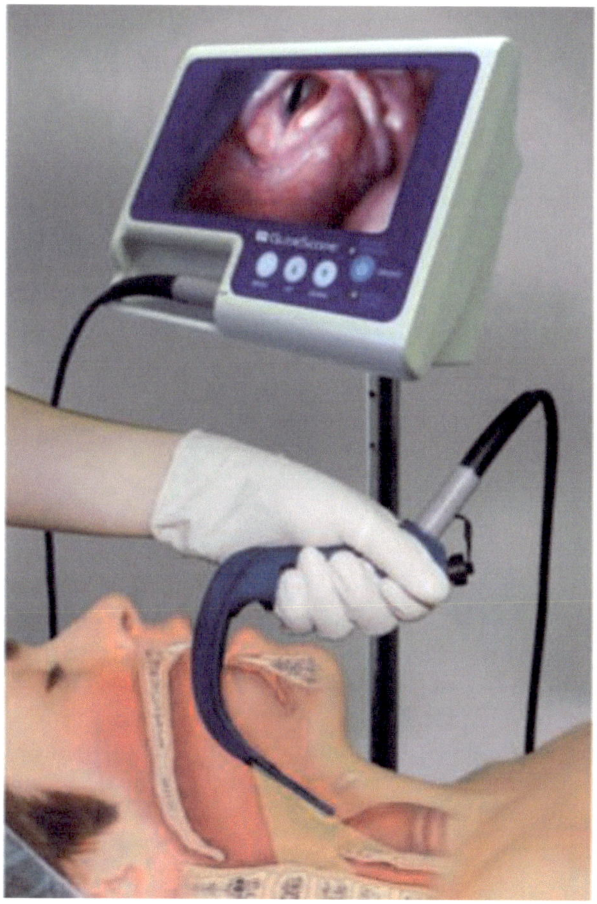

Figure 3.
Indirect videolaryngoscopy with permission from Verathon, Inc., Bothell, WA.

whether oral or nasal and the possibility to do surgical airway should be discussed before starting the procedure between the attending anaesthesiologist and surgeon. The level of experience with airway management should be the highest in the hospital especially with G2 and G3 patients. Nasal intubation is preferred by most of maxillofacial surgeons especially when the mouth is closed at the end of surgery by maxilla-mandibular fixation (MMF) [26]; however it is contraindicated in patients with mid-face and base of the skull fractures [27]. Decongestant nasal drops have to be used to reduce nasal vascularity before insertion of nasotracheal tube, secure the tube position by a loose stitch to the columella of the nose [28], oral insertion of the tube is fixed strongly by tape with tincture benzoin or by submental insertion as both anaesthesia and surgery teams share the same work space (**Figure 4**).

5.6 Submental orotracheal tube intubation

The technique was described to give the surgeon full access to the oral cavity and is indicated in patients with mid-face comminuted fracture, when nasal intubation is contraindicated, or in those patients who require restoration of the occlusion and their condition permits extubating patients at the end of surgery [29].

The technique is contraindicated in inpatients with comminuted mandibular fractures [29].

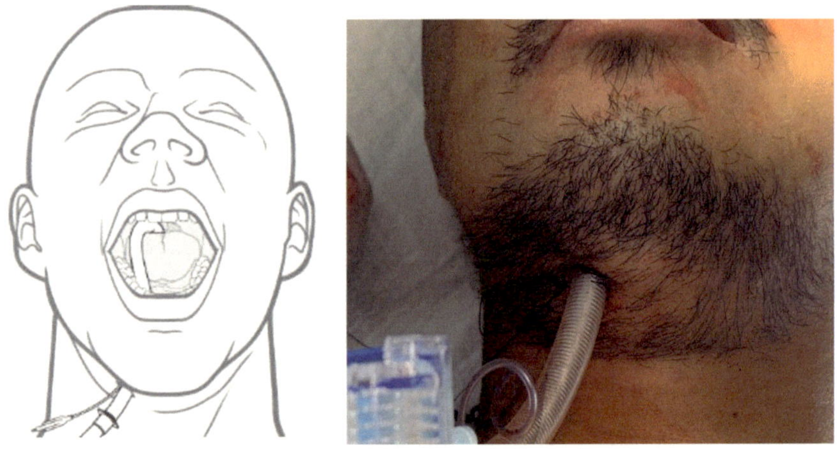

Figure 4.
Submental intubation.

A reinforced, armored, endotracheal tube is used in this technique, in order to prevent the tube from kinking during its usage. After a regular orotracheal intubation, the tube is passed by blunt dissection through the floor of the mouth at halfway between the chin and the angel of the mandible, and then sutured to the skin to secure position (**Figure 4**).

Complications from submental endotracheal intubation include bleeding, damage to the lingual and mandibular branch of the facial nerve and damage to the submandibular gland and/or its duct [30, 31].

6. Airway control in emergency situations

The securing of a patent airway for maxillofacial trauma patients in emergency situations whether inside or outside the hospital carries a considerable risk of failure and death due to airway obstruction. An additional risk is added when most of those patients are managed by inexperienced medical staff. This was shown in a study where there was 97% of trauma patients who were managed by unexperienced physicians in airway management. Most maxillofacial trauma patients who are acutely desaturating are intubated via orotracheal route by direct laryngoscopy [32].

1. Additional choices for managing the emergent airway include the Fastrach intubating laryngeal mask airway (ILMA Fastrach) (**Figure 5**), placed blindly through the mouth to seals off the hypopharynx via a circumferential inflatable cuff; this may prevent aspiration of blood [32, 33].

2. Intubation through LMA using Aintree exchange catheter (**Figure 6**).

   Aintree intubation catheter (Cook Medical, Bloomington, IN, USA) permits intubating patients via any LMA (sizes 3,4,5) with ETT 6–8 mm ID without interruption of oxygenation [34].

   Despite weak reports, blind endotracheal intubation (ETI) with blind use of either gum elastic bougie or tube exchange catheter is not advisable in critically ill patients as it's associated with tracheal injury and has been the cause for positive pressure ventilation-related pneumomediastinum.

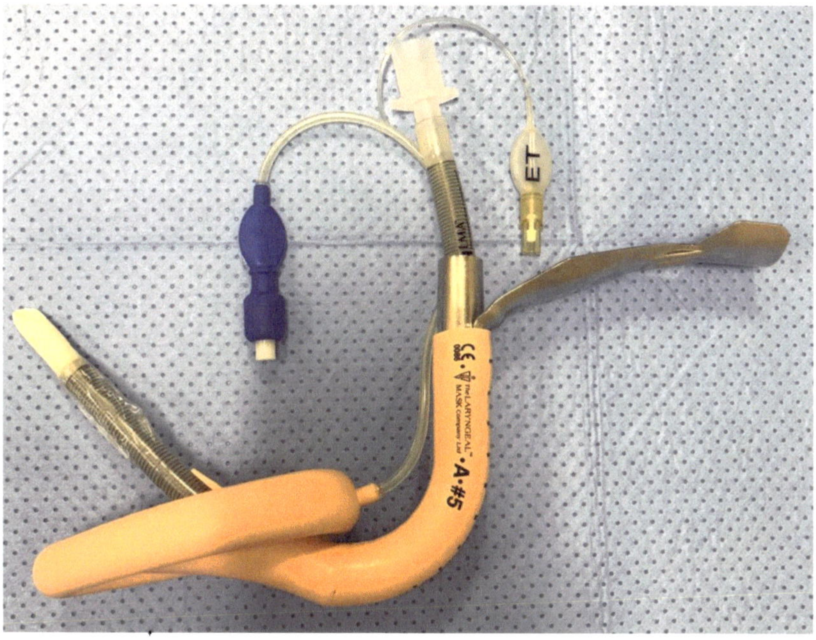

Figure 5.
The intubating laryngeal mask airway.

3. The double lumen airway (Combitube, Tyco Healthcare Group LP, Pleasanton, CA or the laryngeal tube and also known as the King LT (VBM Medizintechnik, Sulz, Germany)), is a dual lumen tube, with dual cuff that is blindly inserted into the oesophagus (**Figure 7**). The distal balloon is smaller and inflated within the oesophagus to prevent gastric reflux. The proximal one is a larger balloon which seals off the oropharynx and allows ventilation via perforations between the two cuffs [35, 36].

   This tube is always inserted by paramedics at the scene due to ease of insertion in comparison of endotracheal intubation [37].

4. Finally, the cricothyroidotomy is indicated in failed attempts at intubation or ventilation [32].

   Other reported indications include airway obstruction by excessive emesis or haemorrhage, known cervical spine fracture, and inability to visualize the vocal cords [38].

   Cricothyroidotomy was reported in 0.4% of emergent airway control patients in total of 8320 trauma admissions [39], and in 0.1–3.3% of patients with maxillofacial trauma [40]. Other studies showed that 15–23% of emergent cricothyroidotomies was used as the first and only means of airway control [41, 42].

6.1 Scalpel cricothyroidotomy

Scalpel cricothyroidotomy is the rapid and most suitable method of securing the airway in the emergency situation. A cuffed endotracheal tube in the trachea prevents the airway from aspiration, provides a secure route for expiration, permits low-pressure ventilation using traditional breathing systems and allows end-tidal CO_2 monitoring. A number of surgical techniques have been described, but there is a lack of evidence of the superiority of one over another. The techniques all have common steps in general: neck extension, identification of the cricothyroid membrane, cutting through the skin and

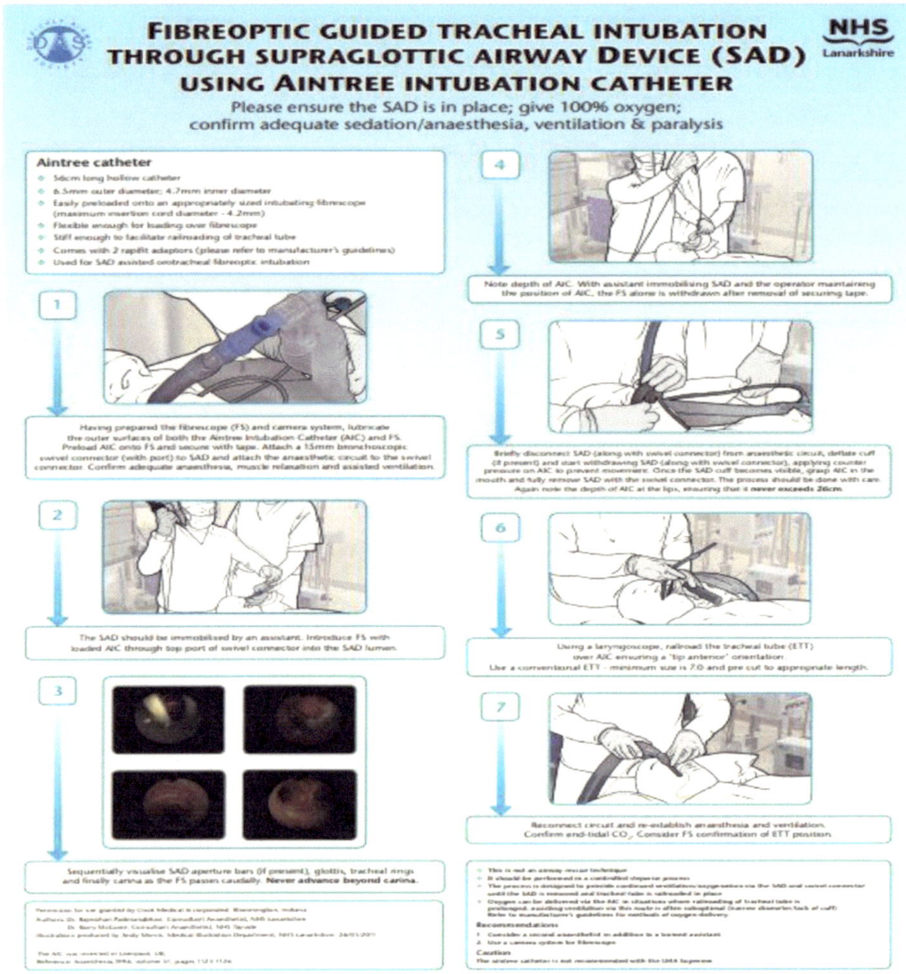

Figure 6.
Fiberoptic guided tracheal intubation through supra-glottic airway device (SAD) using Aintree intubation catheter (DAS guideline with written permission).

cricothyroid membrane and insertion of a cuffed endotracheal tube. In some instances, the skin and cricothyroid membrane are cut sequentially; in others, a single incision is recommended. Many include a placeholder to keep the wound open until the endotracheal tube is in place. Some use special equipment like cricoid hook, tracheal dilators, etc. A single stab incision through the cricothyroid membrane is appealing in terms of its simplicity, but this approach may fail in the thick neck patient or if the anatomy is difficult, and a vertical skin incision is recommended in this situation [43].

6.2 Narrow cannula technique

Narrow-bore cannula techniques are effective in the elective setting; however, their limitations have been well known. Ventilation can be achieved only by using a high-pressure machine, and this is associated with a high risk of barotrauma. Failure because of kinking, obstruction, malposition, or displacement of the cannula can occur even with predesigned cannulae, such as the Ravussin™ (VBM, Sulz, Germany). High-pressure ventilation equipment may not be available in all facilities, and most anaesthesiologists do not use them on a regular basis. Their use in these situations should be restricted to experienced clinicians who use them in routine clinical practice [43].

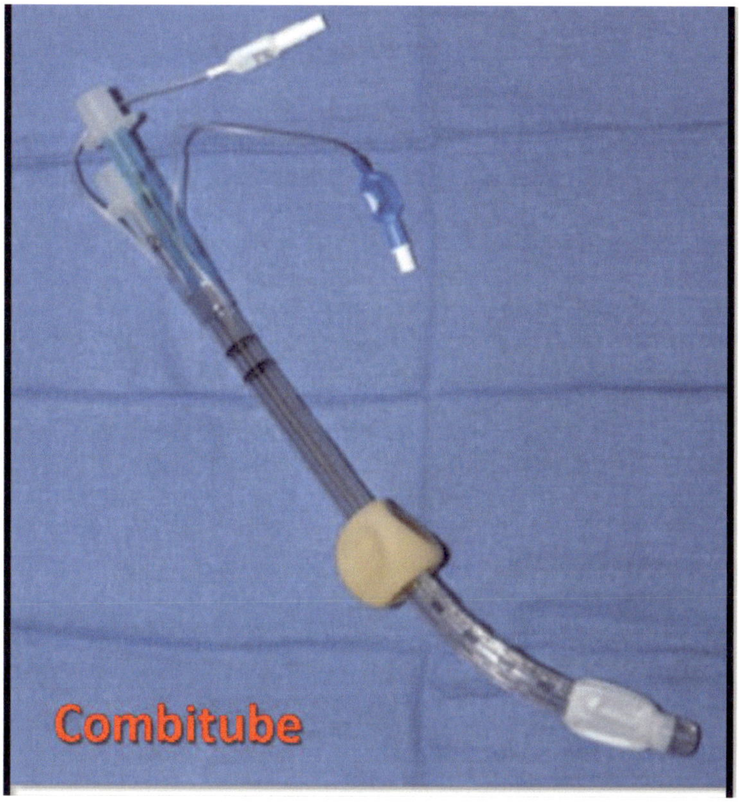

Figure 7.
Oesophageal/tracheal Combitube.

6.3 Wide-bore cannula

Wide-bore cannula over the guidewire: some wide-bore cannula kits, such as the Cook Melker® emergency cricothyrotomy set, use a wire-guided (Seldinger) technique. This approach is less invasive than a surgical cricothyroidotomy and decrease the need for special machine for ventilation. The skills required are familiar to anaesthesiologists and intensivists because they are common to central line insertion and per-cutaneous tracheostomy method; however, these techniques require fine and smooth motor control, making them less suited to stressful situations. However, a wire-guided technique may be a reasonable alternative for anaesthetists who are experienced with this method, the evidence suggests that a surgical cricothyroidotomy is both faster and more reliable.

Non-Seldinger wide-bore cannula: A number of non-Seldinger wide-bore cannula-over-trochar devices are available for airway rescue. Although successful use has been reported in Cannot intubate, cannot oxygenate (CICO), there have been no large studies of these devices in clinical practice [43].

7. Postoperative management

7.1 Extubation

Extubating patients at the end of surgery should be discussed between anaesthesia and surgery teams. Patients with severe trauma to the airway, those with pan facial fracture fixation, prolonged surgery and airway oedema should be kept ventilated in intensive care unit. Extubating patients should be done carefully with all equipment for reintubation ready. Some patients may be extubated in operating theater over airway exchange catheters (AEC) (**Figure 8**).

AEC is a long hollow bougie that comes in several sizes and can be placed into the trachea through the tracheal tube. The tracheal tube is then removed, and the AEC left in the airway with the tip at the level of the mid trachea. It is important that the catheter remains above the carina, and it should not be inserted beyond 25 cm in an adult patient. The AEC can then be used in the same way as a bougie to help reintubate the trachea in case of deterioration. It has been used in the recovery unit and on critical care unit after head and neck surgery. Usually, the AEC can be left in for few hours after extubation but is can be tolerated for up to 72 h [44].

While transferring the patient to intensive therapy unit (ITU), it is safer to keep the patient asleep with tracheal tube in place, but extra care to be taken to avoid tube dislodgment.

7.2 Prepare for unplanned extubation

Notify the team providing ongoing care if the patient had a difficult airway, and have advanced airway equipment and a surgical airway tray at the patient's bedside in case of an unplanned extubation.

7.3 Bailey manoeuvre for extubation

This manoeuvre can be performed by several ways, but it must be done with an adequate depth of anaesthesia (and muscle relaxation) to minimize the risk of laryngospasm. The patient should be properly positioned and preoxygenated, and the oropharynx should be gently suctioned. A deflated SGA is introduced behind the endotracheal tube, its position is confirmed and its cuff is inflated.

The cuff of the endotracheal tube is deflated and the tube is removed, taking care not to remove the SGA with the tube (**Figure 9**).

7.4 Staged extubation set with wire

Staged extubation uses a staged extubation wire (**Figure 10**) to maintain continuous airway access and a staged reintubation catheter to facilitate a successful reintubation if required. Soft, tapered and kink-resistant wire is coated in a polymeric jacket to assure minimal irritation while in position [45].

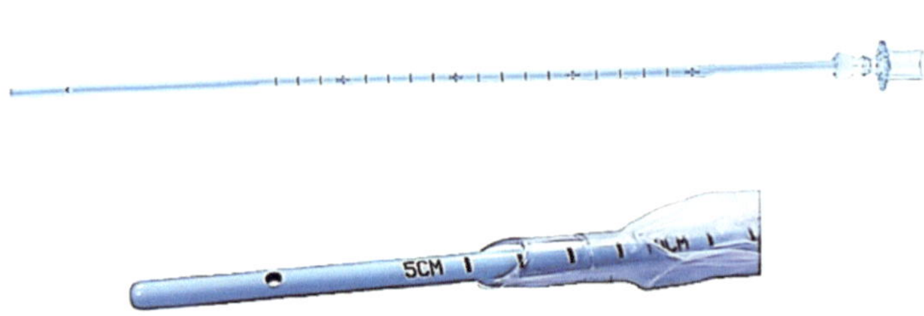

Figure 8.
Airway exchange catheter.

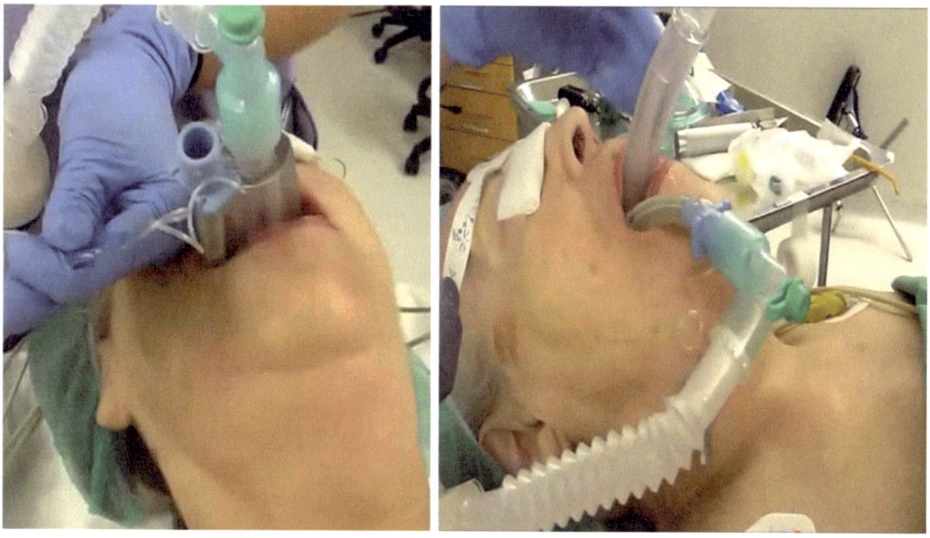

Figure 9.
Bailey manoeuvre.

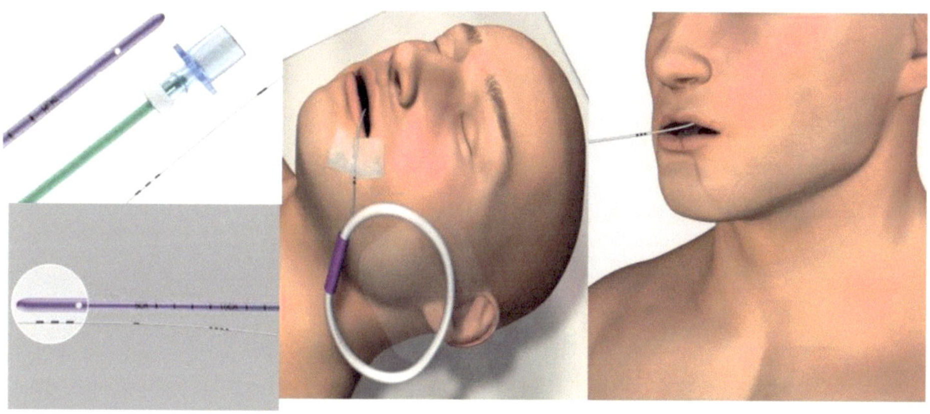

Figure 10.
Staged extubation set with wire.

8. Conclusion

Establishing a secure airway in a trauma patient is one of the primary essentials of treatment. Maxillofacial trauma directly impacts on the airway resulting in compromise and hindering attempts to secure the airway and any delays in securing the airway may lead to morbidity and mortality. So, multiple approaches to securing the airway are possible; each has advantages and disadvantages. Every airway manager has a different set of skills, experience and availability of airway equipment, so management details will vary based on these factors. It is useful to understand common facial injury patterns that affect airway management and then consider how each injury pattern will interfere with common emergency airway manoeuvres. The time available to accomplish the task is short and the patient's condition may deteriorate rapidly. Both decision-making and performance are impaired in such circumstances. In this chapter, we discussed the complexity of the situation and presented a treatment approach.

Author details

Yasser Mahmoud Hammad Ali Hammad[1,2*] and Nabil A. Shallik[1,2,3,4]

1 Department of Anaesthesia, ICU and Perioperative Medicine, HMC, Doha, Qatar

2 Weill Cornell Medical College in Qatar, Doha, Qatar

3 Qatar University, Doha, Qatar

4 Tanta Faculty of Medicine, Tanta, Egypt

*Address all correspondence to: YHammad@hamad.qa

References

[1] Kummer C, Netto FS, Rizoli S, Yee D. A review of traumatic airway injuries: Potential implications for airway assessment and management. Injury. 2007;**38**:27-33 2

[2] Bhojani RA, Rosenbaum DH, Dikmen E, Paul M, Atkins BZ, Zonies D, et al. Contemporary assessment of laryngotracheal trauma. The Journal of Thoracic and Cardiovascular Surgery. 2005;**130**:426-432

[3] Hutchison ML, Skinner D. ABC of major trauma. major maxillofacial injuries. British Medical Journal. 1990;**301**(6752):595-599

[4] Jain U, McCunn M, Smith CE, Pittet J-F. Management of the traumatized airway. Anesthesiology. 2016;**124**:199-2

[5] De Angelis AF, Barrowman RA, Harrod R, Nastri AL. Review article: Maxillofacial emergencies: Maxillofacial trauma. Emergency Medicine Australasia. 2014;**26**:530-537

[6] Ng M, Saadat D, Sinha UK. Managing the emergency airway in Le Fort fractures. The Journal of Cranio-Maxillofacial Trauma. 1998;**4**:38-43

[7] Britt LD, Peyser MD. Penetrating and blunt neck trauma. In: Mattox KL, Feliciano DV, Moore EE, editors. Trauma. New York: McGraw-Hill; 2000. pp. 437-449

[8] Crosby ET. Airway management in adults after cervical spine trauma. Anesthesiology. 2006;**104**:1293-1318

[9] Bhojani RA, Rosenbaum DH, Dikmen E, Paul M, Atkins BZ, Zonies D, et al. Contemporary assessment of laryngo-tracheal trauma. The Journal of Thoracic and Cardiovascular Surgery. 2005;**130**:426

[10] Committee on Trauma American College of Surgeons. Advanced Trauma Life Support for Doctors ATLS. 8th ed. Chicago, Ill: American College of Surgeons; 2008. p. 69

[11] Schaefer SD. Management of acute blunt and penetrating external laryngeal trauma. Laryngoscope. 2014;**124**:233-244

[12] American College of Surgeons. Advanced Trauma Life Support Manual. 9th ed. Chicago: American College of Surgeons; 2012. pp. 2-28

[13] Gruen RL, Jurkovich GJ, McIntyre LK, Foy HM, Maier RV. Patterns of errors contributing to trauma mortality: lessons learned from 2594 deaths. Annals of Surgery. 2006;**244**(3):371-378

[14] Kheterpal S, Healy D, Aziz MF, et al., Multicenter Perioperative Outcomes Group Perioperative Clinical Research Committee. Incidence, predictors, and outcome of difficult mask ventilation combined with difficult laryngoscopy: A report from the multicenter perioperative outcomes group. Anesthesiology. 2013;**119**:1360-1369

[15] Reardon R, Martel M. Airway management in facial trauma. In: Berkow L, Sakles J, editors. Cases in Emergency Airway Management. Cambridge: Cambridge University Press; 2015. DOI: 10.1017/CBO9781139941471.022

[16] Mir F, Patel A, Iqbal R, et al. A randomised controlled trial comparing transnasal humidified rapid insufflation ventilatory exchange (THRIVE) pre-oxygenation with facemask preoxygenation in patients undergoing rapid sequence induction of anaesthesia. Anaesthesia. 2017;**72**:439

[17] Haslam N, Parker L, Duggan JE. Effect of cricoid pressure on the view at laryngoscopy. Anaesthesia. 2005;**60**(1):41-47

[18] Ellis DY, Harris T, Zideman D. Cricoid pressure in emergency department rapid sequence tracheal intubations: A risk benefit analysis. Annals of Emergency Medicine. 2007;**50**(6):653-665

[19] Bhatia N, Bhagat H, Sen I. Cricoid pressure: Where do we stand? Journal of Anaesthesiology Clinical Pharmacology. 2014;**30**(1):3-6

[20] Beckers SK, Brokmann JC, Rossaint R. Airway and ventilator management in trauma patients. Current Opinion in Critical Care. 2014;**20**(6):626-631

[21] Jamal BT, Diecidue R, Qutub A, Cohen M. The pattern of combined maxillofacial and cervical spine fractures. Journal of Oral and Maxillofacial Surgery. 2009;**67**(3):559-562

[22] Rahman SA, Chandrasala S. When to suspect head injury or cervical spine injury in maxillofacial trauma? Dental Research Journal. 2014;**11**(3):336-344

[23] Kill C, Risse J, Wallot P, Seidl P, Steinfeldt T, Wulf H. Videolaryngoscopy with glidescope reduces cervical spine movement in patients with unsecured cervical spine. Journal of Emergency Medicine. 2013;**44**(4):750-756

[24] Robitaille A, Williams SR, Tremblay M-H, Guilbert F, Theriault M, Drolet P. Cervical spine motion during tracheal intubation with manual in-line stabilization: direct laryngoscopy versus GlideScope videolaryngoscopy. Anesthesia and Analgesia. 2008;**106**(3):935-941

[25] Bhardwaj N, Jain K, Rao M, Mandal AK. Assessment of cervical spine movement during laryngoscopy with Macintosh and Truview laryngoscopes. Journal of Anaesthesiology Clinical Pharmacology. 2013;**29**(3):308-312

[26] Robertson G, Doucet JC. Helping anesthesiologists understand facial fractures. Oral and Maxillofacial Surgery Clinics of North America. 2013;**25**(4):561-572

[27] Halland CEJ, Shutt LE. Nasotracheal intubation for head and neck surgery. Anaesthesia. 2003;**58**(3):249-256

[28] Ota Y, Karakida K, Aoki T. A secure method of nasal endotracheal tube tabilization with suture and rubber tube. The Tokai Journal of Experimental and Clinical Medicine. 2001;**26**(4-6):119-122

[29] Barak M, Bahouth H, Leiser Y, El-Naaj IA. Airway Management of the Patient with Maxillofacial Trauma: Review of the Literature and Suggested Clinical Approach. BioMed Research International;**2015**, Article ID: 724032:9

[30] de Toledo GL, Bueno SC, Mesquita RA, Ama-ral MBF. Complications from submental endotracheal intubation: a prospective study and literature review. Dental Traumatology. 2013;**29**(3):197-202

[31] Mittal G, Mittal RK, Katyal S, Uppal S, Mittal V. Airway management in maxillofacial trauma: do we really need tracheostomy/submental intubation. Journal of Clinical and Diagnostic Research. 2014;**8**(3):77-79

[32] Dunham CM, Barraco RD, Clark DE, et al. Guidelines for emergency tracheal intubation immediately after traumatic injury. The Journal of Trauma. 2003;**55**:162-179

[33] Rollert MK. The case against the laryngeal mask airway for anesthesia in oral and maxillofacial surgery. Journal of Oral and Maxillofacial Surgery. 2004;**62**:739-741

[34] Difficult Airway Society. Guidelines for Fiberoptic guided tracheal intubation using through SAD using

Aintree intubation catheter. Visited on 21st of July 2020

[35] Blostein PA, Koestner AJ, Hoak S. Failed rapid sequence intubation in trauma patients: Esophageal tracheal Combi-tube is a useful adjunct. The Journal of Trauma. 1998;**44**:534-537

[36] Davis DP, Valentine C, Ochs M, Vilke GM, Hoyt DB. The Combitube as a salvage airway device for paramedic rapid sequence intubation. Annals of Emergency Medicine. 2003;**42**:697-704

[37] Smith CE, DeJoy SJ. New equipment and techniques for airway management in trauma. Current Opinion in Anaesthesiology. 2001;**14**:197-209

[38] Kellman RM, Losquadro WD. Comprehensive airway management of patients with maxillofacial trauma. Craniomaxillofacial Trauma & Reconstruction. 2008;**1**:1

[39] Salvino CK, Dries D, Gamelli R, et al. Emergency cricothyroidotomy in trauma victims. The Journal of Trauma. 1993;**34**:503-505

[40] Taicher S, Givol N, Peleg M, Ardekian L. Changing indications for tracheostomy in maxillofacial trauma. Journal of Oral and Maxillofacial Surgery. 1996;**54**:292-295

[41] Isaacs JH Jr, Pedersen AD. Emergency cricothyroidotomy. The American Surgeon. 1997;**63**:346-349

[42] Tung TC, Tseng WS, Chen CT, et al. Acute life-threatening injuries in facial fracture patients: a review of 1,025 patients. The Journal of Trauma. 2000;**49**:420-424

[43] Frerk C, Mitchell VS, McNarry AF, Mendonca C, Bhagrath R, Patel A, et al. Difficult Airway Society intubation guidelines working group, Difficult Airway Society 2015 guidelines for management of unanticipated difficult intubation in adults. BJA: British Journal of Anaesthesia. 2015;**115**(6):827-848. DOI: 10.1093/bja/aev371

[44] Cooper RM. The use of an endotracheal ventilation catheter in the management of difficult extubations. Canadian Journal of Anaesthesia. 1996;**43**:90-93

[45] Biro P, Priebe HJ. Staged extubation strategy: Is an airway exchange catheter the answer? Anesthesia and Analgesia. 2007;**105**(5):1182-1185

Chapter 5

Airway Management in Accident and Emergency

Kemal Tolga Saracoglu, Gul Cakmak and Ayten Saracoglu

Abstract

Accidents are associated with airway complications. Tracheobronchial injury, pneumothorax, pneumomediastinum, atelectasis, and subcutaneous emphysema can be observed. Therefore airway management in emergency medicine requires skills and equipment. Rapid-sequence intubation, effective preoxygenation, apneic oxygenation, manual inline stabilization technique should be used properly. Rapid-sequence intubation consists of sedation, analgesia, and muscle paralysis components. Videolaryngoscopes, supraglottic and extraglottic airway devices, bougie and surgical airway tools are among training materials. A range of training materials have been described to improve providers' understanding and knowledge of patient safety. In conclusion providing oxygenation, minimizing the risk of complications and choosing the appropriate devices constitute the airway management's pearls.

Keywords: airway management, emergency medicine, accident

1. Introduction

Approximately 0.5-1% of patients in the emergency medicine department require tracheal intubation for various reasons [1]. Respiratory failure, diseases that cause mental state changes, and cardiac arrest are the leading causes among these reasons. Airway management requires a systematic approach (**Table 1**). This section aims to evaluate the factors such as airway providing methods in emergency conditions, the challenges encountered in the success of these methods, and the training and teamwork required to overcome them.

2. Incidence

While the frequency of difficult intubation in operating rooms is 1.15% –3.8%, this rate varies between 3.0% and 5.3% in the emergency department [2]. Difficult intubation significantly decreases the success rate of the first attempt. The risk of complications accompanies this condition. Therefore, difficult airway management preparation should be performed effectively.

Accidents can cause airway complications. Tracheobronchial injury is one of the least common injuries in blunt chest trauma, but it has a high mortality rate. Approximately 81% of the patients die at the accident site or before reaching the emergency department [3]. Pneumothorax, pneumomediastinum, atelectasis, and subcutaneous emphysema can be seen in radiological imaging. Surgical airway incidence has been reported to be 0.1–7.7% [4].

1. Patients with increasing respiratory failure should be evaluated frequently. The underlying causes of frequently accompanying acidosis should be treated.
2. Effective preoxygenation should be applied.
3. Apneic window duration should be extended with apneic oxygenation techniques
4. Since ketamine has bronchodilator effects; it should be considered in the induction of patients with obstructive pulmonary disease.
5. The presence of conditions such as hypoxemia, hypercapnia, and acidosis that increase Pulmonary Vascular Resistance should be avoided in patients with cardiac disease.
6. First of all, airway clearance should be provided and maintained with basic airway management tools. These include chin lift, jaw thrust, recovery position.
7. The oral or nasal airway should be used in an unconscious patient.
8. Suction should be used to prevent aspiration of secretions, mucus, or vomit residues.
9. RSI should be considered for tracheal intubation, while care should be taken against the risk of hemodynamic deterioration, prolonged apnea, and pulmonary aspiration.
10. Direct or indirect laryngoscopy can be applied. However, video-laryngoscopes have some advantages.
11. Tracheal intubation should be confirmed by capnography. Postintubation hypocapnia is associated with poor outcome.
12. Oxygenation with tracheal intubation, laryngeal mask, and bag valve mask should be tried before invasive techniques such as surgical airway. However, in case of failure, cricothyrotomy should not be delayed.
13. Airway management should be provided with teamwork, and critical situations should be overcome by sharing the work.
14. Recommendations for difficult airway guidelines should be transferred to clinical practice.
15. It should be ensured that the acquired knowledge and skills are made permanent by planning periodical training.

Table 1.
Pearls of airway management in the emergency room.

3. Airway providing methods

Airway management in emergency medicine requires skills and equipment. The Rapid-sequence intubation (RSI) technique is used in the rate of 99% for tracheal intubations performed under emergency conditions [5]. RSI consists of sedation, analgesia, and muscle paralysis components. For this purpose, rocuronium or succinylcholine is used as a muscle relaxant. Rocuronium is increasingly in use due to its advantages such as rapid onset effect, minimal side effects, greater availability than succinylcholine, and rapid reverse ability using sugammadex. In a retrospective study of 215 patients, West et al. [6] reported that rocuronium was chosen to provide muscle relaxation predominantly in the patient group with higher early mortality. The use of rocuronium in this study resulted in hypoxemia more often before RSI and VL. A recent large observational study reported no difference in first-pass success rate and intubation-related adverse events between the use of succinylcholine and rocuronium for RSI in the emergency department [7].

Airway management in emergency conditions is complicated due to several factors including facial and neck trauma, risk of vomiting and aspiration, cervical spinal immobilization, or chest compressions applied for resuscitation. It decreases the success of intubation. During difficult tracheal intubation, prolonged apnea results in a sudden decrease in pH, hemodynamic collapse, dysrhythmia, and bradycardia. PaO_2 decreases as oxygen are suspended from the lungs. Therefore, effective preoxygenation should be performed before the procedure, and apneic oxygenation should be considered throughout the procedure to lengthen the apneic window. Recommended preoxygenation techniques include tidal volume ventilation for 3 min with high FiO_2, 8 min ventilation with 100% FiO_2, or oxygen inhalation until etO_2 reaches 90% and above [8]. Low flow or high flow oxygen is used for apneic oxygenation. Insufflation can also be performed through the venturi mask, nasal cannula, and oxygen cannula or catheters. However, oxygen up to 15 L/min can be given with these techniques. FiO_2 can be given in the range of 0.21-1 with 60-70 L/min flow through high flow systems. In these systems, it is possible to reach high flow rates as oxygen is given by humidifying and heating [9]. The manual inline stabilization (MILS) technique is used in patients with cervical trauma, and direct laryngoscopy worsens the vision in 50% of the cases [10]. C-spine collars and MILS limit the mouth opening. The use of video-laryngoscopes during MILS increases the first attempt success rate by increasing the viewing angle.

4. Psychological barriers

Psychological barriers complicate emergency airway management. This situation causes delays in the application of invasive techniques such as emergency cricothyroidotomy. The Vortex Approach has been defined to increase airway management's success rate applied under emergency conditions [11, 12]. It evaluates the steps of airway management in two parts as preparation and implementation. On the one hand, it is aimed to provide oxygenation successfully without the need for surgical techniques (**Figure 1**). On the other hand, invasive techniques are prepared before the patient is desaturated. Vortex provides effective teamwork. It is thought that this approach can increase the clinical applicability of difficult airway guidelines.

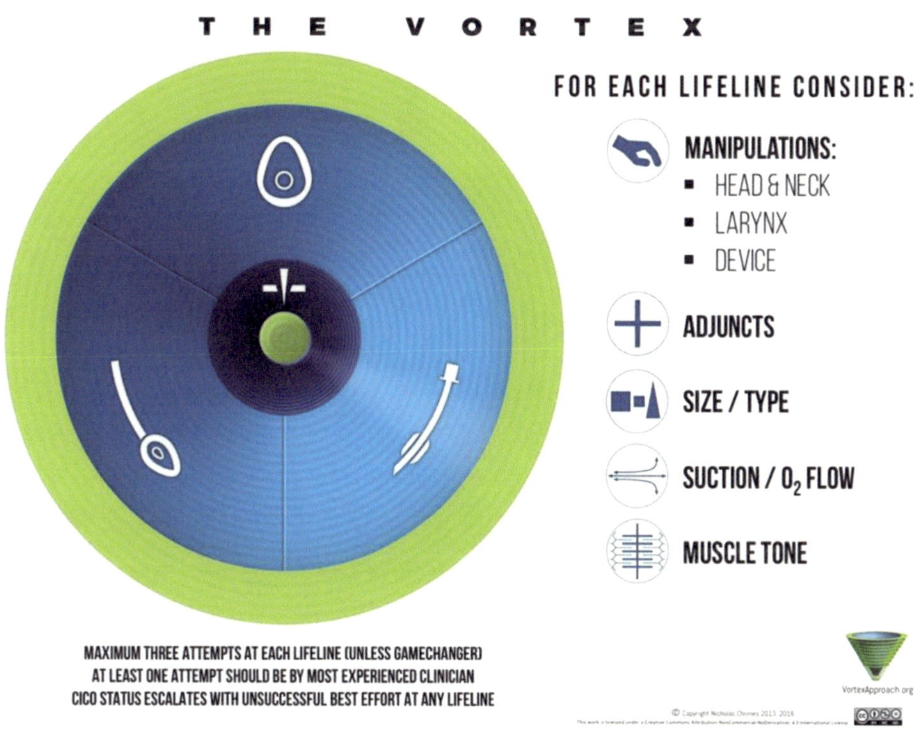

Figure 1.
The Vortex Approach action plan available from: http://vortexapproach.org.

5. Surgical airway

Surgical airway intervention is applied in case of unsuccessful tracheal intubation and cannot intubate-cannot oxygenate situation. Percutaneous cricothyrotomy is the most commonly used procedure. Laceration development in the posterior tracheal wall is a mortal complication. Life-threatening tension pneumothorax, pneumomediastinum, mediastinitis, and progressive respiratory failure can occur when the posterior membranous part of the trachea is injured. Ultrasonography reduces the developmental risk of these complications [13]. However, Siddiqui et al. reported that airway damage might develop despite ultrasound guidance. Also, ultrasound-guided cricothyrotomy takes longer than the conventional technique [14].

6. Training

On the one hand, the continuity of airway providing skills should be ensured through intermittent training, and on the other hand, knowledge about the use of newly developed devices should be obtained. Training requirements in airway

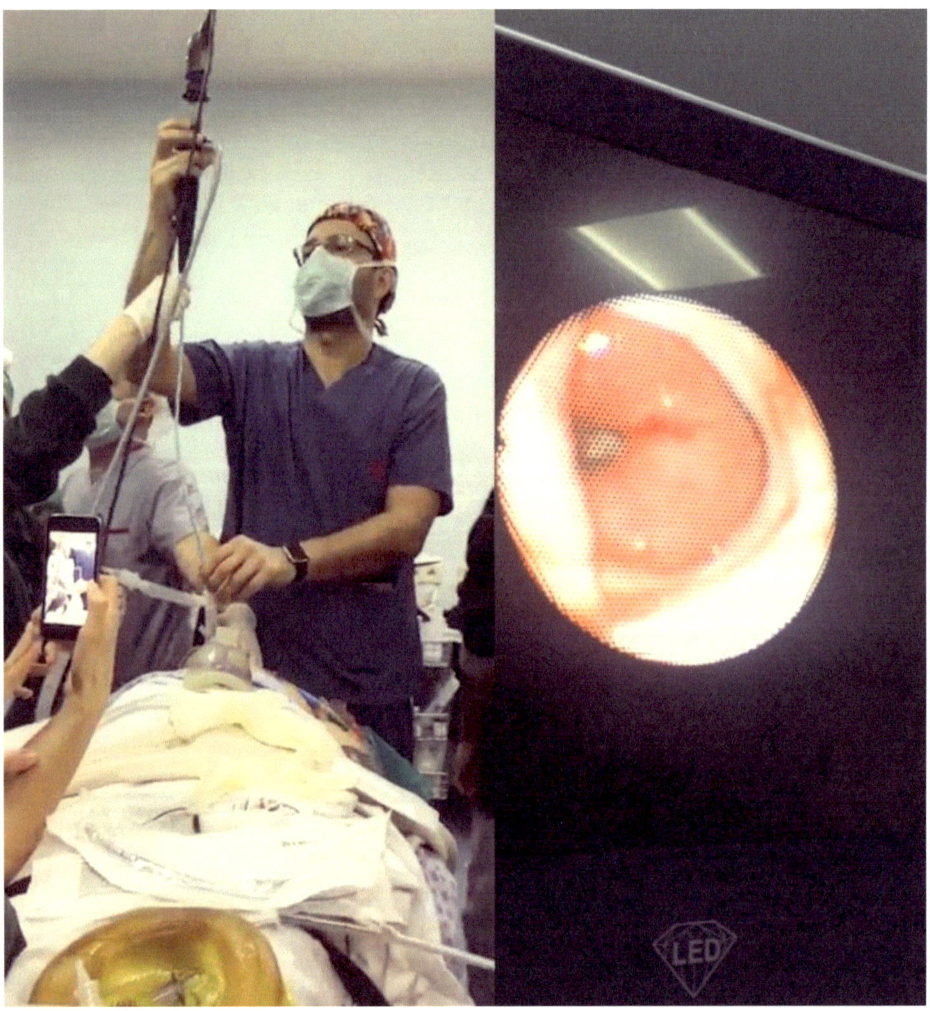

Figure 2.
Intubation through supraglottic airway devices.

management can be divided into airway evaluation, technical aspects of tracheal intubation and alternative airway techniques, and rapid sequential intubation. Fiberoptic intubation and the use of laryngeal masks are among the most common trainings (**Figure 2**) [15]. Simulation-based airway training is also widely used. Both technical and non-technical skills of the participants can be improved with simulators [16]. However, the important fact in training is the intermittent repetition of the acquired skills and permanence. Besides, the transfer of acquired knowledge and skills to the clinical environment should form the basis of training on this subject. For this purpose, different training methods were used to teach airway management to residents and novice users. It has been reported that teaching on cadavers and expression techniques such as Pecha Kucha is effective in achieving success [17].

7. Pre-hospital setting

Pre-hospital settings are often associated with airway management challenges. Although the team is well trained, the frequency of morbidity and mortality is high due to the high risk of complications. Tracheal intubation is the ideal technique [18]. Direct and indirect laryngoscopy can be used for tracheal intubation. It has been reported that the use of video-laryngoscope by emergency medical residents resulted in less esophageal intubation than direct laryngoscopy. In a study analyzing six years retrospectively, data of 2.677 patients were examined [19]. 1.530 intubations (44.7%) were performed with a direct laryngoscope, and video-laryngoscopy was used during 1.895 intubation attempts (55.3%). While esophageal intubation incidence with direct laryngoscope was 5.1%, this ratio was 1.0% with the video-laryngoscope. It has been shown that the use of a checklist in the airway management of patients with severe trauma leads to a decrease in the rate of intubation-mediated complications [20]. Many studies have been conducted in the pre-hospital setting. The success rate and risk of complications of pre-hospital tracheal intubation depend on the experience of healthcare professionals. Intubation performed by healthcare professionals who are not skilled enough to do this significantly increases mortality. A meta-analysis, including 733 studies and data of 4772 patients, reported that tracheal intubation should be performed in emergency medical services [21].

8. Video-laryngoscopes

In recent years, video-laryngoscopes have become a popular tool for the intubation of trauma patients (**Figure 3**). Many studies are comparing direct laryngoscopy and video-laryngoscopy in trauma patients. A systematic review in which nine different studies covering 1329 patients was evaluated, the first attempt success rate was significantly higher with video-laryngoscopes [22]. Besides, the use of video-laryngoscope caused a significant reduction in Cormack and Lehane grades, improving glottic vision. Mucosal trauma decreased with the use of video-laryngoscopy ($p = 0.02$). In another study, data of 150 patients who underwent RSI were analyzed [23]. Better visualization was obtained in the Emergency department through video-laryngoscope than direct laryngoscopy, but the first-attempt success rate did not increase. A recent study conducted with the GlideScope, laryngoscopic grade, and the number of intubation attempts were found to be similar, and it was concluded that intubation could be performed slightly faster [24].

On the other hand, in some studies, using a video-laryngoscope is associated with lower force application to oral structures [25, 26]. More researches are needed regarding the use of video-laryngoscopes in emergency conditions. In a study that

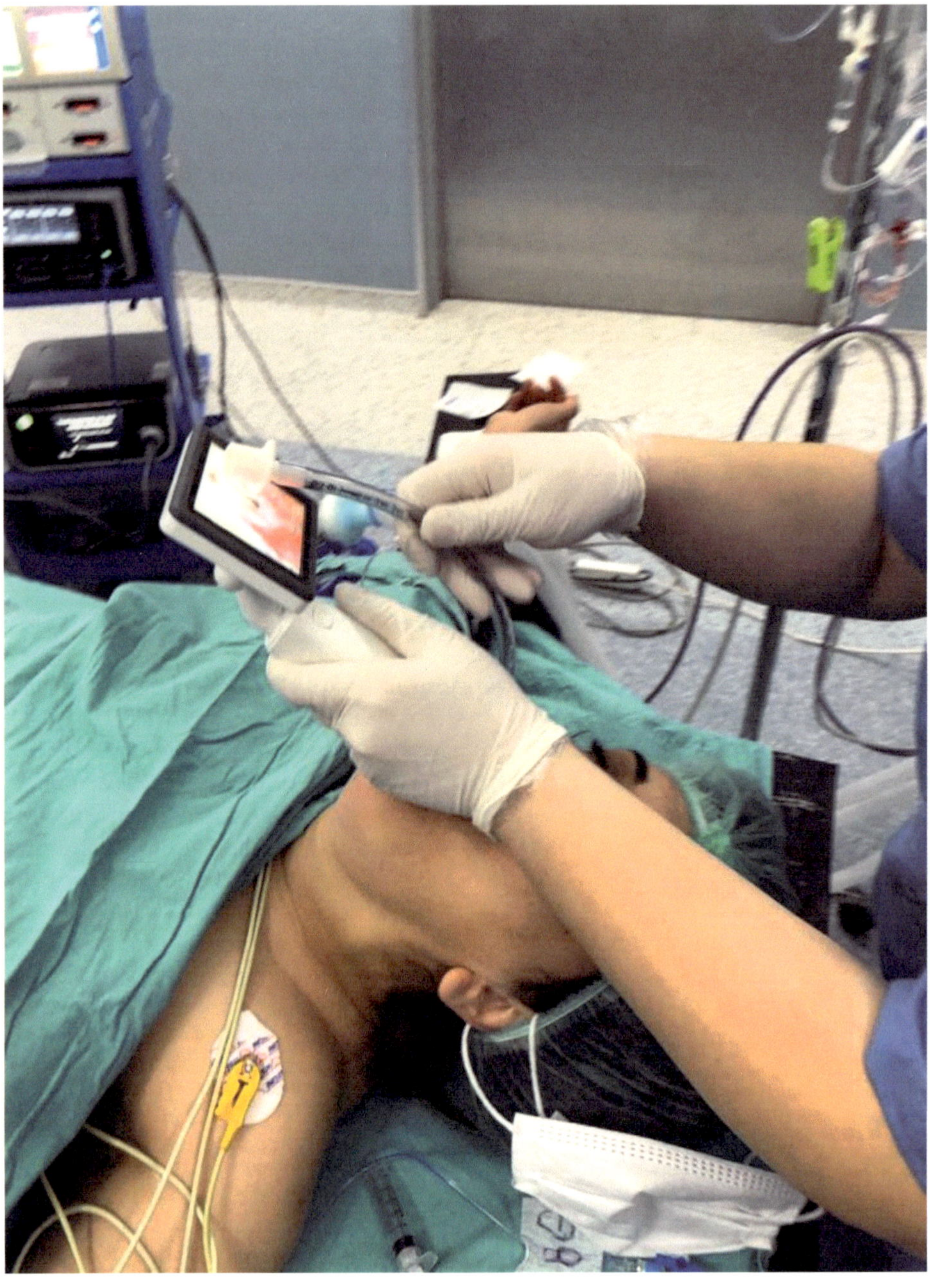

Figure 3.
Tracheal intubation using video-laryngoscopes.

included 4041 emergency room patients over three years, the GlideScope was used for tracheal intubation in 540 patients. It was reported that there was no significant difference in the success rate and unsuccessful tracheal intubation rates in the first attempt when compared with the conventional method [27].

9. Bougie

It is also known as a tracheal tube introducer. It is used to increase the success of tracheal intubation in cases with a poor laryngoscopic view. It is especially useful

DOI: http://dx.doi.org/10.5772/intechopen.96477

when epiglottis can be seen, but vocal cords cannot be visualized. In the studies conducted recently, it has been shown that when compared with the combination of the stylet and tracheal tube, the bougie significantly increases the first pass success rate [28, 29].

10. Conclusion

Management of critical patients in need of airway management in the emergency medicine department requires experience. Providing oxygenation, minimizing the risk of complications, and choosing the appropriate devices constitute the management's pearls.

Author details

Kemal Tolga Saracoglu[1], Gul Cakmak[2] and Ayten Saracoglu[2*]

1 Department of Anesthesiology and Intensive Care, Health Sciences University Kartal, Dr. Lutfi Kirdar Training and Research Hospital, Istanbul, Turkey

2 Department of Anesthesiology and Intensive Care, Marmara University Pendik Training and Research Hospital, Istanbul, Turkey

*Address all correspondence to: anesthesiayten@gmail.com

References

[1] Goto T, Goto Y, Hagiwara Y, Okamoto H, Watase H, Hasegawa K. Advancing emergency airway management practice and research. Acute Med Surg. 2019 May 21;6(4): 336-351. doi: 10.1002/ams2.428.

[2] Clancy M, Nolan J. Airway management in the emergency department. Emerg Med J. 2002 Jan;19(1):2-3. doi: 10.1136/emj.19.1.2.

[3] Díaz C, Carvajal DF, Morales EI, Sangiovanni S, Fernández-Trujillo L. Right main bronchus rupture associated with blunt chest trauma: a case report. Int J Emerg Med. 2019 Dec 10;12(1):39. doi: 10.1186/s12245-019-0258-3.

[4] Lockey D, Crewdson K, Weaver A, Davies G. Observational study of the success rates of intubation and failed intubation airway rescue techniques in 7256 attempted intubations of trauma patients by pre-hospital physicians. Br J Anaesth. 2014 Aug;113(2):220-225. doi: 10.1093/bja/aeu227.

[5] Lentz S, Grossman A, Koyfman A, Long B. High-Risk Airway Management in the Emergency Department: Diseases and Approaches, Part II. J Emerg Med. 2020 Jun 23:S0736-4679(20)30407-8. doi: 10.1016/j.jemermed.2020.05.009.

[6] West JR, Lott C, Donner L, Kanter M, Caputo ND. Peri-intubation factors affecting emergency physician choice of paralytic agent for rapid sequence intubation of trauma patients. Am J Emerg Med. 2018 Jul;36(7):1151-1154. doi: 10.1016/j.ajem.2017.11.038.

[7] April MD, Arana A, Pallin DJ et al. Emergency department intubation success with succinylcholine versus rocuronium: a national emergency airway registry study. Ann Emerg Med 2018; 72: 645-653.

[8] Taş Z, Hoşten T, Kuş A, Cesur S, Türkyılmaz N, et al. Comparison of tidal volume and deep breath preoxygenation techniques undergoing coronary artery bypass graft surgery: Effects of hemodynamicresponse and arterial oxygenation. Turk J Med Sci 2017;47:1576-1582.

[9] Pence HH, Yilmaz M, Saracoglu KT. Apneic oxygenation and high flow. Int J Anesthetic Anesthesiol 2018, 5:081.

[10] Kovacs G, Sowers N. Airway Management in Trauma. Emerg Med Clin North Am. 2018 Feb;36(1):61-84. doi: 10.1016/j.emc.2017.08.006.

[11] Chrimes N. The Vortex: a universal 'high-acuity implementation tool' for emergency airway management. Br J Anaesth. 2016 Sep;117 Suppl 1:i20-i27. doi: 10.1093/bja/aew175.

[12] Saracoglu KT, Saracoglu A. The Vortex Approach for Difficult Airway Management. Clin Med. 2019;1(3):CIM-01-1014.

[13] Asai T. Emergency Cricothyrotomy: Toward a Safer and More Reliable Rescue Method in "Cannot Intubate, Cannot Oxygenate" Situation. Anesthesiology. 2015 Nov;123(5):995-996. doi: 10.1097/ALN.0000000000000849.

[14] Siddiqui N, Arzola C, Friedman Z, Guerina L, You-Ten KE: Ultrasound improves cricothyrotomy success in cadavers with poorly defined neck anatomy: A randomized control trial. Anesthesiolog y 2015; 123:1033-1041.

[15] Graham CA. Advanced airway management in the emergency department: what are the training and skills maintenance needs for UK emergency physicians? Emerg Med J. 2004 Jan;21(1):14-19. doi: 10.1136/emj.2003.003368.

[16] Saracoglu KT, Saracoglu A. Airway management education: an update. Acta Anaesth Belg 2017;68:175-186.

[17] Saracoglu KT, Yilmaz M, Turan AZ, Kus A, Colak T, Saracoglu A. Pecha Kucha with part task training improves the airway management in fresh frozen cadavers: case-control observational study. Med Princ Pract. 2020 Feb 19. doi: 10.1159/000506597. Epub ahead of print.

[18] Gellerfors M, Larsson A, Svensén CH, Gryth D. Use of the Airtraq® device for airway management in the pre-hospital setting--a retrospective study. Scand J Trauma Resusc Emerg Med. 2014 Feb 3;22:10. doi: 10.1186/1757-7241-22-10.

[19] Sakles JC, Javedani PP, Chase E, Garst-Orozco J, Guillen-Rodriguez JM, Stolz U. The use of a video laryngoscope by emergency medicine residents is associated with a reduction in esophageal intubations in the emergency department. Acad Emerg Med. 2015 Jun;22(6):700-707. doi: 10.1111/acem.12674.

[20] Smith KA, High K, Collins SP, Self WH. A preprocedural checklist improves the safety of emergency department intubation of trauma patients. Acad Emerg Med. 2015 Aug;22(8):989-992. doi: 10.1111/acem.12717.

[21] Bossers SM, Schwarte LA, Loer SA, Twisk JW, Boer C, Schober P. Experience in Prehospital Endotracheal Intubation Significantly Influences Mortality of Patients with Severe Traumatic Brain Injury: A Systematic Review and Meta-Analysis. PLoS One. 2015 Oct 23;10(10):e0141034. doi: 10.1371/journal.pone.0141034.

[22] Pieters BMA, Maas EHA, Knape JTA, van Zundert AAJ. Videolaryngoscopy vs. direct laryngoscopy use by experienced anaesthetists in patients with known difficult airways: a systematic review and meta-analysis. Anaesthesia. 2017 Dec;72(12):1532-1541. doi: 10.1111/anae.14057.

[23] Sulser S, Ubmann D, Schlaepfer M, Brueesch M, Goliasch G, Seifert B, Spahn DR, Ruetzler K. C-MAC videolaryngoscope compared with direct laryngoscopy for rapid sequence intubation in an emergency department: A randomised clinical trial. Eur J Anaesthesiol. 2016 Dec;33(12):943-948. doi: 10.1097/EJA.0000000000000525.

[24] Turkstra TP, Turkstra DC, Pavlosky AW, Jones PM. Simultaneous en bloc endotracheal tube insertion with GlideScope® Titanium™ video laryngoscope use: a randomized-controlled trial. Can J Anaesth. 2020 Aug 19. English. doi: 10.1007/s12630-020-01778-2. Epub ahead of print.

[25] Goto T, Koyama Y, Kondo T, Tsugawa Y, Hasegawa K. A comparison of the force applied on oral structures during intubation attempts between the Pentax-AWS airwayscope and the Macintosh laryngoscope: a high-fidelity simulatorbased study. BMJ Open 2014; 4: e006416.

[26] Nakanishi T, Shiga T, Homma Y, Koyama Y, Goto T. Comparison of the force applied on oral structures during intubation attempts by novice physicians between the Macintosh direct laryngoscope, Airway Scope and C-MAC PM: a highfidelity simulator-based study. BMJ Open 2016; 6: e011039.

[27] Choi HJ, Kim YM, Oh YM, Kang HG, Yim HW, Jeong SH; Korean Emergency Airway Management Registry (KEAMR) investigators. GlideScope video laryngoscopy versus direct laryngoscopy in the emergency department: a propensity score-matched analysis. BMJ Open. 2015 May 11;5(5):e007884. doi: 10.1136/bmjopen-2015-007884.

[28] Driver BE, Prekker ME, Klein LR et al. Effect of use of a bougie vs endotracheal tube and stylet on first-attempt intubation success among patients with difficult airways undergoing emergency intubation: a randomized clinical trial.

[29] Driver B, Dodd K, Klein LR et al. The bougie and first-pass success in the emergency department. Ann. Emerg. Med. 2017; 70: 473-8. e471.

Chapter 6

Airway Management in Critical Settings

ELSayed Elkarta and Magdy Eldegwy

Abstract

Airway management continues to be a challenging task for healthcare practitioners and when it comes to critical settings; it carries more challenges even for the skilled persons. Critical settings could be in fact of suits; where intervention takes place, equipment or practitioners taking care of airway management. Critically ill patients with multiple comorbidities, increasing oxygen demand and high respiratory work; that may require elective airway securing. Various protocols, guidelines and recommendations advocated for this task with the prospects of less hemodynamic alteration and prevention of pulmonary aspiration. In the former, starting oxygen therapy for all critical patients on admission was a routine following the concept; if some is good, more must be better. Nowadays excess oxygen may be unfavorable in some acute critical conditions e.g. ischemic strokes, post-acute myocardial infraction and those with hypercapnic respiratory failure. However, still high flow inspired oxygen concentration is the protocol until they are stable then its reduction to reach the targeted arterial oxygen saturation. Oxygen devices used for oxygen delivery are plenty and its selection depends on the many factors; airway patency, patient's conscious level and compliance, and assessment of gas exchange based on arterial blood sample which is recommended for all critically ill patients. Early prompt evaluation of the airway and assessment of gas exchange using arterial blood sample analysis is curial in all critically ill patients to guide for subsequent oxygen supply and whether the patient needs ventilatory support or not. This chapter will focus on airway management, oxygen therapy and types of ventilatory support required for adult critically ill patients, while other situations' airway management's tools and skills will be discussed in another ones.

Keywords: airway, management, critical, hemodynamic, hypoxemia, guidelines, FONA

1. Introduction

Airway patency is crucial and vital for maintenance of life occurs naturally in the awake and conscious individuals or can be accomplished artificially in those becoming unable to maintain it. Incapacity of this might be intentional; as in medical procedures requiring deep sedation and/or general anesthesia or in pathological conditions; where there is an alteration in sensorium or elective airway protection needed.

Airway management is defined as an intervention using a technique, maneuver or a device to keep its patency, consequently its normal physiological functions have been achieved; providing oxygen and removing carbon dioxide.

 IntechOpen

Critical illness is a clinical condition belong to a group of medical situations sharing the need of intensive care unit (ICU) admission and have either single or multiple organ dysfunction. Critically ill patients showing different gradations of snags to maintain the airway and subsequently derangement of aerobic metabolism exists. Optimization of oxygen supply is needed, as dramatic rise of both work of breathing and oxygen demand exist.

Hypoxemia is a medical condition where the partial pressure of oxygen in the arterial blood (P_aO_2) is lower than normal. A P_aO_2 value of less than 60 mmHg in normal individuals with healthy lungs; corresponds to arterial oxygen saturation (SpO_2) of 90%, is used as a cut point for hypoxemia treatment initiation. There are many causes and mechanisms of hypoxemia which required management via oxygen administration. Critically ill patients commonly showing hypoxemic status on the time of admission and oxygen supplementation should be considered in all with high flow delivery system (15 L/min) until becoming stable then reduction of inspired oxygen concentration (FIO_2) to achieve a target of SpO_2 of 94–98% or 88–92% for patients with risk of hypercapnic respiratory failure [1].

1.1 Physiological consideration

Airway is the natural passages of the airflow, inaugurated by nose and mouth downwards to the alveoli in the lungs, where the gas exchange takes place involuntary. Airway patency is mandatory for life and it's the responsibility of pharyngeal-laryngeal muscles tonic control and muco-ciliary system's clearance of mucus and foreign particles.

The airflow via the airway is intermittent and biphasic; inwards during inspiration and outwards during expiration. The work of breathing is a potential energy stored in the lung tissues during inspiration that exists by the work of overcoming the elastic forces and resistance in the airway to be enough for subsequent expiration. In compliant, healthy lung this work of breathing does not consume a portion of the body's energy needs and its daily fraction is less than 3% of total body energy requirement [2].

Impaired consciousness, associated cervical spine trauma, burns and pulmonary shunt causing rapid desaturation and impedes preoxygenation. Besides, limited time for airway management before life-threatening hypoxia, hemodynamically (HD) unstable, imminent risk of collapse before intubation, tricky standard induction drugs effects provoke time pressure environment.

Cessation of the desirable airflow in critically ill patients could be due to a variety of reasons, foremost of those is the airway obstruction. Airway obstruction might occur at any, upper parts; due to foreign body, mucus, secretions, blood and decreased sensorium or lower parts; due to aspiration, infection and spasm of bronchial muscles. Different maneuvers and devices used to eliminate the airway obstruction thus maintenance of airflow will be gained.

Airway management in critically ill patient aimed for:

1. Improving the oxygenation.

2. Airway protection and prevention of pulmonary aspiration.

3. Adjunct for procedures; diagnostic e.g. bronchoscopy or therapeutic e.g. banding of bleeding esophageal varices.

4. Relieve the distress of dyspnea.

5. Reduce the work of breathing.

6. Improve CO_2 clearance.

7. Altered sensorium, required airway protection.

8. Others in ICU.

1.2 Anatomical consideration

Critical illness and its management protocols might hinder the airway anatomy, fluid resuscitation and capillary leak makes the airway edematous and distorted. Furthermore, the patient demography, body mass index (BMI), associated neurological and cardiopulmonary comorbidities, and the indication of ICU admission contribute to anatomical difficulties.

1.3 Devices of oxygen delivery

Oxygen (O_2); is an inert gas essential for life, being inspired through the airway and transported via the lungs towards the blood to be used in cellular respiration and delivery of energy needed for body metabolism. Human body uptake of oxygen in concentration of 20.95% from air by natural airways; nose and mouth, transported down along the conductive airways to be resting in the alveoli where the gas exchange happening. Physiological and pathological conditions required an increased FIO_2 to meet the body oxygen requirement and its high demand. Devices are designed to facilitate oxygen delivery from artificial oxygen sources in correspond to the target of FIO_2, patient's breathing effort and patient's device compliance [3].

All critically ill patients must have high-flow oxygen delivery device (15 L/min), until stable status achieved, then oxygen requirement could be individually determined depending on the existing pathology. Patient's breathing effort is the primary determinant for the oxygen delivery device selection. Critically ill patients might be one of two groups; spontaneous breathing group or assisted ventilation one and each group has a preference in oxygen delivery system [4].

1.3.1 Spontaneous- breathing group

Patients with breathing effort requiring O_2 delivering device matched for their breathing power (**Table 1**).

	O_2 flow rate (L/min)	**FIO_2**	**Example**
Fixed-Performance Devices	2 - 15	Unknown; depend on patient's effort and O_2 flow rate	Simple face mask, face mask with reservoir bag, nasal cannula. (**Figure 1**)
Variable-Performance Devices	High, up to 45	Well-known, fixed.	All obey a principle of high airflow O_2 enrichment (HAFOE). (**Figure 2**)

Table 1.
Oxygen delivery devices [3].

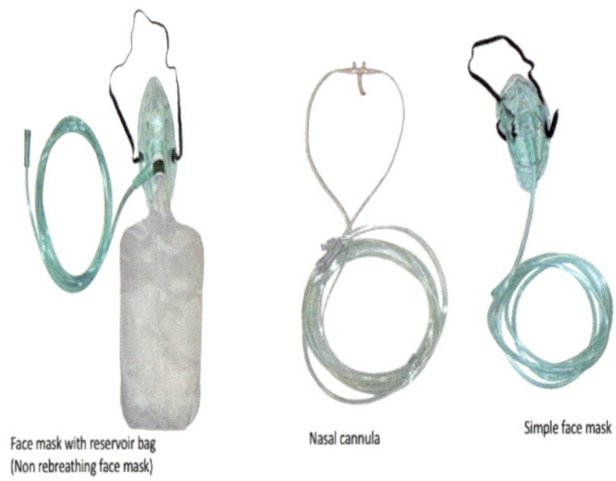

Figure 1.
Oxygen delivery devices (simple face mask with reservoir bag & nasal cannula).

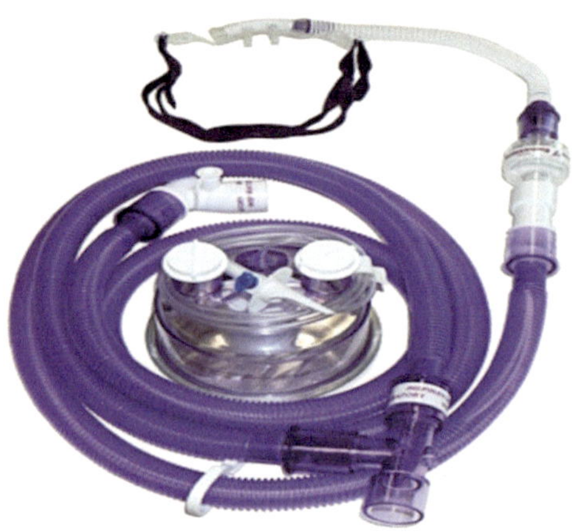

Figure 2.
Oxygen delivery devices (HAFOE).

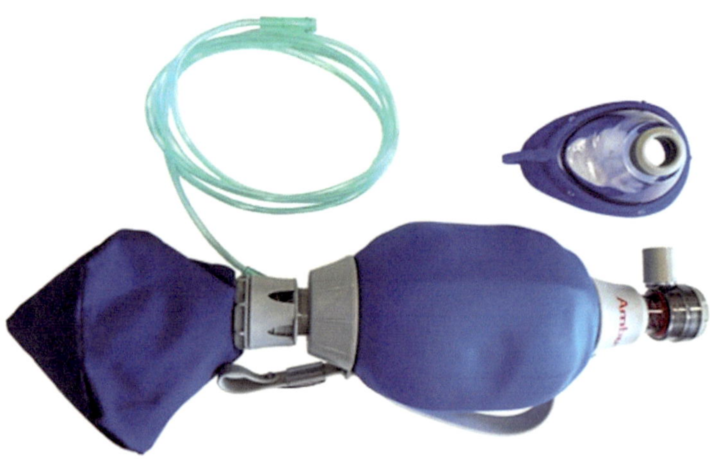

Figure 3.
Oxygen delivery devices. (bag-mask with self-inflating reservoir bag).

1.3.2 Assisted ventilation group

In this group of critically ill patients, failure to maintain oxygenation and/or ventilation despite an increase in FIO_2 or development of apnea and indicated mechanical ventilation (MV), airway supporting device might be perpetual or temporary as a bridge till the steady one is fixed. Noninvasive positive pressure ventilation (NIPPV), could have both properties as it might be a tie till improvement or securing definitive airway securing device suitable for MV.

Bag-mask with self-inflating reservoir bag; (**Figure 3**) is considered the simplest and commonest O_2 delivery device used in critically ill patients for oxygenation until an airway securing device fixed. It provides FIO_2 close to 100% while the only O_2 delivery device able to provide 100% FIO_2 is the anesthetic breathing system.

2. Airway management in ICU

Airway management in ICU is unlike that carried out in operation theater (OT) and higher in its complications; brain damage and death, and most of it is done on urgent and emergency basis in lack of experienced airway management professionals. In addition; critically ill patients showing limited cardiopulmonary reserve, this increases their risk of hypoxemia and hypotension upon exposure to airway management medications. Subsequently, tracheal intubation for those categories of patients could be life-threatening condition; up to 40% of patients are associated with increase in complication rates of hypoxemia (25%) [5] and hypotension (10–25%) [6], arrhythmia, cardiac arrest and death [7] upon exposure to airway stimulation or pharmacological agents used for it.

Incapacity to perform tracheal intubation at the first attempt "first pass success" has higher risk than that in OT and occurs in 30% of ICU intubations [8]. Many factors contribute to that; lack of competent and expert professional for intubation, patient's factors and pharmacological agents' dosage choices. This came with the conclusion of Fourth National Audit Project (NAP4), as it showed around 25% of airway management done in ICU & ED are associated with major adverse effects mostly due to the aforementioned factors [9]. Moreover, equipment unavailability, unfamiliarity and inadequate planning resulting in more stressful environment and subsequently delay in airway management with increasing morbidity and mortality.

ICU settings are not suitably planned for airway management due to several reasons. Limited access to the patient as the bed space is crowded by monitoring, ventilator and other equipment, (**Figure 4**) in addition of the ICU bed is less maneuverable compared to the OT table with unavailability of advanced airway management equipment making it more challenging. Moreover, varying team members of multi-professional backgrounds with non-enough time, experience, accompanying medical devices (collars, masks) and sensorium alteration lead to improper airway assessment beside and inability to ensure adequate preoxygenation necessary to avoid the hypoxia during airway instrumentation. Moreover, unavailability of trained assistance such as anesthesia nurse or technician and lack of structured airway management for ICU staff.

Communication and proper documentation of the airway assessment and its management throughout different hospital facilities is crucial and it might affect the workflow performance. Checklist is the best method of communication among the healthcare professionals from different medical background. Equipment, medications preparation checklist and proper assignment of human forces could make the airway management scenario less stressful and empower its success among critically ill patients.

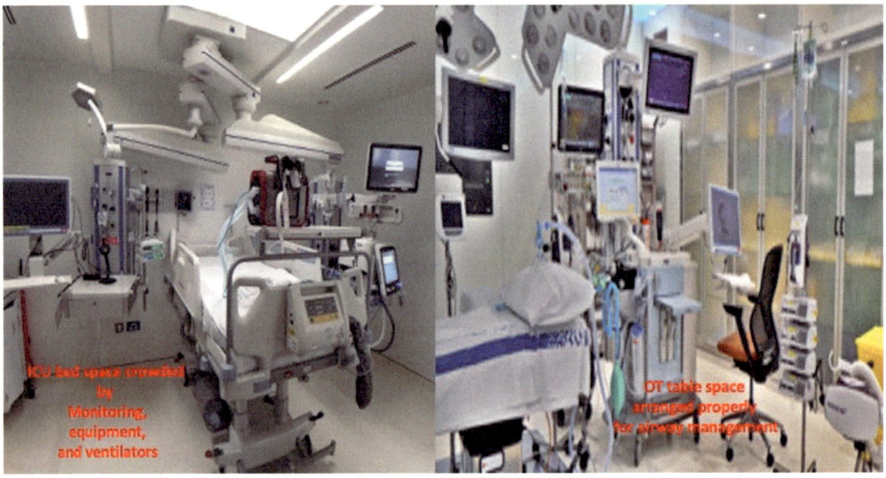

Figure 4.
ICU bed vs. OT space (showed crowding with monitoring, equipment and ventilators).

Quite few challenges could be integrated in airway management for ICU adults, so we can wrap up the considerations and specific precautions that must be accomplish making it less pressure and successfully performed procedure (**Table 2**).

2.1 Pre-intervention stage

Thorough clinical assessment and prediction of threats that may limit the success of airway management of critically ill patients could be addressed in this time. Also, optimization of all factors; position, preparation and preoxygenation, accentuates the accomplishment of proper airway management intervention.

2.1.1 Airway assessment challenges

Not only thorough assessment of the airway in critically ill patient is vital for successful and safe management but it is unique and carries challenges as compared to that done for patients undergoing daily elective or emergency airway management. Varieties airway assessment modalities, techniques and scoring system had been proposed to allow its safe and easy practice management. Despite the anesthesiologists' or intensivists'predictions of anticipated airway difficulties are a strong diagnostic modality with high positive ratio, but the high proportion of unanticipated difficult endotracheal intubation and its low positive predictive values limits its reliability as a diagnostic test in medical practice [9].

Moreover, the proposed airway assessment scales vary from the simple, that often fail to address the many factors associated with a difficult airway, to the complex, which are impractical as a clinical tool. None have been shown to be accurate in predicting airway management problems, and none have been assessed in the ED setting [10].

NAP4 reports identified frequent airway management failure rate and the high-risk airway patient's identification was not managed through an appropriate airway management approach [9].

Standard airway assessment in critically ill patients is usually unfeasible and difficult to be done especially in those dependent on oxygen delivery devices; face mask or nasal cannula, to avoid hypoxia and provide adequate preoxygenation. The only validated airway assessment scoring system reliable for critically ill patients is the MACOCHA score

Challenge	Consideration		Precaution
ICU environment	ICU space;		• Ideal stuff positioning
	Equipment;		• Standard airway trolley availability • Advanced airway; VL, FOB, Bougie available
	Team member;		• Team members briefing and specific task assignment
Patient-related	Physiological;	• HO instability	• Optimization & vasopressors proactively use.
		• Pulmonary shunt	• Optimal preoxygenation with O_2 delivery devices.
		• Limited reserve & time for airway management	• Systematic, logical, and strategic airway management techniques escalation.
	Anatomical;		Anticipation and plan for failure.
	Difficult airways;		• Recognition and readiness for difficulties. • MACOCHA score use. • Reduce number of attempts. • Appropriate induction medications, NMBS is routine. • Plan for failure. • Consider FONA.
	Urgency;		• Checklist in preparation and communication. • Follow up guidelines & standardized protocols.
	Pharmacological agents;		• Ketamine is recommended. • Avoid over sedation. • Routine use of NMBS. • Consider induction time longer than traditional.
	Aspiration risk;		• Modified RSI with cricoid pressure or DSI. • Head-up position.
Postintubation care	Red flag recognition;		• ETT obstruction, displacement. • Ventilators mechanics and Monitoring: ETT related.

Abbreviations definition; **VL**: *video-laryngoscope.* **FOB**: *fiberoptics laryngoscope.* **MACOCHA**: *Mallampati score, Apnea syndrome, Cervical spine limitation, Opening mouth, Coma, Hypoxia, Anesthesiologist non-trained.* **FONA**: *front of neck airway.* **NMBS**: *neuromuscular blockers.* **RSI**: *rapid sequence induction.* **DSI**: *delayed sequence induction*

Table 2.
ICU airway management challenges, considerations and precautions.

(**Table 3**) [11]. It has the advantage of being created with easy identifiable and clinically appropriate variables. Additionally, its used objectives are close to those identified in OT and include risk factors associated with difficult tracheal intubation [12]. Considering any investigations of the airway that already done; such as chest x-ray, CT scan and 3D and Virtual Endoscopy (VE) could be helpful in airway evaluation and might be derive the plan for airway management in critically ill patients [13].

It's recommended to define the cricothyroid membrane for possible front of neck airway (FONA) as a strategy of a plan for failure. This could be done by manual palpation; laryngeal handshake technique [14] (**Figure 5**) or using ultrasound that is accurately defining cricothyroid membrane site, measurements and surrounding structures such as thyroid gland and its vessels [15].

2.1.2 Preparation and preoxygenation challenges

Formerly it's mentioned that; checklist, proper communication, documentation and team briefing with specific task assignment is a key for successful airway management in critical settings. Standard pre-intubation checklist has been developed via Difficult Airway Society (DAS), Intensive Care Society (ICS), Faculty of Intensive Care Medicine (FICM) and Royal College of Anesthetists (RCoA), United Kingdom solving this high-pressure situation (**Figure 6**).

Efficient preoxygenation with end-tidal oxygen concentration of more than 85% is the target [16] must be done in parallel to assessment and preparation. Traditional techniques are somewhat doing this task [17] and the choice of oxygen delivery device depends on the patient's comfort, device availability and the indication for intervention. Although use FIO_2 of 100% with high flow rate; 10–15 L/min

Factors		Points
Factors related to patient	Mallampati score III or IV	5
	Obstructive sleep apnea syndrome (OSA)	2
	Reduced mobility of cervical spine.	2
	Limited mouth opening <3cm.	1
Factors related to pathology	Coma	1
	Sever hypoxemia (<80%)	1
Factors related to operator		1
Total:		**12**

Abbreviations definition: MACOCHA= Mallampati score III or IV, Apnea syndrome, Cervical spine limitation, Opening mouth <3cm, Coma, Hypoxia, Anesthesiologist non-trained.
Score: 0-12 =easy; 12=difficult.

Table 3.
MACOCHA score [11].

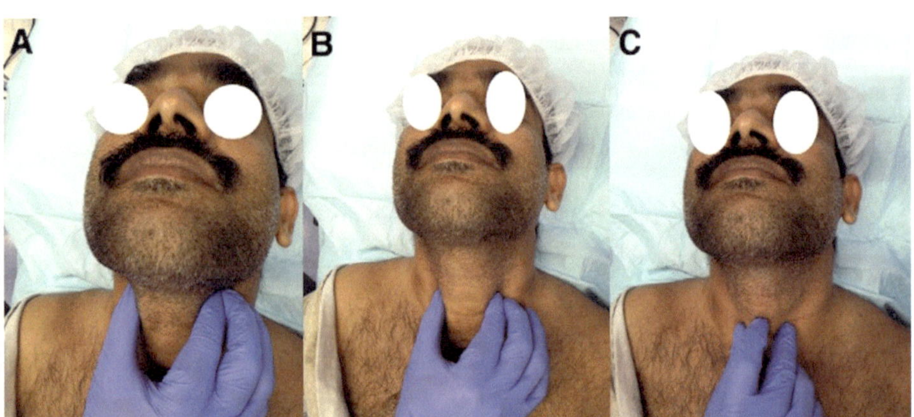

Figure 5.
Laryngeal handshake technique.

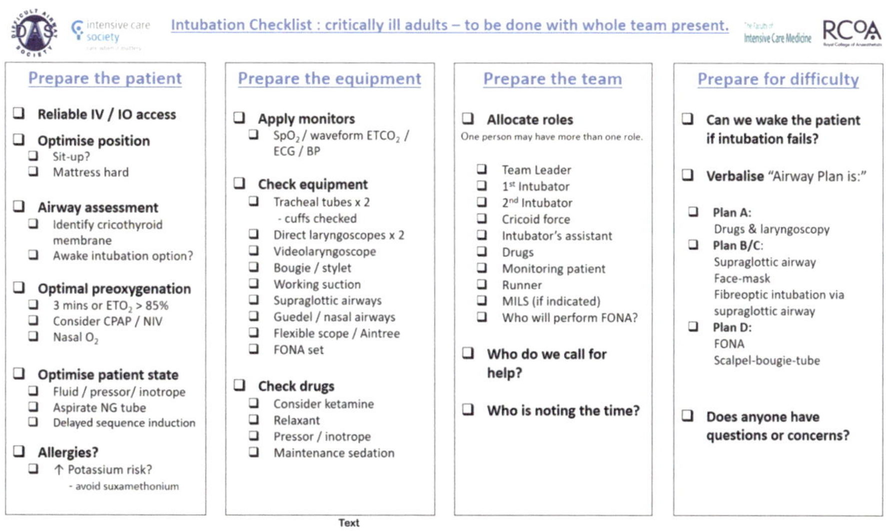
Intubation Checklist : critically ill adults – to be done with whole team present.

Prepare the patient
- ❑ Reliable IV / IO access
- ❑ Optimise position
  - ❑ Sit-up?
  - ❑ Mattress hard
- ❑ Airway assessment
  - ❑ Identify cricothyroid membrane
  - ❑ Awake intubation option?
- ❑ Optimal preoxygenation
  - ❑ 3 mins or ETO_2 > 85%
  - ❑ Consider CPAP / NIV
  - ❑ Nasal O_2
- ❑ Optimise patient state
  - ❑ Fluid / pressor/ inotrope
  - ❑ Aspirate NG tube
  - ❑ Delayed sequence induction
- ❑ Allergies?
  - ❑ ↑ Potassium risk? - avoid suxamethonium

Prepare the equipment
- ❑ Apply monitors
  - ❑ SpO_2 / waveform $ETCO_2$ / ECG / BP
- ❑ Check equipment
  - ❑ Tracheal tubes x 2 - cuffs checked
  - ❑ Direct laryngoscopes x 2
  - ❑ Videolaryngoscope
  - ❑ Bougie / stylet
  - ❑ Working suction
  - ❑ Supraglottic airways
  - ❑ Guedel / nasal airways
  - ❑ Flexible scope / Aintree
  - ❑ FONA set
- ❑ Check drugs
  - ❑ Consider ketamine
  - ❑ Relaxant
  - ❑ Pressor / inotrope
  - ❑ Maintenance sedation

Prepare the team
- ❑ Allocate roles
  One person may have more than one role.
  - ❑ Team Leader
  - ❑ 1st Intubator
  - ❑ 2nd Intubator
  - ❑ Cricoid force
  - ❑ Intubator's assistant
  - ❑ Drugs
  - ❑ Monitoring patient
  - ❑ Runner
  - ❑ MILS (if indicated)
  - ❑ Who will perform FONA?
- ❑ Who do we call for help?
- ❑ Who is noting the time?

Prepare for difficulty
- ❑ Can we wake the patient if intubation fails?
- ❑ Verbalise "Airway Plan is:"
  - ❑ Plan A: Drugs & laryngoscopy
  - ❑ Plan B/C: Supraglottic airway, Face-mask, Fibreoptic intubation via supraglottic airway
  - ❑ Plan D: FONA, Scalpel-bougie-tube
- ❑ Does anyone have questions or concerns?

Text

Figure 6.
Pre-management preparation; patient, equipment, team assignment.

in a tight-sealed facemask for 3 minutes could be enough in intact spontaneously breathing derive [18] but the use of simple face mask even with reservoir bag is not recommended [19]. Moreover, non-invasive positive pressure ventilation (NIPPV) and continuous positive pressure ventilation (CPAP) could be alternatives for pre-oxygenation in seriously hypoxic patients resulting in improved oxygenation and prevention of atelectasis associated with FIO_2 of 100% via supporting the minute volume ventilation (MVV) [20].

High flow nasal oxygenation (HFNO) between 30 and 70 L/min is a suitable method for preoxygenation that showed safety to extend the safe apnea time during airway instrumentation and effectiveness when combined with NIPPV use [21]. Not only, continuous positive airway pressure (CPAP) delivery with a tight-sealed facemask of 5–10 cm H_2O is recommended for preoxygenation, but also, the use of nasal oxygen with a flow of 5 L/min throughout airway management [19] and might be achieved by NIPPV especially in patients with respiratory failure [20].

Plan for failure must be the strategy of airway management planning, allowing logical and prepared expectations for different scenarios that might occur during the procedure. The guidelines resulted from collaborations of DAS/ICS/FICM/RCoA in United Kingdom with the aim of providing structured, standard and systematic approach of airway management in critically ill patients with the concern of not being a replacement of clinical judgment but rather an organizational and individual framework for clinical practice preparation and health care professionals training [19] (**Figure 7**).

Providing the patient's comfort, upper airway patency, optimizing functional residual capacity and decreasing aspiration risk; sniffing position is desirable as an initial position for airway management in critical settings, [22] while titration of bed head-up if cervical spine injury was suspected or confirmed [22, 23] and with prevalence of obesity among population, ramping position could be an alternative [24].

All airway management in critical settings must be carried out in presence of standard ASA monitoring; electrocardiogram (ECG)/heart rate (HR), non-invasive blood pressure (NIBP), pulse oximetry with oxygen saturation (SPO_2), end-tidal carbon dioxide ($EtCO_2$) [25]. Invasive blood pressure (IBP) is desirable either vasopressors in-use or HD instability is most likely expected and end-tidal oxygen concentration (EtO2) monitoring; if available.

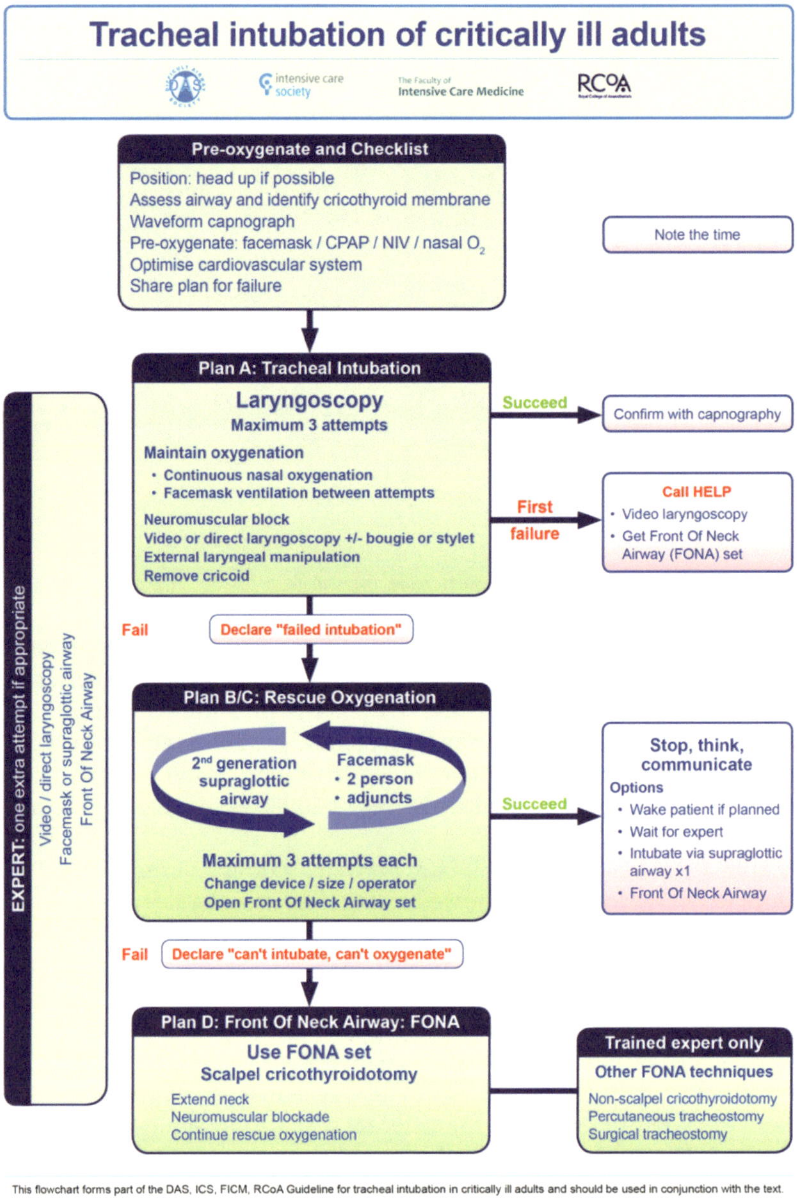

Figure 7.
DAS/ICS/FICM/RCoA guidelines for ETI in critically ill patients.

2.1.3 Anesthesia induction and pharmacological considerations

Hypnosis, analgesia and skeletal muscle relaxation is a triad to commence general anesthesia required for airway management and instrumentation. A variety of pharmacological agents are described to achieve this task with specific considerations in dosing titration, delayed onset and extended effect duration.

Airway management of critically ill patients is mostly carried out in ICU while the risk to be done in non-ICU suites still considerable. Non-ICU suites include pre-hospital area, emergency department, radiology department and inpatient ward which carry the risk of difficultly and hence increase in adverse consequences of airway management, that will be discussed separately in corresponding chapters.

There are many factors recommended to reach the optimal airway management in critically ill patients including; intravenous induction agents, use of fast onset neuromuscular blocking agent (NMBA), precautions against pulmonary aspiration, laryngoscopic techniques aimed at first-pass success, and confirmation of successful tracheal intubation by waveform capnography.

Rapid sequence induction and intubation (RSII) is a technique commonly used to protect the airway against gastric contents aspiration and modified to be implemented in some clinical circumstances. A classic RSII consists of oxygen administration, application of cricoid pressure, and the avoidance of mask ventilation before insertion of an endotracheal tube (ETT) for airway securement [26].

A modified RSII in comparison to a classic RSII is to attempt for lung ventilation using positive-pressure ventilation via a facemask [27] before airway securement by ETT.

Delayed sequence intubation (DSI) seems to be safe, effective and could offer an alternative of rapid sequence induction in patients requiring emergency airway management who cannot tolerate preoxygenation or peri-intubation procedures [28]. The ideal DSI induction agent is Ketamine as it preserves airway reflexes and respiratory drive permitting preoxygenation and procedural sedation. DSI technique steps are; ensure the patient has a patent airway, place standard nasal cannula at 5 liters/min in awake patient and increases to 15 liters/min in unconscious one prior to placement of the preoxygenation device. Preoxygenation device choices based on the patient's $SpO2$: if $SpO2 > 95\%$ use bag-valve-mask (BVM) with PEEP valve and a good seal at 15 L/min $O2$, or non-rebreather (NRB) mask and a good seal at 15 L/min $O2$ (or more) while $SpO2 < 95\%$: use BVM with PEEP valve and a good seal and preoxygenate for at least 3 minutes [19].

2.1.3.1 Induction agents

Choice of induction drug is according to hemodynamic status of the patient; Ketamine is increasingly favored in most circumstances [29]. Administration of a rapidly acting opioids enables lower doses of hypnotics to be used, maintaining cardiovascular stability and minimizing changes of intracranial pressure.

Etomidate as an induction agent is not a first line for intubation in the critically ill patients because the other induction agents have been successfully used without risk of adrenal suppression. Its relative value of short-term hemodynamic stability that is accompanied by a potential adverse effect of adrenal suppression making its use as an anesthetic induction agent in critically ill patients is controversial, although it provides excellent intubating conditions [30]. Another meta-analysis also investigating non-intubation-related adverse effects of Etomidate in critically ill patients stated that its use is not worsening of mortality, organ dysfunction or resource utilization, even if it's adverse effects on adrenal gland function [31]. It's found that hypotension was more prevalent in patients receiving Etomidate compared with Ketamine in the first 24 hours after intubation and subsequent mechanical ventilation [32].

Moreover, Propofol has temporary hypotension episodes as compared to Etomidate, but there is no difference in patients requiring vasopressors after 24 hours [33]. Propofol and Ketamine mixture may have an improved hemodynamic profile compared with Etomidate. Few studies evaluated Etomidate versus Ketamine, finding no difference between them [34].

Dexmedetomidine, Remifentanil and Droperidol have been suggested as induction agents for DSI, but these agents do not have the same pattern of Ketamine as rapid onset, preservation of airway reflexes, intact respiratory drive and safety profile. Fentanyl have a significant sedative effect in addition to analgesia, that may be helpful when titrated to the desirable effect and to avoid over sedation.

NMBA improves intubating conditions, facemask ventilation, nasogastric tube insertion hence, reduction in the number of intubations attempts and optimizing chest wall compliance [35]. Succinylcholine has many side-effects including life-threatening hyperkalemia and its short duration of action can spared for difficult intubation scenarios. Rocuronium could be the choice in the critically ill patients, providing similar intubating conditions to Succinylcholine and can be antagonized using Sugammadex [36].

Graded sedation intubation without use of NMBA has also been proposed and clinically considered for technique of choice of airway management in critically ill patients [37].

2.2 Intervention stage

This is the subsequent stage, that follows patient's optimization achieved through concomitant preoxygenation, positioning and preparation of staff, equipment and medications. It is a highly stressful time and must be carried out in a strictly controlled and strategic manner.

Current guidelines state four main routes or plans as standard practice and should be done in sequence. From practical point, we believe that algorism might be modified or interchanged according to the given circumstances, such as in ED and prehospital critical settings, health care professionals could go for plan B/C straight away bypassing plan A because of limited facilities and unsuitable environment that mandate minimal airway manipulation with accomplishment of securing airway patency, proper oxygenation and/or ventilation.

2.2.1 Plan A

Plan A stresses on maintenance of oxygenation either via continuous nasal cannula or interrupted facemask application between laryngoscopic attempts and allowing enough time for desirable effect of pharmacological agents, laryngoscopy attempts using direct (DL) or video-laryngoscope (VL).

With a maximum of three trials, confirmed endotracheal intubation (ENI) through capnography with waveform trace and direct visualization of ETT pass beyond the vocal cords, the call for help of the appropriate help once failed first attempt is a must. Absence of wave trace capnography is a confirmation of failed ETI after exclusion of other causes such as ETT obstruction, pulmonary edema and cardiac arrest. Chest auscultation and its rise during inspiration are rarely used as indicator for successful ETI in critically ill patients [38].

First attempt of ETI, must be done by the most trained, proficient available and must have all team support and consideration of manoeuvers or manipulations with the aim of improving laryngoscopy is recommended after failed first attempt [19]. Operator replacement and equipment change; use of a different blade, addition of others; bougie and external laryngeal manipulation might be reasonable and helpful.

Despite of fulfilling all the available recourses to achieve an optimal laryngoscopic view, with failure of the ETI attempts, either three done or not, the team leader must swiftly proceed to the next airway management plan. DL is the standard use in ETI during daily clinical practice hence its use experience is granted. On the other hand, VL should be in preparation for difficult situation; MACOCHA score > 3 [11] and ensure its availability for critically ill patient management. DL versus VL is the choice of the professionals involved in the airway management scenario and could be the device selected for first attempt according to the institutional policy and training preferences [39].

2.2.2 Plan B/C: (backup plan)

Critically ill patients' lifesaving by maintaining oxygenation during airway management is the priority and failed ETI [8] in the preceding plan A could resulted in sever hypoxemia [6, 40] that has several serious consequences. It's the responsibility of the team leader to ensure maintenance of adequate oxygenation throughout the stages of airway management. ETT considered as a standard and definitive airway securing device while alternatives used to provide oxygenation in scenarios of failed ETI such as supraglottic airway (SGA) devices and facemask ventilation device.

SGA is considered as a plan B rescue device which consist of variety of devices used for the same purpose; securing upper airway patency that does not require long experience. Facemask ventilation used as a plan C with the purpose of providing O_2 till an alternative being fixed. DAS/ICS/FICM/RCoA guidelines use SGA (plan B) and facemask ventilation (plan C) alternatively to ensure oxygenation after plan A failure confirmation with maximum three turn attempts [19].

Second-generation laryngeal mask airways (LMA) not only possess a design of providing oxygenation, reduce the aspiration risk and conduit for fiberoptic intubation (FOI) [40], but also, promising successful performance in critical areas have been reported [41] so, it's the model of SGA devices to be considered in standard practice and should be available in the difficult airway management trolley. Provision of oxygenation, airway securing, avoidance of aspiration with minimal airway trauma, constantly remain the goals throughout the intervention and subsequent plan to awake patient, wait for airway expert, Fiberoptic Intubation (FOI) through LMA attempt for once or proceed to FONA remains the area of discussion among the airway management team [19].

Basically, it's not recommended to proceed for blind ETI via LMA, [42] on the other hand, FOB accessibility in ICU should be granted [14, 43]. There are alternatives to perform LMA/FOI-guided either using small ETT 6.0 mm inner diameter mounted over the FOB to be advanced through LMA or using Aintree intubation catheter (Cook Medical, Bloomington, IN, USA), that permits ETT > 7.0 mm inner diameter without interruption of oxygenation. Blind ETI with use of either gum elastic bougie or tube exchange catheter (Frova catheter; Cook Medical, Bloomington, IN, USA) is not advisable in critically ill patients as it's associated with tracheal injury, pharyngeal perforation, bronchial bleeding and accused for subsequent positive pressure ventilation-related pneumomediastinum [44].

2.2.3 Plan D; life-saving front of neck airway (FONA)

Life-threatening hypoxemia development in critically ill patients is frequent [45] and might be encountered at any stage of airway intervention, hence its prevention though ETI (plan A), SGA and facemask (plan B/C) use is emphasized. Not only, plan of failure with serious hypoxemia elaboration could drive towards FONA (**Figure 8**) but also, inadequate minimal oxygenation, aspiration, difficult ventilation and failure of LMA/FOI are potential indications [46]. Forever, efforts to eliminate cannot intubate cannot oxygenate (CICO) scenario must be maintained and its causes must be corrected while preparation of FONA is being proposed. The possible reasons for CICO might be related to patient's (airway; impacted foreign body or laryngeal narrowing either from inside as laryngeal edema or from outside as high cricoid pressure), cardiovascular collapse or related to equipment failure.

Late FONA during airway management scenario is common and is responsible for its associated morbidity and mortality [43, 47]. FONA setup prior to and at declaration of CICO occurred in three steps; immediate availability of FONA set, opening the set after one failed attempt of plan B/C and immediate FONA set use on CICO declaration [19].

FONA either scalpel cricothyroidotomy or other techniques; which need experience, specific preparations and include non-scalpel cricothyroidotomy, percutaneous tracheostomy and surgical tracheostomy. Scalpel cricothyroidotomy recommended in DAS guidelines offers the following advantages; timesaving, reliable, conducted in few steps with well-known immediately available equipment,

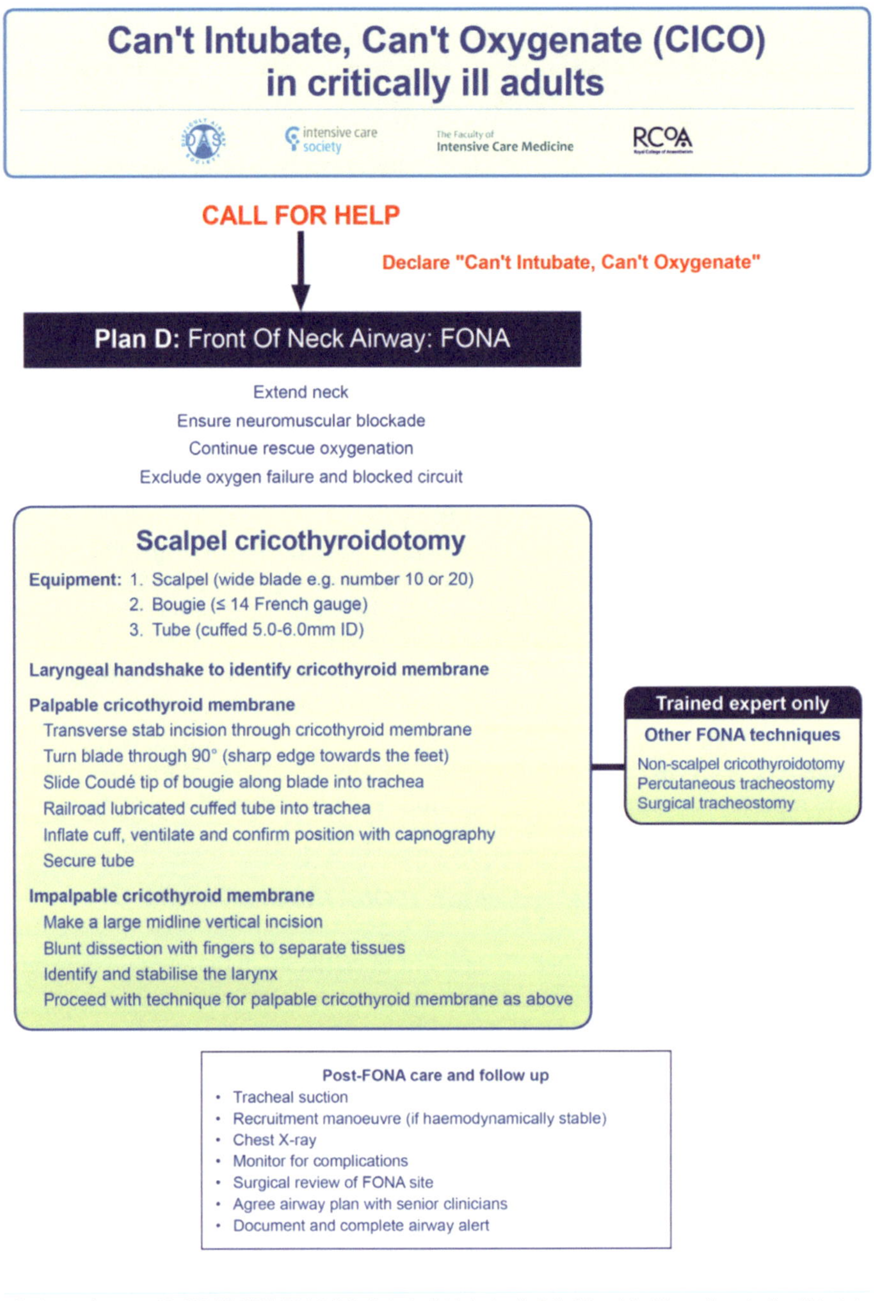

Figure 8.
Plan D protocol in DAS/ICS/FICM/RCoA guidelines.

high success rate, fitting for most of patients and providing definitive airway device [48]. For a brief technique steps of scalpel cricothyroidotomy and tracheostomy in ICU, will be discussed in another chapter.

Plan D (FONA) failure means a bad scenario that carries poor prognosis and must be avoided by follow-up FONA steps in a proper way as once it encountered, non-scalpel cricothyroidotomy by experienced professional, percutaneous dilatable tracheostomy and surgical tracheostomy have to be proposed immediately without delay.

2.3 Post-intervention stage

2.3.1 Post-intubation care

Not only providing airway securing device in critically ill patients is highly challenging, but post airway securing maintenance is also important to prevent airway displacement or obstruction. In addition of airway care, sedation and/or muscle relaxation are typically administered. They are not only having high-risk during intubation but also afterwards in rates of 82%; airway displacement and blockage, with 25% leading to death [49].

Furthermore; postintubation hypoxia occurred from multiple attempts, interruption of oxygenation, alveolar de-recruitment and collapse, and changes in the alveolar gas exchange may indicate an increase in initial lung volumes settings and benefiting from recruitment manoeuvers [38].

Attention payed towards recognition of red flag in intubated patients such as absent air entry on auscultation, abnormal $EtCO_2$, increasing peak airway pressure (PAP), unattained inhaled tidal volume and abnormal chest x-ray findings, mandate immediate management.

2.3.2 Weaning and extubation

Airway securing device in critically ill patients might be temporary for bridging a reversible and treatable medical disorder or permanent for irreversible and long-term pathology that demanding it. The former, long-term medical conditions, alternative tracheostomy have to be considered with a debate of its timing, On the other hand in reversible and corrected medical conditions; weaning and extubation must be considered in due time to avoid complications of prolonged ETT. Critically ill patients' intubation is challenging and extubation does too.

Tracheostomy might be an alternative of ETT as a definitive airway in critically ill patients in incidence of 7–19% [50] while extubation is the plan once the circumstances permit. Extubation is an elective procedure and mandates careful evaluation, preparation with the target of maintenance of oxygenation and stand-by intubation plan if extubation failure takes place.

DAS incorporated extubation guidelines in anesthesia practice and could derive that in ICU and summarized in four steps; [51].

Step 1: Plan for extubation:

i. Considering the reasons for intubation in addition of the complications of prolonged dependence on ETT and its anatomical and physiological consequences.

ii. "At-risk" extubation is a term used to describe the possible hazards associated with extubation process and must be considered in the plan step, especially the pre-existing factors.

iii. A difficult airway trolley equipment and monitors should be immediately available for use.

Step 2: Prepare the extubation:

i. Target for optimization of airway and spontaneous ventilation to ensure the success of extubation.

ii. This could be carried out by different methods such as ETT cuff leak test; to exclude laryngeal edema, spontaneously breathing trial (SBT), gastric decompression; as gastric distension results in diaphragmatic splint and breathing restriction. The plan for airway rescue must be considered and discussed in preparation.

Step 3: Perform extubation:

i. Avoid interruption of oxygenation by pre-extubation oxygenation via FIO2 of 100% O2.

ii. Patient's position; without adequate supporting evidence any one over the other, it's advisable extubation in head-up or semi-recumbent position especially in obese patients.

iii. Gentle suctioning of oropharyngeal cavity and extubation in fully awake state or conscious-sedation state using Remifentanil [52] might be alternatives.

Step 4: post-extubation care:

i. Beware of Warning signs of early airway compromise; stridor, obtunded breathing and agitation.

ii. Standard monitoring should be continued in post-extubation phase.

iii. Standard respiratory care for patients with airway compromise.

iv. Upright position, and high-flow humidified oxygen administration.

v. Documentation and recommendations for future management.

vi. Clinical details and instructions for extubation and post-extubation care should be recorded focusing on difficulties and details of airway management and future recommendations should be recorded.

2.4 Special circumstances

1. Airway management for ICU procedures like bronchoscopy, please refer to other chapters.

2. Full stomach in ICU, will be discussed in another chapter.

3. Previous tracheostomy that recently disconnected, it's advisable to re-cannulate the stoma but proceed for FONA should not be delayed [19].

4. ETT exchange in ICU remains common for many reasons that happening frequently such as ETT displacement or occlusion by crusted mucus, cuff rupture or surgical procedures mandate other ETT type. This task has to be taken seriously and reviewing the initial ETI documentation is essential and will provide a logical ETT exchange plan. Tube-exchange catheter is designed for that, providing its use with DL or VL which has superior glottic view, greater success rate and fewer complications [53]. New ETI could be another alternative but with the previous ETI documentation, all precautions and recommendations discussed earlier must be considered.

5. Varieties of abnormal clinical status might be accompanying the airway management in critically ill patients such as obesity, burn, pregnancy etc.... and required specific considerations, please review the book chapters for more details.

6. Specific alteration in airway management in COVID19 might be considered despite few data available. High Flow Nasal Cannula (HFNC) suggested to reduce the requiring supported ventilation [54] and NIV might reduce the rate of tracheal intubation [55]. Tracheal intubation in COVID 19 patients is considered as highest risk for health care professionals cross-infection and could be carried out in controlled environment [56]. More details about this topic will be available in specific chapter.

3. Training and skills maintenance

Critically ill patients usually are underestimated as specific airway difficulty and being at high risk of failure. Not only due to infrequent training of focused airway and crisis management but also, physicians may neither have anesthesia rotation nor airway skills required for difficult airway management. Training on sole skills performance is unsatisfactory to achieve maximum safety [57] and ineffective teamwork that includes poor communication, lack of shared targets, situational awareness, role assignment, leadership, coordination, mutual respect and post-event debriefings is associated with poor patients' outcome [58].

Focused risk assessment training, prevention of hypoxia, airway red flags, early call for help and request for advanced airway skills in concomitant with specific protocols and guideline presented. Team training, focused airway management training courses and workshops including simulation-based education are crucial and step up for airway management in both ED and ICU suites.

The crisis resource management (CRM) techniques from aviation industry has been advocated for use in ICU to promote a team approach to patient care and safety in critical settings [59]. The committee on quality of healthcare in America believes that health care organization should accomplished team training programs for health care professionals in critical care areas using demonstrating message such as crew resources management techniques employed in aviation, including simulation as people make fewer errors when they work in teams [60].

4. Conclusion

Airway management in critically ill patient continues to be challenging for health care professionals even for expertise requiring implementation of specific guidelines and protocols to eliminate the its adverse consequences. Airway management tools and skills needed, could be attained through formal training by anesthesia clinical rotation, airway management courses, workshops and simulation training.

Teamwork is a key for success and must be proceeded by debriefing and specific task assignments. Plan of failure in a step wise approach for success and airway management should be considered early without delay that will be associated with more difficulties and unwanted outcome.

Optimization of oxygen delivery throughout the airway intervention is mandatory and should not be compromised for any reason. FONA should be considered in primary preparation and must be done in appropriate time without delay. Documentations and records must involve all stages of airway management and include details of difficulties.

Author details

ELSayed Elkarta[1*] and Magdy Eldegwy[2]

1 Al-Azhar University, Faculty of Medicine in Damietta, New Damietta, Egypt

2 Al-Azhar University, Faculty of Medicine in Cairo, Cairo, Egypt

*Address all correspondence to: salkarta@hotmail.com

References

[1] Watts ER, Walmsley SR. Inflammation and Hypoxia: HIF and PHD Isoform Selectivity. Trends Mol Med. 2019 Jan; 25(1):33-46

[2] West, J.B.: Respiratory Physiology: 2011, The Essentials, 9th edn. Philadelphia: Lippincott, Williams and Wilkins.

[3] O'Driscoll, B.R., Howard, L.S., Davidson, A.G: Guidelines for emergency oxygen use in adult patients. Thorax; 2008,63(Suppl VI): vi1-73.

[4] Nolan, J., Soar, J., Lockey, A. et al.: Advanced Life Support, 2011, 6th edn. London: Resuscitation Council.

[5] Griesdale DE, Bosma TL, Kurth T, Isac G, Chittock DR. Complica- tions of endotracheal intubation in the critically ill. Intensive Care Med 2008; 34: 1835-42

[6] Jaber S, Amraoui J, Lefrant JY, et al. Clinical practice and risk factors for immediate complications of endotracheal intubation in the intensive care unit: a prospective, multiple-center study. Crit Care Med 2006; 34: 2355-61

[7] Bowles TM, Freshwater Turner DA, Janssen DJ, Peden CJ, on behalf of the RTIC Severn Group. Out-of-theatre tracheal intubation: prospective multicentre study of clinical practice and adverse events. Br J Anaesth 2011; 107: 687-92

[8] Nolan JP, Kelly FE. Airway challenges in critical care. Anaesthesia 2011; 66: 81e92

[9] Cook TM, Woodall N, Harper J, Benger *J. major* complications of airway management in the UK: results of the Fourth National Audit Project of the Royal College of Anaesthetists and the Difficult Airway Society. Part 2: intensive care and emergency departments. Br J Anaesth 2011; 106: 632-42

[10] A K Nørskov 1, C V Rosenstock, J Wetterslev, G Astrup, A Afshari, L H Lundstrøm. Diagnostic Accuracy of Anesthesiologists' Prediction of Difficult Airway Management in Daily Clinical Practice: A Cohort Study of 188064 Patients Registered in the Danish Anaesthesia Database. Anaesthesia 2015; 70(3):272-81

[11] De Jong A, Molinari N, Terzi N, et al. Early identification of patients at risk for difficult intubation in the intensive care unit: development and validation of the MACOCHA score in a multicenter cohort study. Am J Respr Crit Care Med 2013; 187: 832e9

[12] Yildiz TS, Korkmaz F, Solak M, Toker K, Erciyes N, Bayrak F, Ganidagli S, Tekin M, Kizilkaya M, Karsli B, et al. Prediction of difficult tracheal intubation in Turkish patients: a multicenter methodological study. Eur J Anaesthesiol 2007; 24:1034-1040.

[13] Shallik N, Labib A, Ganaw A, Shaikh N, Moustafa A, Hammad Y. Virtual bronchoscopy and 3D reconstruction in the critical care setting. Qatar Medical Journal. 2020 Feb 6;2019(2-Qatar Critical Care Conference Proceedings):81

[14] Frerk C, Mitchell VS, McNarry AF, et al. Difficult Airway Society 2015 guidelines for management of unanticipated difficult intubation in adults. Br J Anaesth 2015; 115: 827e48

[15] Kristensen MS, Teoh WH, Rudolph SS. Ultrasonographic identification of the cricothyroid membrane: best evidence, techniques, and clinical impact. Br J Anaesth 2016; 117: i39e48

[16] Tanoubi I, Drolet P, Donati F. Optimizing preoxygenation in adults. Can J Anaesth 2009; 56: 449e66

[17] Mort TC. Preoxygenation in critically ill patients requiring emergency tracheal intubation. Crit Care Med 2005; 33: 2672e5

[18] Pandey M, Ursekar R, Aphale S. 3 minutes tidal breathing a gold standard technique of pre-oxygenation for elective surgeries. Innov J Med Health Sci 2014; 4: 194e7

[19] Higgs A, McGrath B.A, Goddard C, Rangasami J, Suntharalingam G, Gale R, Cook T.M and on behalf of Difficult Airway Society, Intensive Care Society, Faculty of Intensive Care Medicine, Royal College of Anesthetists. Guidelines for the management of tracheal intubation in critically ill adults. BJA, 2018; 120 (2): 323e352

[20] Delay JM, Sebbane M, Jung B, et al. The effectiveness of noninvasive positive pressure ventilation to enhance preoxygenation in morbidly obese patients: a randomized controlled study. Anesth Analg 2008; 107: 1707e13

[21] Jaber S, Monnin M, Girard M, et al. Apnoeic oxygenation via high-flow nasal cannula oxygen combined with non- invasive ventilation preoxygenation for intubation in hypoxaemic patients in the intensive care unit: the single center, blinded, randomized controlled OPTINIV trial. Intensive Care Med 2016; 42: 1877e87

[22] Brindley PG, Simmonds MR, Needham CJ, Simmonds KA. Teaching airway management to novices: a simulator manikin study comparing the 'sniffing position' and 'win with the chin' analogies. Br J Anaesth 2010; 104: 496e500

[23] Weingart SD, Levitan RM. Preoxygenation and prevention of desaturation during emergency airway management. Ann Emerg Med 2012; 59: 165e75

[24] Dixon BJ, Dixon JB, Carden JR, et al. Preoxygenation is more effective in the 25 degrees head-up position than in the supine position in severely obese patients: a randomized controlled study. Anesthesiology 2005; 102: 1110e5

[25] Association of Anaesthetists of Great Britain and Ireland. Recommendations for standards of monitoring during anaesthesia and recovery 2015. Anaesthesia 2016; 71: 85e93

[26] Koerber JP, Roberts GE, Whitaker R, Thorpe CM. Variation in rapid sequence induction techniques: current practice in Wales. Anaesthesia. 2009; 64:54-59.

[27] Schlesinger S, Blanchfield D. Modified rapid-sequence induction of anesthesia: a survey of current clinical practice. Aana J. 2001; 69:291-298.

[28] Scott D. Weingart, Seth Trueger, Nelson Wong, Joseph Scofi, Neil Singh, Soren S., Rudolph: Delayed Sequence Intubation; A Prospective Observational Study. Ann Emerg Med. 2014;1-8.

[29] Upchurch CP, Grijalva CG, Russ S, et al. Comparison of etomidate and ketamine for induction during rapid sequence intubation of adult trauma patients. Ann Emerg Med 2017; 69: 2433.e2.

[30] Kaushal RP, Vatal A, Pathak R. Effect of etomidate and propofol induction on hemodynamic and endocrine response in patients undergoing coronary artery bypass grafting/mitral valve and aortic valve replacement surgery on cardiopulmonary bypass. Ann Card Anaesth 2015; 18:172178.

[31] Jabre P, Combes X, Lapostolle F, Dhaouadi M, Ricardhibon A, Vivien B, et al. Etomidate versus ketamine for rapid sequence intubation in acutely ill patients: a multicenter randomized controlled trial. Lancet. 2008; 374:293-300.

[32] Seisa MO, Gondhi V, Demirci O, et al. Survey on the current state of endotracheal intubation among the critically ill. Journal of Intensive Care Medicine 2016; 40:17.

[33] Rocchio MA, Sylvester K, Beik N, et al. Retrospective review of propofol versus etomidate during rapid sequence intubation in the emergency department at a tertiary academic center. Pharmacol Pharm 2017; 8: 23141.

[34] Bruder EA, Ball IM, Ridi S, Pickett W, Hohl C. Single induction dose of etomidate versus other induction agents for endotracheal intubation in critically ill patients. Cochrane Database Syst Rev. 2015;1:CD010225.

[35] Heuer JF, Barwing TA, Barwing J, et al. Incidence of difficult intubation in intensive care patients: analysis of contributing factors. Anaesth Intensive Care 2012; 40: 120e7

[36] Marsch SC, Steiner L, Bucher E, et al. Succinylcholine versus rocuronium for rapid sequence intubation in intensive care: a prospective, randomized controlled trial. Crit Care 2011; 15: R199

[37] Reynolds SF, Heffner J. Airway management of the critically ill patient. Chest. 2005; 127:1397-412.

[38] Frova G, Tuzzo D. Anesthesia accidents: accidental esophageal intubation. Minerva Anestesiol 1999; 65: 362e6

[39] Kelly FE, Cook TM. Randomized controlled trials of video-laryngoscopy vs. direct laryngoscopy on intensive care are needed. Intensive Care Med 2014; 40. 765e5

[40] Amathieu R, Combes X, Abdi W, et al. An algorithm for difficult airway management, modified for modern optical devices (Airtraq laryngoscope; LMA CTrach TM): a 2- year prospective validation in patients for elective abdominal, gynecologic, and thyroid surgery. Anesthesiology 2011; 114: 25e33

[41] Grier G, Bredmose P, Davies G, Lockey D. Introduction and use of the ProSeal laryngeal mask airway as a rescue device in a pre-hospital trauma anaesthesia algorithm. Resuscitation 2009; 80: 138e41

[42] Halwagi AE, Massicotte N, Lallo A, et al. Tracheal intubation through the I-gel TM supraglottic airway versus the LMA FastrachTM: a randomized controlled trial. Anesth Analg 2012; 114: 152e6

[43] Cook TM, Woodall N, Frerk C, on behalf of the Fourth National Audit Project. Major complications of airway management in the UK: results of the fourth national audit project of the Royal College of Anesthetists and the Difficult Airway Society. Part 1: anaesthesia. Br J Anaesth 2011; 106: 617e31

[44] Mehmet Sahin 1, Daniel Anglade, Martine Buchberger, Adrien Jankowski, Pierre Albaladejo, Gilbert R Ferretti. Case Reports: Iatrogenic Bronchial Rupture Following the Use of Endotracheal Tube Introducers. Can J Anaesth. 2012 Oct;59(10):963-7.

[45] Grimaldi, D., Hraiech, S., Boutin, E. et al. Hypoxemia in the ICU: prevalence, treatment, and outcome. Ann. Intensive Care 2018; 8, 82.

[46] Carron M, Freo U, Michielan F, Ori C. Effects of tracheal intubation on ventilation with LMA classic for percutaneous dilation tracheostomy. Minerva Anestesiol 2010; 76: 181e7

[47] ANZCA Airway Management Working Group. Transition from supraglottic to infra-glottic rescue in the 'can't intubate can't oxygenate' (CICO) scenario. 2014. Available from: http://www.anzca.edu.au/documents/

report-from-the- anzca-airway-management-working-gr.pdf. [Accessed 17 February 2017]

[48] Hubble MW, Wilfong DA, Brown LH, Hertelendy A, Benner RW. A meta-analysis of prehospital airway control techniques part II: alternative airway devices and cricothyrotomy success rates. Prehosp Emerg Care 2010; 14: 515e30.

[49] Mort TC, Braffett BH. Conventional versus video laryngoscopy for tracheal tube exchange: glottic visualization, success rates, complications, and rescue alternatives in the high-risk difficult airway patient. Anesth Analg 2015; 121: 440e8

[50] Shah RK, Lander L, Berry JG, Nussenbaum B, Merati A, Roberson DW. Tracheotomy outcomes and complications: a national perspective. Laryngoscope 2012; 122: 25e9

[51] Popat M, Mitchell V, Dravid R et al. Difficult Airway Society Guidelines for the management of tracheal extubation. Anaesthesia. 2012;67(3):318-340.

[52] Nishina K, Mikawa K, Maekawa N, Obara H. Fentanyl attenuates cardiovascular responses to tracheal extubation. Acta Anaesthesiologica Scandinavica 1995;39: 85-9.

[53] Thomas AN, McGrath BA. Patient safety incidents associated with airway devices in critical care: a review of reports to the UK National Patient Safety Agency. Anaesthesia 2009; 64: 358e65

[54] Rochwerg B, Solo K, Darzi A, et al. Update Alert: Ventilation Techniques and Risk for Transmission of Coronavirus Disease, Including COVID-19. Ann Intern Med 2020.

[55] Schünemann HJ, Khabsa J, Solo K, et al. Ventilation Techniques and Risk for Transmission of Coronavirus Disease, Including COVID-19: A Living Systematic Review of Multiple Streams of Evidence. Ann Intern Med 2020; 173:204.

[56] El-Boghdadly K, Wong DJN, Owen R, et al. Risks to healthcare workers following tracheal intubation of patients with COVID-19: a prospective international multicentre cohort study. Anaesthesia 2020.

[57] Gaba DM. Structural and organizational issues inpatient safety: a comparison of health care to other high-hazard industries. Calif Manag Rev. 2000; 43:83-102

[58] McGaghie WC, Issenberg SB, Petrusa ER, Scalese RJ. A critical review of simulation-based medical education research: 2003-2009. Med Educ. 2010; 44:50-63

[59] Gaba DM, Fish KJ, Howard SK. Crisis management in anesthesia. New York: Churchill Livingstone; 1994

[60] Kohn LT, Corrigan JM, Donaldson MS, editors. To err is human: building a safer health system. Washington (DC); 2000

Chapter 7

Airway Management in Full Stomach Conditions

Saba Al Bassam, Ahmed Zaghw, Muhammad Jaffar Khan, Neethu Arun and Arunabha Karmakar

Abstract

Pulmonary aspiration in the perioperative period is one of the well-known complications under anesthesia and procedural sedation. A full stomach condition either due to non-adherence to fasting guidelines or due to various other factors that delay gastric emptying are the most common causes. Following aspiration, a patient may develop a wide spectrum of clinical sequelae. The key factors in preventing aspiration include proper pre-operative assessment, appropriate premedication and operating room preparations. Rapid sequence induction and intubation is the recommended technique for securing the airway in cases of full stomach. Management of aspiration depends on the nature of the aspirate. Pre-operative fasting guidelines have been established by various medical societies which may be modified in special circumstances of high risk of aspiration. Prediction of difficult airway in certain cases of full stomach necessitates clinical expertise in airway management.

Keywords: pulmonary aspiration, full stomach, gastric volume, rapid sequence induction, negative pressure pulmonary edema

1. Introduction

Full stomach is a condition when a patient has ingested a certain amount of food or drink within a certain period prior to anesthetic induction or believed to have an anatomical, hormonal, metabolic or pathological condition that delays the gastric emptying. The amount of food or Full stomach poses a risk of pulmonary aspiration of gastric contents during the perioperative period more than if the patient had been fasting or definitive time has passed to allow the gastric emptying. Pulmonary aspiration poses a significant risk to each individual surgical patient, affecting the outcome of the surgical care and poses high costs for healthcare system. The incidence of pulmonary aspiration during anesthesia is around 1 in every 2000–3000 surgeries. The National Audit Project 4 (NAP4) by the Royal College of Anesthetists in the UK showed that aspiration was 23% among all reported cases to NAP4 either as a primary or secondary event. Unfortunately, more than 50% of the death related to anesthesia in NAP4 was because of aspiration [1].

2. History

The first case descriptions of aspiration under anesthesia had been reported in the late 19th century. In 1861, out of the first 51 reported cases that died under Chloroform, Dr. Sanom reported two cases died following sudden vomiting under anesthesia with an estimate of aspiration related mortality of 2%. In 1876 at the Guy's Hospital in UK, the first reported case of death related aspiration after recovery from anesthesia was reported, when a patient turned cyanotic after vomiting in the recovery area, later undigested meat was retrieved from the upper pharynx and trachea was full of vomitus. In U.S.A., the first case was reported in 1898, a 6-year-old boy who had his dinner 3.5 h before anesthesia, has died from aspiration in the recovery. The autopsy confirmed undigested spinach material in the main bronchus [2].

In the 50s of the twentieth century, the danger of a full stomach was realized based on high aspiration rate, but optimum fasting time was insufficiently recognized. The observational studies have found esophageal pooling of incomplete swallowing of fluid are very common under anesthesia. Aspiration risks were found in early 1950 to be high in hemorrhage, bowel obstruction, peritonitis and multiple abdominal surgeries, using of both narcotics and the belladonna alkaloids, and under obstetrics anesthesia, especially if pain and delivery are prolonged. In 1951, aspiration accounts for 4% of overall maternal death, and have reported that aspiration contributed to more than 50% of the mortality [3]. Surprisingly, the aspiration was not limited to inhalation anesthesia; but also, during spinal anesthesia. In 1946, Dr. Mendelson describes the relationship between aspiration of solid and liquid matter, and pulmonary sequelae in obstetric patients. Another tracer dye-based aspiration study 1950 by Dr. Weiss found the minor regurgitations were very common. Interestingly, the incidence rate of blue dye regurgitation was 26% in the pharynx, 16% in the bronchus as confirmed by bronchoscopy, but the frank vomiting occurred in only 8% [4].

Out of the historical recommendations were stomach decompression by a stomach tube pre induction, hyperventilation, head-up position during induction and recovery in lateral position, but no reliable and safe method has been recommended. Sellick's technique of cricoid pressure was introduced in 1961 to prevent regurgitation and aspiration during induction.

3. Physiology of regurgitation and aspiration

The physiological mechanisms preventing gastric content from regurgitation and aspiration are **lower esophageal sphincter, upper esophageal sphincter** and **protective airway reflex.**

Upper esophageal sphincter is the cricopharyngeal muscle acting on the transition zone between esophagus and hypopharynx. **Lower esophageal sphincter (LES)** is composed of circular muscle fiber at the junction of esophagus and stomach, acting as a true sphincter. The difference between Lower esophageal pressure (LOP) and gastric pressure is called the esophageal barrier pressure. Intragastric pressure is less than 7 mmHg, LOP in conscious patient is 15–25 mmHg higher than intragastric pressure. An incompetent LOS reduces barrier pressure and increase the risk of regurgitation. When esophageal pressure equals intragastric pressure, this will lead to a common cavity which in turn causes spontaneous gastroesophageal reflex. LOP decreases during peristalsis, vomiting, pregnancy and various drugs for instance anticholinergic, inhalational anesthetics, Thiopentone and opioids. Intragastric pressure increases if gastric volume is more than 1000 ml and with raised intra-abdominal pressure. Gastric volume is influenced by the rate of gastric secretion; approximately 0.6 ml/kg/h, swallowing of saliva 1 ml/kg/h, ingestion of solid and food and the rate of gastric emptying. LES can be affected by food as (Chocolate, Ethanol and Caffeine), hormones (as Progesterone, Glucagon, Secretin, Cholecystokinin, and Somatostatin), drugs (as Anticholinergic, alpha-adrenergic antagonist, Beta adrenergic agonist, Calcium channel blocker, Diazepam and Morphine) and smoking. All anesthetic agents except Ketamine as well as muscle relaxants decrease upper esophageal sphincter tone.

Protective upper airway reflexes

1. Coughing which is forceful expiration after brief inspiration.

2. Laryngospasm is a closure of both false and true vocal cords with apnea.

3. Expiration reflex which lead to sudden opening of the glottis and the closure of the false cord.

4. Spasmatic panting which involve a rapid closing and opening of the glottis and shallow breathing of around 60 breath per minute for less than 10 seconds.

Opioids can blunt all these reflexes except laryngospasm. Reduced consciousness level in perioperative period including after emergence will affect these reflexes increasing the risk of aspiration [5].

3.1 Pathology of lung aspiration

Pulmonary aspiration is defined by the inhalation of oro-pharyngeal or gastric contents into the larynx and the respiratory tract or the presence of bilious secretions or particulate matter in the tracheobronchial tree. Time frame of perioperative pulmonary aspiration starts from preoperative period until 2 h after termination of anesthesia. Diagnosis of perioperative pulmonary aspiration is made by direct examination of the oral-pharynx, bronchoscopy assessment of the tracheobronchial tree, or postoperative chest X-rays showing new infiltrates [6, 7].

During the induction of anesthesia, as the patient loses consciousness and the protective airway reflexes are obtunded, the gastric contents, in case of full stomach, may regurgitate through the esophagus and get aspirated into the lungs. Clinical outcomes of pulmonary aspiration range from benign hypoxia and desaturation, to fatal course of Acute Respiratory Distress Syndrome (ARDS), respiratory failure, cardiopulmonary collapse and death (**Figure 1**). The severity of these pulmonary complications depends on the acidity and the volume of gastric contents as well as the immune response of the patient. Small particulate aspiration induces a foreign body reaction of inflammation and consequently results in granuloma formation. Aspiration of acidic content induces acute inflammatory response and progresses rapidly to pneumonitis over 24–48 h. Hypoxia is common due to either upper airway obstruction or obstructed lower airway by debris, thus leading to high airway resistance and vicious cycle of alveolar collapse, alveolar edema and reflex bronchospasm [8].

3.2 Pathophysiology of pulmonary aspiration

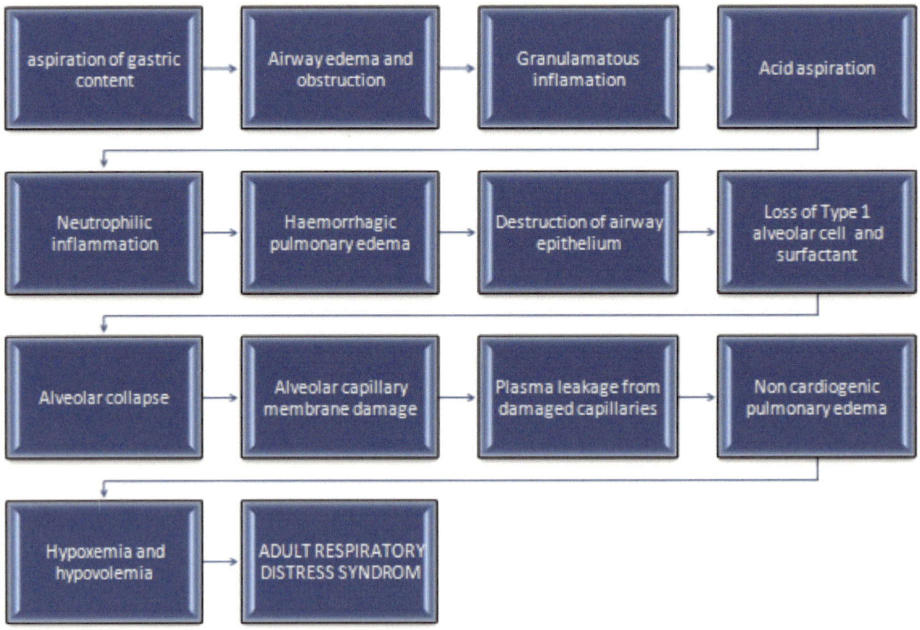

Figure 1.
Summary of pathophysiology of pulmonary aspiration, modified from Dal Santo et al. [8].

3.3 Types of aspiration-related pulmonary complications

1. Aspiration pneumonitis or chemical pneumonitis
2. Bacterial pneumonia
3. Particle-associated aspiration

3.3.1 Aspiration pneumonitis or chemical pneumonitis

Chemical pneumonitis, the most common type of pulmonary aspiration, was first described by Curtis Lester Mendelson in 1946 as inflammation of the lung parenchyma resulting from aspiration of sterile gastric contents. The morbidity and mortality associated with aspiration pneumonitis can be attributed to the acidity and volume of the aspirate. If the pH of the aspirate is less than 2.5 and the volume is >0.3 ml/kg (20–25 ml in adults), it can lead to fatal pneumonitis [9].

The acidity of the aspirate can cause chemical injury to the tracheobronchial tree and the lung parenchyma which can trigger a series of immune responses. The direct corrosive effect of gastric acid on the alveolar-capillary epithelium peaks in 1–2 h. This is followed by an inflammatory response which peaks in 4–6 h which involves neutrophilic invasion of the alveoli and lung parenchyma. This phase is also characterized by the involvement of a spectrum of inflammatory mediators, inflammatory cells, adhesion molecules, and enzymes, including tumor necrosis factor α, interleukin-8, cyclooxygenase and lipoxygenase products, and reactive oxygen species, though the major role in the mechanism of lung injury is played by neutrophils & complement activation [9].

The clinical course may have either of the 3 outcomes [10]:

1. Clinical and radiological improvement.

2. Initial improvement then gradual clinical and radiological deterioration.

3. Refractory severe course.

3.3.2 Bacterial pneumonitis

A contaminated aspirate can lead to bacterial infection of the lung parenchyma, with a course of complete recovery or progress to lung abscess formation, exogenous lipoid pneumonia or chronic interstitial fibrosis. The most common pathogens are *Staphylococcus aureus*, *Pseudomonas aeruginosa*, Enterobacter species, Klebsiella species and *Escherichia coli*. The major anaerobes that have been isolated from pulmonary infections include Pepto streptococcus, Fusobacterium nucleatum, Fusobacterium necrophorum, Prevotella, Bacteroides melaninogenicus [11].

3.3.3 Particle-associated aspiration

If particulate matter is present in the aspirate it can lead to variable degrees of airway obstruction. The severity of airway obstruction depends upon the size of the particle and the caliber of the airways. Aspiration of a larger particle can even lead to complete airway obstruction with subsequent sudden respiratory distress, cyanosis, and aphonia that may lead to sudden death if the obstruction is not immediately relieved. Smaller particles in the distal airways cause less severe obstruction and gradual course of respiratory symptoms as irritative cough, wheezing, dyspnea and superimposed bacterial pneumonia if the distal obstruction persists for more than 1 week. Chest X-Ray could show atelectasis or obstructive emphysema with a mediastinal shift and elevated diaphragm as shown in **Figure 2** below.

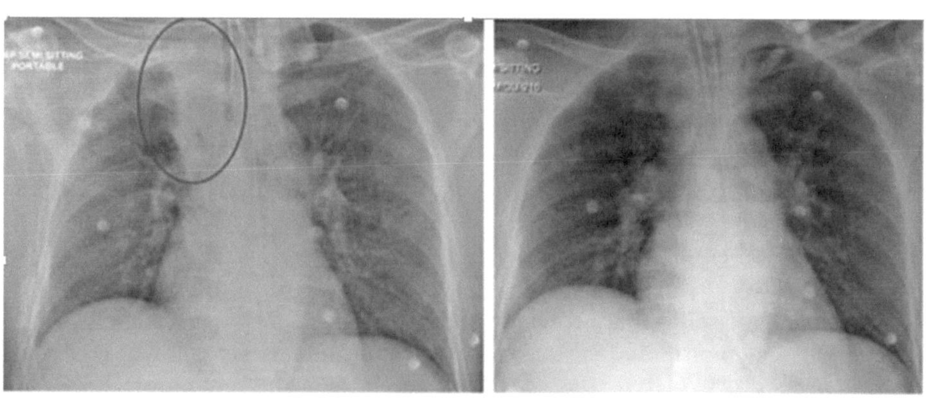

Figure 2.
A chest radiograph (on the left) for a patient with a witnessed aspiration of food particles after neuro-intervention procedure under sedation, showing right upper lobe atelectasis and bilateral pulmonary edema and infiltrates. (On the right), the resolution of collapse and infiltrates after 2 days of respiratory support with invasive ventilation and Tazocin antibiotics in ICU. Picture courtesy of Dr. El Sayed E lKarta with his permission, Hamad Medical Corporation, Doha, Qatar.

4. Outcome-driven anesthesia related morbidity and mortality

In American Society of Anesthesiology (ASA) closed claims, the three leading respiratory events related to death or brain damage before 1990 were all non-aspiration related as; inadequate oxygenation/ventilation, difficult intubation and undetected esophageal intubation. Fortunately, the overall proportion of other non-aspiration respiratory-related death or brain death events have dramatically decreased over time, from 30% of the claims in the 1970s to 15% in the 1990s, possibly, due to incorporation of pulse oximetry, capnography and advent of supraglottic device and videoscopes into general clinical practice [12].

In ASA closed claims, the occurrence of aspiration has remained constant over time around 3.5%, with reduction of other non-aspiration respiratory claims. The mortality and brain death related to non-aspiration respiratory events have been decreasing since 1970 to 1990 from 50–30%. Surprisingly, to date still 60% of death and brain injury was attributed to aspiration compared to 43% for the remainder of the ASA claims [12].

In NAP4, among all respiratory claims, pulmonary aspiration contributed to only 5% of all claims. The topmost contributors to the NAP4 respiratory claims as 60% of the whole claims; were Inadequate ventilation, esophageal intubation and difficult intubation, all are considered as common risk factors for aspiration pneumonia. Still, the aspiration in NAP4 constitutes over 50% of airway-related deaths in anesthesia exceeding the feared consequence of cannot intubate cannot ventilate (CICV) scenario. 23% of all NAP4 claims have aspiration as either primary or secondary event. Cases not leading to mortality commonly resulted in significant morbidity and prolonged stay on intensive care [1].

4.1 Risk factors of aspiration

Risk factors cannot be ignored or easily overlooked in the preoperative assessment as 93% of aspiration cases in NAP4 have identifiable risk factors however the aspiration risk have been identified in only 40% of the primary anesthesia related aspiration. Thus, it mandates more judicious preoperative assessment [13] (**Table 1**).

4.1.1 Poor airway assessment

Poor assessment could lead equally to difficult airway scenarios and aspiration.

4.1.2 Poor planning and prophylaxis

Unstructured, inorganized and unplanned sequence for airway management.

4.1.3 First generation supraglottic airway devices (SAD)

Numerous cases of aspiration occurred during use of a first-generation SAD in patients who had multiple risk factors for aspiration and in several in whom the aspiration risk was so high that rapid sequence induction and intubation (RSII), should have been used [14].

4.1.4 Obesity and after bariatric surgery

Obesity is an independent risk factor for full stomach and airway management may be difficult in these patients, preoperative gastric ultrasound is recommended to assess the risk of aspiration. Complications in obese patient included an increased

Surgical factors
• Emergency surgery (trauma) • Upper abdominal or laparoscopic surgery • Positioning (lithotomy or Trendelenburg) • Prolonged surgery >2 h
Patient factors
• Hiatal hernia • Gastrointestinal obstruction/abdominal distension • Pregnancy • Morbid obesity • Upper gastrointestinal hemorrhage • Intracranial hypertension • ICU patients • Diabetes mellitus or those with gastroparesis • Gastroesophageal reflux / Incompetent lower Esophageal Sphincter • Opioids
Patient factors
• Light depth of anesthesia • 1st Generation of Supra Glottic Device "SGA" • Insufflation of stomach with bag mask ventilation or LMA • Anesthesia delivered by Trainees

Table 1.
Summary of the factors for aspiration pneumonia per Asai's risk factors [12].

frequency of aspiration and other complications during the use of SAD, difficulty at tracheal intubation and airway obstruction during emergence or recovery [15].

4.1.5 Difficult airway and failure of airway management

The 13% of the ASA aspiration claims have occurred during difficult airway management. In NAP4, still the topmost contributors to respiratory claim were inadequate ventilation, esophageal intubation and difficult intubation report as 60% of the claims, and all that are common risk factors for aspiration pneumonia [1].

4.1.6 Number of intubation attempts

The NAP4 registry has found the number of attempts, and trials are significantly associated with higher rate of aspiration 22% regurgitation, 13% aspiration were reported after the second attempts [1].

4.1.7 Underlying pathologies

4.1.7.1 Diabetes mellitus

Diabetes is a common metabolic and endocrine disease, complicated with diabetic gastroparesis, known as gastric paralysis. It was found that hemoglobin

A1c value of more than 7%, could lead to delayed gastric emptying, by decreasing the frequency of gastric contraction, while the risk score of aspiration increase significantly [16].

4.1.7.2 Advanced age

Old age is an independent risk factor for delayed gastric emptying, as it is common in elderly patient to have anorexia, dyspepsia and impaired gastric peristalsis [17].

4.1.7.3 Gastrointestinal disorder

Functional delayed gastric emptying (FDGE) and Ileus are common complications following abdominal surgeries especially bowel resection, colon and rectal surgery, all lead to impaired contractility, motility and gastric emptying [18].

4.1.7.4 Specific anesthesia time

ASA closed claims have identified that aspiration cases were associated with anesthesia induction in 60%, maintenance in 18% and during emergence in 11% and in PACU in 5% anesthesia related claims, indicating that aspiration commonly occurs during induction, but the risk is still high even till PACU [12].

4.1.8 Type of anesthesia

Mainly the aspiration is during general anesthesia; however, 7% of aspiration in ASA closed claims have occurred during regional anesthesia or monitored anesthesia care. 18% of the aspiration that occurred during maintenance of anesthesia was either by facemask, laryngeal mask [12].

4.1.9 Gastric volume

It was found that when gastric volume (GV) was less than 0.4 ml/kg, the incidence of vomiting was only 6.7%. Once the volume exceeded 0.8 ml/kg, the incidence of vomiting was as high as 44.1%. In supine position, patients with cross-section area (CSA) less than 340 mm^2 was considered as fasting. On the contrary, CSA was greater than 340 mm^2 indicates GV of greater than 0.8 ml/kg [19].

4.1.10 Determination of critical volume of gastric contents

A critical volume of gastric contents required to produce severe aspiration pneumonitis has been even more debatable than determining critical PH. In one study, pulmonary injury became independent of pH as the volume of aspirate was increased from 0.5 to 4.0 ml/kg in dogs. Nevertheless, it was generally accepted that the volume of gastric fluid of 0.4 ml/kg places a subject at risk for developing aspiration pneumonitis based on experimental instillation of gastric fluid into the right main stem bronchus of a single Rhesus monkey [20].

However, The ASA Task Force on Preoperative Fasting, despite extensive screening of the current data, has been unable to establish a link between residual gastric volume and pulmonary aspiration [21].

5. Perioperative anesthesia management in full-stomach patients

Identification of patients who are at risk for pulmonary aspiration is the first step toward minimizing the incidence of perioperative pulmonary aspiration. Two patient risk categories exist: those with a full stomach (i.e., history of ingestion of a meal with less than 6 h fasting time) and those designated as having a full stomach despite a prolonged preoperative fast. **Aspiration prophylaxis goals in preoperative period** are summarized in **Table 2**.

5.1 Fasting recommendations

Guidelines for preoperative fasting are formulated in order to reduce the risk of aspiration under general anesthesia or procedural sedation. They apply to all patients undergoing elective surgeries or procedures under general anesthesia, regional anesthesia, procedural sedation and monitored anesthesia care (MAC). Aspiration can happen during all the above-mentioned types of anesthesia as the anesthetic and sedative drugs can obtund the protective airway reflexes which can in turn result in aspiration of gastric contents. It is not applicable to patients undergoing minor surgeries or procedures solely under local anesthesia.

2017 American Society of Anesthesiology (ASA) task force fasting recommendations are summarized in the **Table 3**. For certain procedures like intragastric balloon removal or repositioning, fasting time up to 12 h is recommended. (Please refer to other chapter for more details). Other circumstances and comorbidities as listed in 4.1 might necessitate certain modifications in the fasting guidelines.

Gastrointestinal factors
• Enhancing gastric emptying • Decreasing gastric volume • Minimize the volume of gastric contents • Increasing pH of gastric contents • Reduce gastroesophageal reflex
Fasting time
• Adequate preoperative fasting based on age and food type specific recommendation
Pharmacologic therapies
• Decrease gastric acidity • Facilitating gastric emptying/drainage • Maintenance of competent lower esophageal sphincter tone
Anesthesia techniques
• Preoperative (History – Optimization of risk factors) • Intraoperative (Preoxygenation + RSI + Cricoid maneuver) • Postoperative and recovery (awake during extubation)

Table 2.
Summary of aspiration prophylaxis goals in preoperative period.

Consumed meal/drink	Minimum hours of fasting required
1.Clear fluids	2 h
2.Breast milk	4 h
3.Infant formula/non-human milk	6 h
4.Light meal	6 h
5.Heavy meal (fried food, fatty food, meat)	8 h

Table 3.
2017 ASA fasting guidelines recommendations.

5.2 Pharmacologic therapies

To increase gastric pH, **Histamine antagonist (H2)** and **proton pump inhibitors (PPIs)** are commonly used. H_2 antagonists as Ranitidine, Famotidine, and Cimetidine, act by blocking the H_2 receptors of gastric parietal cells inhibiting the stimulatory effect of histamine on gastric acid secretion. **Proton Pump Inhibitors (PPIs)** as Omeprazole, Lansoprazole and Pantoprazole, irreversibly blocking the Hydrogen/Potassium ATPase of parietal cells and prevent the release of hydrochloric acid [22].

The goal for enhanced gastric emptying is achieved by **prokinetics** such as Metoclopramide [23]. It stimulates the motility of upper GI and is used in risk patient to reduce gastric volume such as Gastroesophageal reflux disease (GERD), Diabetic and pregnant patients and in emergency patients who had no time to be NPO. It also has a peripheral and central Dopamine receptor antagonist activity and might reduce the risk of postoperative nausea and vomiting. Oral antacid can be used in patients with risk of regurgitation and aspiration. Antacids work by neutralization of gastric acid content, single dose 15–30 min before surgery will increase PH above 2.5. Sodium Citrate 0.3 M is non-particulate antacid that itself will not cause pulmonary damage if aspirated with the gastric fluid. Antacids increase gastric volume especially in repeated doses, but this side effect is less important than its action on increasing gastric pH. Decrease gastric volume can be achieved by 6 h fasting before surgery, naso-gastric (NG) tube used to aspirate the gastric content before anesthesia or the use of PPI like Omeprazole to inhibit gastric acid secretion.

5.3 Role of preoperative point of care ultrasound

Ultrasonography has been recommended as a reliable, noninvasive, bedside tool to determine gastric volume and content in the perioperative period based on many studies [24, 25]. A cutoff of antral cross-sectional area of 340 mm^2 correlates with fluid volume gastric contents greater than 0.8 ml/kg, a high risk of aspiration [19]. However, most studies to date deal with validity considerations and propose that bedside ultrasound accurately determines gastric volume rather than contents [26]. Thus, the use point-of-care ultrasonography in the preoperative period as a screening tool has been recently advocated especially in vulnerable population.

5.4 Anesthesia technique for full stomach

Anesthesia management of patient with full stomach commences from preoperative period through intraoperative and concludes postoperatively.

5.4.1 Preoperative

5.4.1.1 Pre-anesthesia history

A full preoperative history is a critical step for risk assessment. Predisposing factors as Gastroesophageal reflux disease (GERD), esophageal dysmotility, diabetes, bloating and any condition that delay gastric emptying, history of bariatric surgery or any pathological conditions in upper GI could increase risk of volume regurgitation.

5.4.1.2 Preoperative fasting

Generally, it is recommended to take clear fluid for up to 2 h preoperatively and stop solid food for 6 h before the surgery as per ASA recommendations described in detail in (**Table 2**) [21].

5.4.1.3 Preemptive nasogastric tube placement

No evidence to support routine preoperative gastric emptying to reduce aspiration risk even in emergency cases except patients suspected ileus or obstruction [27].

5.4.2 Intraoperative

The meticulous and skillful airway management is the main goals in preventing gastric aspiration into the lungs during general anesthesia. Airway management techniques intraoperatively involve the following:

1. Adequate preoxygenation with 100% oxygen

   Preoxygenation is administered by face mask for 3 minutes of normal tidal volume breathing that will increase oxygen reserve in the functional reserve capacity (FRC) and provide additional safe apnea time. Passive oxygen insufflation by a nasal canula with 10 l/min during laryngoscopy can prolong the apnea time until desaturation in high risk patient of difficult intubation during airway management [28, 29].
   High frequency nasal canula (HFNC) or trans-nasal humidified rapid insufflation ventilatory exchange (THRIVE) with up to 60 l/min oxygen can be used in critically ill patient that have shorter safe apneic time [30]. It was found that THRIVE will not cause gastric distension or increase the risk of regurgitation. Oxygen flow of 70 l/min will generate a nasopharyngeal pressure of 7 cm H_2O, with this pressure it is unlikely to cause gastric distension. In a study 80 patient underwent RSI with the use THRIVE for preoxygenation, no patient shows any sign of regurgitation [31].

2. Definitive airway device by a cuffed endotracheal tube

3. Use of rapid sequence induction during tracheal intubation (RSII) with effective cricoid pressure application

   All equipment should be ready for intubation as variable size facemask, different types of laryngoscopes, different sizes of endotracheal tubes, oral and nasal airways, video laryngoscope, supraglottic airway of different sizes, and a bougie. Anxiolytic might be used to relieve anxiety; Opioid dose should be used carefully to avoid respiratory depression and loss of airway reflexes [32]. Patient head should be positioned in sniffing position to facilitate intubation, the operating table head part to put it up to make the larynx above the level of lower esophageal sphincter. Short acting Opioids Fentanyl 1–3 mcg/kg IV 3 min before induction will reduce sympathetic response to intubation. Induction of anesthesia can be done by Propofol 1.5–2.5 mg/kg IV, Etomidate 0.2–0.6 mg/kg IV or Ketamine 1–2 mg/kg IV depending on the patient general condition. Intravenous Lidocaine 1 mg/kg can be given 2 min prior to intubation to blunt the sympathetic response of intubation. Succinylcholine 1–1.5 mg/kg provide complete relaxation in 30–60 s or Rocuronium 0.9–1.2 mg/kg achieve maximum neuromuscular block in 55–75 s if Succinylcholine is contraindicated.

Sellick's maneuver or cricoid pressure of approximately 30 N or 3 kg is applied on the cricoid ring against the cervical vertebra to occlude the lumen of the esophagus to prevent regurgitation of the stomach content to the pharynx. It is routinely applied during RSII until confirmation of Endotracheal Tube (ETT) position and inflation of the tube cuff [33]. Assistant should be directed to apply cricoid pressure by the intubating physician either to shift or release the pressure if the laryngeal view is disturbed or active vomiting has happened. It is advised to leave the NG tube in place while doing RSII, connect it to suction to drain stomach contents then leave it open to air and to suction the stomach before emergence [34].

If difficult intubation is expected, or patient might desaturate with apnea e.g. obese patients, patients with high intraabdominal pressure or those with sepsis or fever, it is advised to use **modified RSII.** Modified RSII refers to cricoid pressure and gentle mask ventilation before intubation [35].

Number of studies shows that application of cricoid pressure will prevent gastric insufflation even if mask ventilation pressure is up to 60 cm H2O [36]. Some patients cannot tolerate preoxygenation such as agitated patients due to hypoxia, hypercapnia or underlying medical condition. In those patients it is advisable to intubate them using **delayed sequence intubation (DSI)**. DSI is done under procedure sedation using a dissociative dose of Ketamine (1–1.5 mg/kg) to sedate the patient sufficiently to allow mask preoxygenation with his airway reflexes being reserved. Small observational studies in ICU show some improvement in preoxygenation using DSI [37]. Another study shows that using Ketamine to facilitate preoxygenation will decrease peri-intubation hypoxia from 44 to 3.5% [38].

4. Wide bore suction (Yankeur) must be immediately available

The importance of suction cannot be overemphasized in airway decontamination. It has been incorporated with the laryngoscopy steps in the **Suction Assisted Laryngoscopy Airway Decontamination procedure (SALAD)** which was developed by Dr. James DuCanto. SALAD is performed using a rigid suction catheter to decontaminate the oral cavity and to depress or lift the tongue for better laryngoscope position then further decontamination of the hypopharynx followed by further insertion of the catheter into the proximal esophagus for continuous drain of emesis. The suction catheter is placed to the left corner of the mouth so that it will be easier to be pinned in place by the laryngoscope. Intubation and inflation of the tracheal tube will be performed while the suction catheter in upper part of esophagus so that any pharyngeal soiling or regurgitated contents could be removed instantaneously (**Figure 3**).

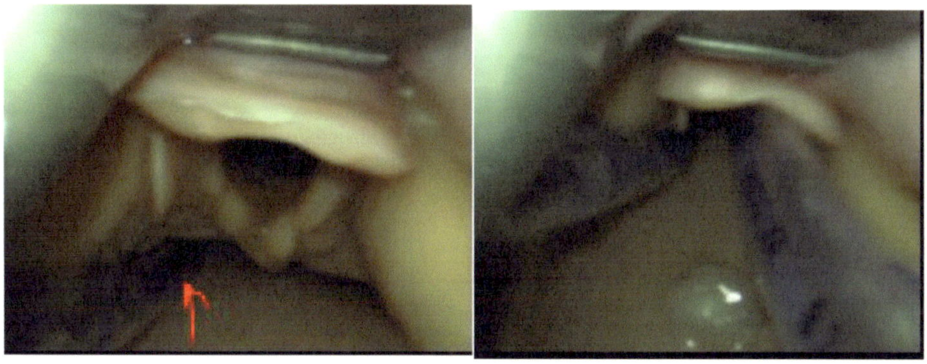

Figure 3.
A videoscope picture showing the SALAD technique. On the left, suction catheter advanced in upper esophagus. On the right, ETT in place while the suction catheter in upper esophagus. Picture courtesy of Dr. Nabil Shallik with his permission, Hamad medical corporation, Doha, Qatar.

Suction of pharyngeal contents decrease the volume of aspirates to the lung, thus could decrease the severity [39].

5. Use of airway adjuvant as optical stylet, or a video laryngoscopy in expected difficult airway

   Optical Stylets (OS) are rigid or semirigid tubular devices that fit inside tracheal tube. OS composed of a fiberoptic bundles or a video chip at distal end to convey the image. Different types of Optical stylets are available for instance Shikani Optical Stylets and Bonfils Retromolar Intubation Fiberscope. Optical stylets are useful mainly in patients with suspected difficult intubation. Airway trauma and technical difficulties due to fogging and secretion limit OS use.

Different kinds of laryngoscopes can be used to assist intubation, many studies recommend the use of video laryngoscope use for higher first attempted intubation rate especially for Mallampati 3 and 4, and better glottic view [40].

5.4.3 Postoperative

On extubation, emptying of the stomach using NG tube is recommended before emergence of the patient from anesthesia and it is advised to extubate the patient in a fully awake state, and a full recovery of the airway reflexes. Patient should be transferred to recovery with the head of the bed elevated to reduce the chance of reflux or in lateral position.

6. Management of aspiration

The first step in aspiration management is to be vigilant for any signs and symptoms of aspiration in patients especially in those who are known to have full stomach. Any witnessed gastric or oropharyngeal contents into the trachea during induction, maintenance or emergence from anesthesia, witnessed vomitus through the nose or mouth or sudden elevation of peak airway pressures during ventilation or cough, persistent hypoxia, bronchospasm or abnormal breath sounds following intubation, sore throat, dyspnea at recovery may suggest that a patient has aspirated (**Table 4**). Management in the intensive care unit includes monitoring and supportive therapy and broad-spectrum antibiotics.

Immediate steps in clinically significant aspiration
1. Call for **help** for **senior** anesthesiologist.
2. **Suction** for the fluid/particulate in the oropharynx and trachea.
3. **Definitive** airway management with a cuffed endotracheal tube with mechanical ventilation.
4. **Continuous monitoring** of vital signs, baseline chest radiograph and arterial blood gas
5. **Hemodynamic support** (two wide bore intravenous cannula, vasopressors with conservative fluid administration to avoid pulmonary edema)
6. **Respiratory support** using lung protective ventilation strategy if required which combined low tidal volume with relatively high respiratory rate along with positive end expiratory pressure.
7. **Lung recruitment** to patients to maintain adequate saturation.
8. Portable **chest radiograph** as a baseline documentation.
9. **Stabilization** before surgical incision If the surgery cannot be postponed
10. **Postponing** the surgery is recommended in significant airway obstruction, impaired oxygenation or ventilation or cardiovascular effects such as hypotension and shock.
11. **Multidisciplinary team** of intensivist, Infection disease and pulmonologist for post-operative intensive care.

Table 4.
Summary for immediate steps in aspiration prophylaxis.

6.1 Chemical pneumonitis

The main stay of treatment in chemical pneumonitis includes immediate tracheal suctioning to remove the aspirated material followed by pulmonary support. Use of antibiotics must be revaluated by the team after 48–72 h and its use discontinued if there are no signs of infection [41].

6.2 Bacterial pneumonia

The antibiotic regimen should include aerobic and anaerobic coverage, especially against gram-negative bacilli and *Staphylococcus aureus*. **Carbapenem** (Imipenem, Meropenem) or Piperacillin Tazobactam in resistant Gram-negative bacilli or in patients who have received intravenous antibiotic coverage in the past 90 days. If anaerobic bacteria are suspected, parenteral antibiotic of Ampicillin-Sulbactam 1.5–3 g intravenous every 6 h or **Amoxicillin Clavulanate** (immediate release 875 mg orally twice daily or extended release 2 g orally twice daily) is an appropriate alternative.

Other alternative regimens include **Metronidazole** 500 mg orally or intravenous three times daily plus either amoxicillin 500 mg orally three times daily or Penicillin G intravenous 1–2 million units intravenous every 4 to 6 hours. In penicillin allergy Clindamycin 600 mg intravenous every 8 h or **Ceftriaxone** 1–2 g intravenous daily or **Cefotaxime** 1–2 g intravenous every 8 h in combination with Metronidazole. Oral antibiotics switch from parenteral antibiotics is based on clinical improvement, hemodynamic stability, tolerance for oral medications [41, 42].

7. Full stomach in special populations

7.1 Difficult airway management in full-stomach patient

If a difficult airway is predicted, the risk of aspiration may be weighed against the risk of difficult or failed airway management. In such a case, modified rapid sequence induction and intubation (RSII), awake fiberoptic intubation or inhalational induction may be considered. The advantages of awake tracheal intubation are maintenance of protective airway reflexes, uncompromised airway oxygenation and ventilation and maintenance of normal muscle tone, which helps in the identification of anatomic landmarks. It is accomplished by adequate preoperative preparation, use of an intravenous anti-sialagogue to reduce oral secretions, cautious use of intravenous sedation and an experienced skill anesthetist. Topicalization of the airway is controversial, as airway reflexes might be abolished after topical anesthesia of lower airways putting the patient at risk of aspiration as the larynx will no longer be "AWAKE". It is recommended to use topical anesthesia on base of tongue, vallecula and epiglottis while spraying the local anesthesia directly to vocal cord, transtracheal anesthesia and anesthesia to recurrent laryngeal nerve should be avoided in high risk of aspiration [43].

Presently, Supraglottic Airway Device (SAD) is recognized in the ASA difficult airway algorithm. It could be used as ventilation device or serves as conduit for intubation, or both. The **Proseal™** Laryngeal mask airway is potentially useful device especially in patient with high risk for gastric regurgitation and pulmonary aspiration as it has been shown to protect adult and pediatric patients from large-volume aspiration in some studies, however no studies have confirmed its effectiveness comparing to cuffed endotracheal tubes at reducing the risk of aspiration [44, 45].

7.2 Pediatric population

The accurate incidence rate of aspiration pneumonitis in pediatric anesthesia is unknown. However, it has been acknowledged as a rare event, it was reported as three times more common than in adults [46]. A prospective survey between 1978 and 1982 found only four aspirations among 40,240 in pediatric general anesthesia reported with no morbidity or mortality was reported. Other studies based on esophageal pH monitoring and barium contrast have stated that silent pulmonary aspiration may be more frequent in pediatric population with no neurological or anatomical abnormalities than in adults, with no respiratory consequences. Diagnosis of aspiration pneumonia in children should be made only if there are swallowing difficulties, known gastro-esophageal reflux or a witnessed aspiration [47].

7.3 Obstetric population

Mendelson was the first to describe 66 cases of aspiration between 1932 and 1945, with an incidence of 1 in 667 parturient and two deaths, both caused by acute upper airway obstruction. The mortality incidence was estimated about 1 in 22,008 [48]. In ASA closed claims, obstetric related aspiration constituted a 21% of all claims. A dramatic decreasing trend over time, in the 1970–1979; 43% of the respiratory claims compared to 20% in the 1980s and only 7% (two claims) of the aspiration claims in the 1990s. This suggests that benefit of the aspiration prevention strategies in the obstetric populations that introduced into clinical practice in the 1980s. A recent literature review found an incidence of failed tracheal intubation of 2.6 per 1000 obstetric general anesthesia (1 in 390) and associated maternal mortality of 2.3 per 100,000 general anesthesia (one death for every 90 failed intubations) [49].

The main recommendation is to adopt the neuraxial blocks as a main anesthetic technique, optimum pharmacological prophylaxis, avoiding of general anesthesia, minimizing airway manipulation and relying on RSII if general anesthesia cannot be avoided [50].

7.4 Trauma and other life saving/organ saving surgeries

Trauma and life-saving procedures have been proved to delay gastric emptying; thus, the fasting time may not be reliable. The volume of the gastric content is related to the nature of the trauma/emergency event, the interval between the last food intake and the time of acute event. Ultrasound studies have demonstrated that 56% of adult emergency cases have full stomach even though they were fasting (median 18 h). A patient for emergency surgery should always be considered as having a full stomach, thus adequate precautionary measures must be assumed to prevent aspiration. In trauma or other emergency events, prokinetics are not recommended. Erythromycin might facilitate gastric emptying in such patients but with a limited available evidence. Preoperative insertion of nasogastric tube is recommended only in cases of acute bowel obstruction but may not ensure adequate gastric emptying and could be associated with complications. Rapid sequence induction and intubation with cricoid pressure must be practiced in such cases in order to prevent aspiration [51].

7.5 Airway management for patient with NG tube in situ

Routine preoperative nasogastric tube (NG) insertion is not recommended except in selected patient with small bowel or gastric outlet obstruction. Usually those patients present to operating theater with nasogastric tube placed preoperatively. Whether to keep the gastric tube in situ, withdraw it to the esophagus, or remove it completely before induction of anesthesia is a debatable issue. The presence of the gastric tube may diminish the function of the upper and lower esophagus sphincter, with no impairment of the efficacy of cricoid pressure during rapid sequence induction based on cadaveric studies [33]. Enteral feeding usually contains carbohydrates, fat and protein, so it is considered as a full meal, thus should be stopped 8 h prior to surgery in patient that do not have endotracheal tube or tracheostomy tube in place and to continue tube feeding in case post pyloric position of the feeding tube for non-abdominal surgery [52]. As prolonged nutritional restriction may result in catabolic state in severely ill patient, however, continuation of enteral feeding might lead to aspiration, the decision to continue enteral feeding or stop it is a case-based decision with assistance of multidisciplinary team of anesthesiologist, surgeon and the primary physician. In conclusion, the current consensus is that a gastric tube, after stomach is decompressed, should not be withdrawn and left in situ during rapid sequence induction based on available literatures [27].

7.6 Airway management in post-bariatric surgery patient

Currently, the laparoscopic gastric banding and the laparoscopic Roux-en-Y gastric bypass are the most performed bariatric procedures that have proven safe, cost effective with fewer complications [53]. The major changes in gastric anatomy and physiology after weight reduction surgeries are decrease in esophageal sphincter relaxation and change in esophageal-gastric peristalsis, thus there is potential risk of esophageal regurgitation and pulmonary aspiration during general anesthesia [54]. Despite dramatic weight loss, the risk of perioperative pulmonary aspiration in post bariatric surgery patient was 6% [55]. Therefore, Post-bariatric patients must be carefully evaluated preoperatively with attention to signs and symptoms of reflux/regurgitation and delayed gastric emptying. Currently, there are no guidelines on airway and anesthetic management for post-bariatric patients. However, such patients should be encouraged to consume only liquid meals the day before the operation, prolonged pre-operative fasting period maybe helpful in the preoperative period. Intraoperatively, Rapid-sequence induction and intubation (RSII) with definitive airway as the anesthetic technique of choice and insertion of nasogastric tube must be considered. In patients with an expected difficult airway, an awake intubation should be the technique of choice [56].

7.7 Upper airway bleeding

Upper airway bleeding is a catastrophic event that might cause airway related death even in healthy young patients. Airway management in those patients is extremely challenging. Some of techniques used to secure airway such as video laryngoscope or fiberoptic laryngoscopes might be ineffective because of the soiled hypopharynx and equipment with blood, effective preoxygenation might be difficult in an anxious not tolerated patient, THRIVE and HFNO should be used with extreme caution because blood may force in lower airway, use of SAD has limited effectiveness because of the high risk of aspiration, patient swallow the blood and should be considered as a full stomach case and patient cannot lie supine feeling suffocated and difficult to deal with, are the main problems associated with airway management in these patients [57].

Upper airway bleeding might be idiopathic such as nasal bleeding, bleeding tumor and vascular malformation, trauma to face and neck, post-surgery for instance post tonsillectomy bleeding or cancer surgery or iatrogenic such as traumatic airway manipulation.

Airway management started with airway examination and localizing cricothyroid membrane as an emergency solution of cannot intubate scenario. Out of all the airway management ways, only the placement cuffed ETT using RSII might fulfill the desired goals which are; securing a conduit for patient ventilation, protect the patient from blood aspiration in the lungs, and provide good space for the surgeon to address the source of bleeding and controlling it [57].

In case of failure to intubate the patient, SAD devices, retrograde intubation or blind nasal intubation in case of spontaneous breathing patient could be a solution for airway management.

Failure of the above techniques mandate cricothyroidotomy or tracheotomy with a cuffed tube [57].

7.8 Rapid sequence induction and intubation (RSII) for COVID19 patients

There is a high chance of aerosol spread of the virus during airway management of patient with COVID 19. RSII is the preferred way to intubate those patients. Awake intubation should not be done because coughing during intubation increase virus spread. All standard airway equipment should be available plus bag mask with High Efficiency Particular Air filter (HEPA) filter, video laryngoscope with disposable blades, ventilator and tubing with inline adapter and HEPA filter and smooth clamp for ETT. It is preferred to intubate the patient in negative pressure room if available and to limit staff available during intubation to a maximum of three [58].

After strict donning process with full Personal Protective Equipment (PPE), preoxygenate the patient for 3–5 min using 10–15 l/min of 100% O2 and avoid bag mask ventilation (BMV) if possible. If saturation drops and BMV is needed so assure tight mask fitting with no leaks. Use of high dose of muscle relaxant Rocuronium or Suxamethonium to avoid coughing while intubation, use video laryngoscope if it is available, inflate ETT cuff as soon as possible, clamp the ETT before connecting to ventilator, HEPA filter should be placed between the ETT and the ventilator [59] (for more details, kindly refer to Chapter 1).

8. Perioperative negative pressure pulmonary edema versus pulmonary aspiration

Negative Pressure Pulmonary Edema (NPPE) also known as Post-Obstructive Pulmonary Edema (POPE), is a form of non-cardiogenic pulmonary edema that can occur perioperatively due to laryngospasm during anesthesia or following extubation in adults. NPPE is a potentially life-threatening complication following general anesthesia and is manifested by upper airway obstruction, followed by strong inspiratory effort (negative pressure). This occurs in 0.05–0.1% of cases as a life-threatening complication of general anesthesia with tracheal intubation [60]. NPPE was first hypothesized in 1927 by Morre and was described later by Oswalt in 1977. It is essential to notice the potential causes, make differential diagnosis and determine the effective treatment. NPPE usually presents with respiratory distress, hypoxia, cyanosis, frothy pink sputum, and hemoptysis. It is important to distinguish negative pressure pulmonary edema from pulmonary aspiration at the end of general anesthesia, however the diagnosis requires a strong suspicion as the presentation mimics aspiration pneumonia. In general, NPPE often demonstrates marked bilateral perihilar alveolar infiltrates on chest X-ray. Treatment modality includes supportive care such as careful post-op monitoring, reliving airway obstruction, oxygen supplementation, Bilevel Positive Airway Pressure (BIPAP) and assisted ventilation [61, 62].

9. Conclusion

Patients proceeding for surgery should receive the safest anesthesia experience possible. An anesthesiologist should be prepared to manage a patient with a suspected full stomach which includes meticulous attention to airway management during induction, through emergence, and after extubation.

Pre-operative care should include adequate time for gastric emptying for non-emergent cases; administering non-particulate antacids per orally to increase gastric pH and to identify patients who may have delayed gastric emptying. Rapid sequence induction and intubation with or without cricoid pressure are recommended as per institutional guidelines. They should have a wide bore rigid suction device ready during intubation and emergence. A nasogastric tube may be placed to empty the stomach pre-induction if the patient has a suspected ileus or gastrointestinal obstruction. After surgery is completed patients should be emerged until they are fully awake with return of airway protective reflexes and then extubated. It is also recommended to empty the stomach with a nasogastric or orogastric tube prior to extubation. Postoperatively patients must be transferred to recovery and recovered in a head up position or in a lateral position.

Presence of expertise in advanced airway management is essential for awake tracheal intubation and dealing with difficult or failed airway in a patient with a full stomach. Preoperative counseling for patients with high risk for difficult airway management and pulmonary aspiration of gastric contents regarding alternative anesthesia options other than general anesthesia should be sought out.

Author details

Saba Al Bassam*, Ahmed Zaghw, Muhammad Jaffar Khan, Neethu Arun and Arunabha Karmakar
Department of Anesthesia, Perioperative Medicine and Critical Care Medicine, Hamad Medical Corporation, Doha, Qatar

*Address all correspondence to: smahdi@hamad.qa

References

[1] Cook TM, Woodall N, Frerk C. Major complications of airway management in the UK: Results of the fourth National Audit Project of the Royal College of Anaesthetists and the difficult airway society. Part 1: Anaesthesia. British Journal of Anaesthesia. 2011;**106**:617-631

[2] Gardner AM, Pryer DL. Historical and experimental study of aspiration of gastric and oesophageal contents into the lungs in anaesthesia. British Journal of Anaesthesia. 1966;**38**:370-379

[3] Adriani J, Berson W. Aspiration during anesthesia and surgery. The American Surgeon. 1954;**20**:568-574

[4] Weiss WA. Regurgitation and aspiration of gastric contents during inhalation anesthesia. Anesthesiology. 1950;**11**:102-109

[5] Ng A, Smith G. Gastroesophageal reflux and aspiration of gastric contents in anesthetic practice. Anesthesia and Analgesia. 2001;**93**:494-513

[6] Olsson GL, Hallen B, Hambraeus-Jonzon K. Aspiration during anaesthesia: A computer-aided study of 185 358 anaesthetics. Acta Anaesthesiologica Scandinavica. 1986;**30**:84-92

[7] Sakai T, Planinsic RM, Quinlan JJ, Handley LJ, Kim T-Y, Hilmi IA. The incidence and outcome of perioperative pulmonary aspiration in a university hospital: A 4-year retrospective analysis. Anesthesia and Analgesia. 2006;**103**:941-947

[8] Dal SG. Acid aspiration: Pathophysiological aspects, prevention, and therapy. International Anesthesiology Clinics. 1986;**24**:31-52

[9] Marik PE. Aspiration pneumonitis and aspiration pneumonia. The New England Journal of Medicine. 2001;**344**:665-671

[10] Bynum LJ, Pierce AK. Pulmonary aspiration of gastric contents. The American Review of Respiratory Disease. 1976;**114**:1129-1136

[11] Bartlett JG. Anaerobic bacterial infections of the lung and pleural space. Clinical Infectious Diseases. 1993;**16**(Suppl 4):S248-S255

[12] Metzner J, Posner KL, Lam MS, Domino KB. Closed claims' analysis. Best Practice & Research. Clinical Anaesthesiology. 2011;**25**:263-276

[13] Robinson M, Davidson A. Aspiration under anaesthesia: Risk assessment and decision-making. Continuing Education in Anesthesia, Critical Care and Pain. 2014;**14**:171-175

[14] Asai T II. Who is at increased risk pulmonary aspiration? British Journal of Anaesthesia. 2004;**93**:497-500

[15] Bouvet L, Desgranges F-P, Aubergy C, Boselli E, Dupont G, Allaouchiche B, et al. Prevalence and factors predictive of full stomach in elective and emergency surgical patients: A prospective cohort study. British Journal of Anaesthesia. 2017;**118**:372-379

[16] Szarka LA, Camilleri M. Stomach dysfunction in diabetes mellitus: Emerging technology and pharmacology. Journal of Diabetes Science and Technology. 2010;**4**:180-189

[17] Gangavatiker R, Pal S, Javed A, Dash NR, Sahni P, Chattopadhyay TK. Effect of Antecolic or Retrocolic reconstruction of the gastro/duodenojejunostomy on delayed gastric emptying after Pancreaticoduodenectomy: A randomized controlled trial. Journal of Gastrointestinal Surgery. 2011;**15**:843-852

[18] Yoshizaki T, Obata D, Aoki Y, Okamoto N, Hashimura H, Kano C, et al. Endoscopic submucosal dissection for early gastric cancer on the lesser curvature in upper third of the stomach is a risk factor for postoperative delayed gastric emptying. Surgical Endoscopy. 2018;**32**:3622-3629

[19] Bouvet L, Mazoit JX, Chassard D, Allaouchiche B, Boselli E, Benhamou D. Clinical assessment of the ultrasonographic measurement of antral area for estimating preoperative gastric content and volume. Anesthesiology. 2011;**114**:1086-1092

[20] Raidoo DM, Rocke DA, Brock-Utne JG, Marszalek A, Engelbrecht HE. Critical volume for pulmonary acid aspiration: reappraisal in a primate model. British Journal of Anaesthesia. 1990;**65**:248-250

[21] Practice guidelines for preoperative fasting and the use of pharmacologic agents to reduce the risk of pulmonary aspiration: Application to healthy patients undergoing elective procedures. Anesthesiology. 2017;**126**:376-393

[22] Nishina K, Mikawa K, Takao Y, Shiga M, Maekawa N, Obara H. A comparison of rabeprazole, lansoprazole, and ranitidine for improving preoperative gastric fluid property in adults undergoing elective surgery. Anesthesia and Analgesia. 2000;**90**:717-721

[23] Czarnetzki C, Elia N, Frossard J-L, Giostra E, Spahr L, Waeber J-L, et al. Erythromycin for gastric emptying in patients undergoing general anesthesia for emergency surgery: A randomized clinical trial. JAMA Surgery. 2015;**150**:730-737

[24] Van De Putte P, Perlas A. Ultrasound assessment of gastric content and volume. British Journal of Anaesthesia. 2014;**113**:12-22

[25] Zhang G, Huang X, Shui Y, Luo C, Zhang L. Ultrasound to guide the individual medical decision by evaluating the gastric contents and risk of aspiration: A literature review. Asian Journal of Surgery. 2020. DOI: 10.1016/j.asjsur.2020.02.008

[26] Perlas A, Davis L, Khan M, Mitsakakis N, Chan VWS. Gastric sonography in the fasted surgical patient: A prospective descriptive study. Anesthesia and Analgesia. 2011;**113**:93-97

[27] Salem MR, Khorasani A, Saatee S, Crystal GJ, El-Orbany M. Gastric tubes and airway management in patients at risk of aspiration: History, current concepts, and proposal of an algorithm. Anesthesia and Analgesia. 2014;**118**:569-579

[28] Weingart SD, Levitan RM. Preoxygenation and prevention of desaturation during emergency airway management. Annals of Emergency Medicine. 2012;**59**:165-175.e1

[29] Ramachandran SK, Cosnowski A, Shanks A, Turner CR. Apneic oxygenation during prolonged laryngoscopy in obese patients: A randomized, controlled trial of nasal oxygen administration. Journal of Clinical Anesthesia. 2010;**22**:164-168

[30] Chua MT, Khan FA, Ng WM, Lu Q, Low MJW, Yau YW, et al. Pre- and Apnoeic high flow oxygenation for RApid sequence intubation in the emergency department (pre-AeRATE): Study protocol for a multicentre, randomised controlled trial. Trials. 2019;**20**(1):195. DOI: 10.1186/s13063-019-3305-8

[31] Lodenius Å, Piehl J, Östlund A, Ullman J, Jonsson Fagerlund M. Transnasal humidified rapid-insufflation ventilatory exchange

(THRIVE) vs. facemask breathing pre-oxygenation for rapid sequence induction in adults: A prospective randomised non-blinded clinical trial. Anaesthesia. 2018;**73**:564-571

[32] Mort TC. Complications of emergency tracheal intubation: Hemodynamic alterations--part I. Journal of Intensive Care Medicine. 2007;**22**:157-165

[33] Salem MR, Joseph NJ, Heyman HJ, Belani B, Paulissian R, Ferrara TP. Cricoid compression is effective in obliterating the esophageal lumen in the presence of a nasogastric tube. Anesthesiology. 1985;**63**:443-446

[34] Hagberg CA, Gabel JC, Connis RT. Difficult airway society 2015 guidelines for the management of unanticipated difficult intubation in adults: Not just another algorithm. British Journal of Anaesthesia. 2015;**115**:812-814

[35] Ehrenfeld JM, Cassedy EA, Forbes VE, Mercaldo ND, Sandberg WS. Modified rapid sequence induction and intubation: A survey of United States current practice. Anesthesia and Analgesia. 2012;**115**:95-101

[36] Salem MR, Wong AY, Mani M, Sellick BA. Efficacy of cricoid pressure in preventing gastric inflation during bag mask ventilation in pediatric patients. Anesthesiology. 1974;**40**:96-98

[37] Weingart SD, Trueger NS, Wong N, Scofi J, Singh N, Rudolph SS. Delayed sequence intubation: A prospective observational study. Annals of Emergency Medicine. 2015;**65**:349-355

[38] Jarvis JL, Gonzales J, Johns D, Sager L. Implementation of a clinical bundle to reduce out-of-hospital Peri-intubation hypoxia. Annals of Emergency Medicine. 2018;**72**:272-279.e1

[39] Podcast 196 - Having a Vomit SALAD with Dr. Jim DuCanto - Airway Management Techniques during Massive Regurgitation, Emesis, or Bleeding. Available from: https://emcrit.org/emcrit/having-a-vomit-salad-with-ducanto/ [Accessed: 15 July 2020]

[40] Jungbauer A, Schumann M, Brunkhorst V, Börgers A, Groeben H. Expected difficult tracheal intubation: A prospective comparison of direct laryngoscopy and video laryngoscopy in 200 patients. British Journal of Anaesthesia. 2009;**102**:546-550

[41] Mandell LA, Niederman MS. Aspiration pneumonia. The New England Journal of Medicine. 2019;**380**:651-663

[42] Ott SR, Allewelt M, Lorenz J, Reimnitz P, Lode H, German Lung Abscess Study Group. Moxifloxacin vs ampicillin/sulbactam in aspiration pneumonia and primary lung abscess. Infection. 2008;**36**:23-30

[43] WALTS LF. Anesthesia of the larynx IN the patient with a full stomach. JAMA. 1965;**192**:705-706

[44] Patel M, Swadia V, Bansal G. Prospective randomized comparative study of use of PLMA and ET tube for airway management in children under general anaesthesia. Indian Journal of Anaesthesia. 2010;**54**:109

[45] Wheeler M. ProSeal™ laryngeal mask airway in 120 pediatric surgical patients: A prospective evaluation of characteristics and performance. Paediatric Anaesthesia. 2006;**16**:297-301

[46] Phillips S, Daborn AK, Hatch DJ. Preoperative fasting for paediatric

anaesthesia. British Journal of Anaesthesia. 1994;**73**:529-536

[47] Milross JG, Negus BH, Street NE, Gaskin KJ. Gastro-oesophageal reflux and adverse respiratory events in children under anaesthesia. Anaesthesia and Intensive Care. 1995;**23**:587-590

[48] Mendelson CL. The aspiration of stomach contents into the lungs during obstetric anesthesia. American Journal of Obstetrics and Gynecology. 1946;**52**:191-205

[49] Kinsella SM, Winton AL, Mushambi MC, Ramaswamy K, Swales H, Quinn AC, et al. Failed tracheal intubation during obstetric general anaesthesia: A literature review. International Journal of Obstetric Anesthesia. 2015;**24**:356-374

[50] Lundgren C, Howell V. Education for anaesthesia providers worldwide Obstetric Anaesthesia. 2019. Available from: www.wfsahq.org/resources/update-in-anaesthesia [Accessed: 15 July 2020]

[51] Brown CA, Bair AE, Pallin DJ, Walls RM, Near III Investigators. Techniques, success, and adverse events of emergency department adult intubations. Annals of Emergency Medicine. 2015;**65**:363-370.e1

[52] Nespoli L, Coppola S, Gianotti L. The role of the enteral route and the composition of feeds in the nutritional support of malnourished surgical patients. Nutrients. 2012;**4**:1230-1236

[53] Picot J, Jones J, Colquitt JL, Gospodarevskaya E, Loveman E, Baxter L, et al. The clinical effectiveness and cost-effectiveness of bariatric (weight loss) surgery for obesity: A systematic review and economic evaluation. Health Technology Assessment. 2009;**13**(41). DOI: 10.3310/hta13410

[54] Chen RY, Burton PR, Ooi GJ, Laurie C, Smith AI, Crosthwaite G, et al. The physiology and pathophysiology of gastroesophageal reflux in patients with laparoscopic adjustable gastric band. Obesity Surgery. 2017;**27**:2434-2443

[55] Ardila-Hani A, Soffer EE. Review article: The impact of bariatric surgery on gastrointestinal motility. Alimentary Pharmacology & Therapeutics. 2011;**34**:825-831

[56] Cuomo R, Giardino FR, Nisi G, Brandi C, Zerini I, Voglino C, et al. Aspiration pneumonia: A shadow in post-bariatric patient: Correlation between aspiration and minigrastric bypass. Obesity Surgery. 2019;**29**:3937-3940

[57] Michael Seltz Kristensen MD, Barry McGuire MD. Managing and securing the bleeding upper airway: A narrative review, /published online: 23 September 2019, Canadian anesthesiologists' society 2019. Canadian Journal of Anesthesia. 2020;**67**:128-140

[58] Wax RS, Christian MD. Practical recommendations for critical care and anesthesiology teams caring for novel coronavirus (2019-nCoV) patients. Canadian Journal of Anesthesia. 2020;**67**:568-576

[59] Cook TM, El-Boghdadly K, McGuire B, McNarry AF, Patel A, Higgs A. Consensus guidelines for managing the airway in patients with COVID-19: Guidelines from the difficult airway society, the Association of Anaesthetists the Intensive Care Society, the Faculty of Intensive Care Medicine and the Royal College of Anaesthetists. Anaesthesia. 2020;**75**:785-879

[60] Pathak V, Rendon ISH, Ciubotaru RL. Recurrent negative pressure pulmonary edema. Clinical Medicine & Research. 2011;**9**:88-91

[61] Lemyze M, Mallat J. Understanding negative pressure pulmonary edema. Intensive Care Medicine. 2014;**40**:1140-1143

[62] Liu R, Wang J, Zhao G, Su Z. Negative pressure pulmonary edema after general anesthesia: A case report and literature review. Medicine (Baltimore). 2019;**98**:e15389

Chapter 8

Airway Management in Head and Neck Pathology

Muayad M. Radi Al-Khafaji, Hossam Makki, Hassan Haider, Furat Abbas and Abhishek Menon

Abstract

Studies have demonstrated that poor assessment and planning contribute to airway complications and that current airway assessment strategies have a poor diagnostic accuracy in predicting difficult intubation in the general population. There is a higher risk for difficulties during airway management in patients with pathologies arising from the head and neck region and are more likely to need emergency surgical access. Therefore, thorough assessment and adequate knowledge about the various head and neck pathologies is mandatory. In this chapter, we will briefly go through the preoperative assessment and history & clinical assessment, the investigations. Also we will discuss the airway management at various pathologies involving the head and neck region whether benign/malignant pathologies, OSA (obstructive sleep apnea) and post head & neck operative airway management.

Keywords: head and neck, voice and swallowing, difficult airway, preoperative airway assessment

1. Introduction

Working with our anesthesia colleagues at one place which is the upper airway passages is one of the most important (and often neglected) aspects of successful laryngeal operation. Lack of cooperation and pre-surgical planning with the anesthesiology team can make simple micro-laryngoscopy case into an airway crisis [1]. Airway management for head and neck tumors surgery demands special consideration and high focus. A planned approach and thorough communication across multidisciplinary teams will help in reducing any unwanted outcomes.

2. Preoperative assessment

A thorough pre-operative assessment is the mainstay of any successful anesthetic management of onco-surgery of the head and neck. Appropriate control of any co-morbidity is of paramount importance. A considerable number of these patients may have a difficult airway, which may require utilization of advanced airway management techniques. A planned approach and thorough communication across multidisciplinary teams will help in reducing any unwanted outcomes. A step by step approach is essential during the Preoperative assessment of such patients.

2.1 History and clinical examination

An ideal pre-operative assessment starts with a complete history & physical examination, requisite investigations, analysis of the extent of lesion, considerations for concurrent radio-and/or chemotherapy and a multidisciplinary team discussion on the plan for airway and pain management.

Symptoms suggestive of airway obstruction should be checked during history taking:

- Hoarseness: it can be an early manifestation of glottic carcinoma but is often delayed with supraglottic or subglottic tumors.

- Stridor: inspiratory stridor could be suggestive of a subglottic lesion, expiratory stridor a supraglottic lesion, and biphasic stridor a glottic lesion.

- Dysphagia, or odynophagia: may indicate pharyngeal problem.

- Dyspnea: flow volume loops are very helpful in differentiating between dyspnea caused by upper airway obstruction or due to pulmonary disease.

Some important questions that must kept in mind for every patient coming to the operating room:

1. Mouth opening: mouth opening of around 5–6 cm is considered with in normal limits at least 3 cm mouth opening is required for successful laryngoscopy.

2. Mallampati test: has been correlated with ease of laryngoscopy. This assessment alone can provide valuable and important information about the size of tongue in relation to oral cavity size and is a useful predictor of intubation difficulty (**Figure 1**).

3. Size of the mandibular space: it is the space from the inner side of the submentum to the hyoid bone. A distance greater than 6 cm means that there will

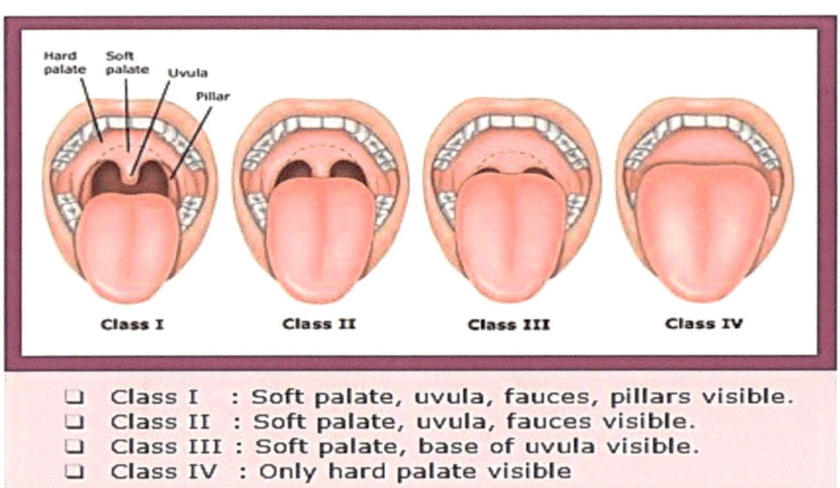

Figure 1.
Mallampati classification.

be enough room for the tongue to move into the mandibular space and direct laryngoscopy will be easy. If this space is small, the larynx is usually located anteriorly, and intubation will be more difficult. In general, 2 fingerbreadths or more indicate easy intubation.

4. Ability to assume sniffing position is a predictive indicator for a relatively straight axis to the glottis. The sniffing position is considered as a moderate flexion of the patient neck on his chest and extension of his neck about the atlantoaxial junction.

A meticulous physical examination of the patient must be done to check for vital parameters, pallor, icterus, and features suggestive of fluid overload, raised jugular venous pressure, generalized lymphadenopathy, metastasis, body mass index and any tenderness in the spine. Appropriate work-up must be done to rule out distant metastasis in the most common sited such as lungs, lymph nodes, spine, brain and liver.

Routine preanesthetic assessment clinic (PAC) tests such as a complete blood workup, ECG, echocardiography, chest radiography, liver & renal function tests and serum electrolytes must be done for all patients. Patient should also be advised for smoking cessation as a high number of patients with head and neck cancer (HNC) have smoking history.

Patients should also be evaluated for any pre/concurrent radio - chemotherapy. Preoperative radiotherapy, this can give rise to difficult laryngoscopy, difficult intubation (**Figure 2**).

2.2 Pre-operative imaging and endoscopy

Computerized tomography (CT) is a very good diagnostic tool with excellent Risk–Benefit Ratio. It is readily accessible, with faster image acquisition. One of the advantages of CT is that it can also be extended to include other sites of the body for staging purposes especially in cancer cases. Thin Slices, high resolution image acquisition allows high quality multiplanar reconstruction (**Figure 3**). Drawbacks of CT include exposure to ionizing radiation, inferior soft tissue contrast when compared to MRI, renal failure secondary to injection of iodinated contrast medium (**Table 1**).

Classification	Description
ASA 1	Healthy patients
ASA 2	Mild to moderate systemic disease caused by the surgical condition or by other pathological processes, and medically well controlled
ASA 3	Severe disease process which limits activity but is not incapacitating
ASA 4	Severe incapacitating disease process that is a constant threat to life
ASA 5	Moribund patient not expected to survive 24 hours with or without an operation
ASA 6	Declared brain-dead patient whose organs are being removed for donor purposes

Figure 2.
AS a grading used for predicting anesthesia risk.

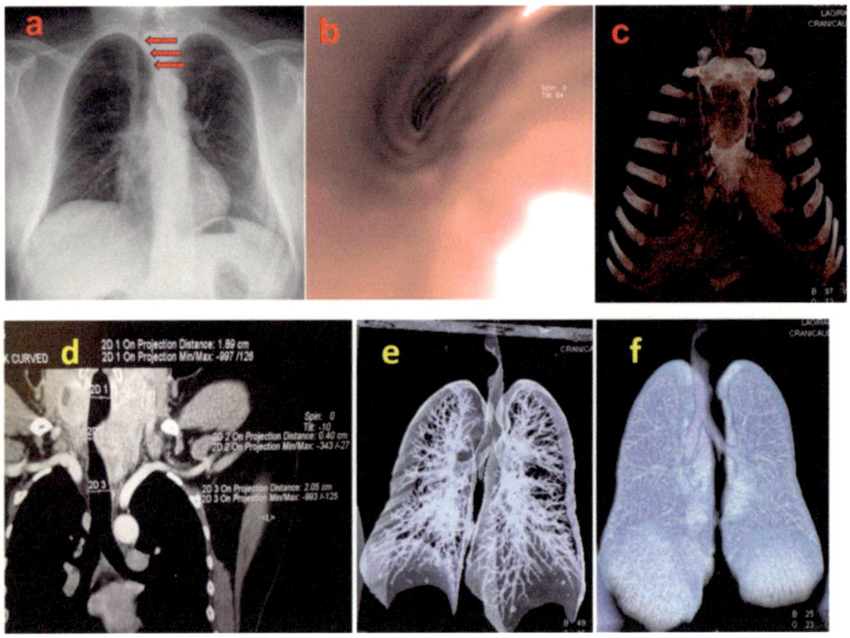

Figure 3.
(a) Chet X-ray showing tracheal deviation at T4-T5 level. (b) 3D reconstruction of MDCT with virtual endoscopy showing tracheal stenosis. (c) Sternum eroded by thyroid cancer metastasis. (d, e, f) coronal cut contrast enhances MDCT showing narrowing at level T4-T5 along with enlarged thyroid.

2.3 CT virtual endoscopy

Virtual endoscopy is an excellent tool used to obtain an anatomically similar representation of the intraluminal geography of the airway, including supraglottic, glottic and subglottic structures without the risk of exposure to ionizing radiation. Compared to conventional 3D reconstructions, the images obtained through virtual endoscopy give a perspective which, when rendered, creates the impression of a true endoscopic image allowing for a tailored approach towards the airway management (**Figure 3b**).

One of the limitations of virtual endoscopy, especially in airway pathologies, is that dynamic airway studies cannot be assessed. Hence, conventional airway endoscopy remains the "gold standard" in most airway assessment and pathologies. Virtual endoscopy can be used to supplement conventional airway endoscopy to help in planning the management of such cases [2].

2.4 MRI

MRI gives excellent contrast resolution compared to CT and is a useful in identifying specific characteristics pertaining to soft tissue masses and complex soft tissue lesions [2]. Even though the unwanted risks of ionizing radiation are absent with the use of MRI as compared to CT, images can be prone to motion artifact due to increased acquisition times that often require the patient to stay still for at least several minutes at a time.

Dynamic MRI is a useful tool in diagnosing certain uncommon airway pathologies such as in diagnosis of tracheo-broncho-malacia in pediatric population, in sleep studies for visualization of upper airway dynamics etc.

Mass effect leading to airway compromise from benign and malignant lesions such as hemangioma and lymphomas are more conspicuous on MRI, with high T2 signal intensity, compared to CT [3].

USG	X-ray	CT	CT reconstruction and virtual endoscopy	MRI	3D-printing
• It is currently one of the most explored and utilized radiological modality. • It is relatively cheap and easily. Accessible. • Can be performed in a non teritiary setting. • It has certain limitation such has in deeper lesions.	• Useful in emergencies for quick diagnosis. • Lateral views are most commonly used. Flexion, extension and frontal views can also be used. • Used for Prediction of difficult airway, size and depth of left double lumen endotrachial tube (DLT). • Used for confirmation of ET tube position. • For diagnosing tracheal lesions.	• Has been used extensively in evaluation and planning of pediatric airway. More precise and superior compared to X-ray. • Tracheal lesions are characterized better compared to X-ray. • Conditions such as tracheomalacia, fistula, etc. not seen in X-ray can be picked up on CT. • Study of static and dynamic airway anatomy possible with CT. • Can also be used for Evaluation of airway narrowing and deviation, for predicting left DLT size and difficult airway	• Images are reconstructed using data from helical CT. • Virtual endoscopy can be compared to real airway endoscopic evaluation as it saves administration of local or general anesthesia and improves patient compliance. • One of the drawbacks of virtual endoscopy is that it is not useful in dynamic airway studies. • Then can also be easily extended to involve the bronchus.	• Limited use due to increased cost and time consuming. • Defines soft tissue lesions better when compared to CT. • It is non ionizing when compared to CT hence can be considered for certain pediatric conditions. • Dynamic MRI is a Useful tool in diagnosing certain uncommon airway pathologies such as in diagnosis of tracheobronchomalacia in pediatric population, in sleep studies for visualization of upper airway dynamics etc.	• It is upcoming revolutionary technology in which 3D models are printed using 3D printers with the data acquired from CT scans. • Can be used in simulation of airway for precision Preoperative planning. • Has potential for vast applications in anesthesia training, planning and management. • The technology is presently in its nascent stage and hence not a viable option for a majority of cases.

Table 1.
Comparing the different radiological modalities.

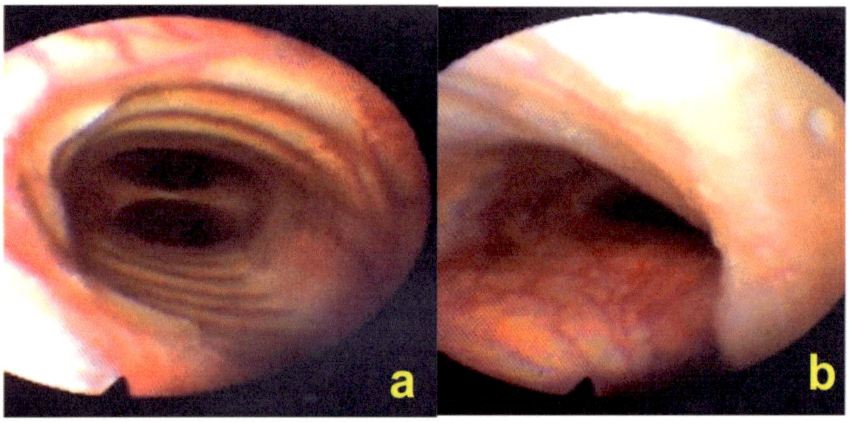

Figure 4.
Example of fiber optic tracheoscopy on a tracheal stenosis patient under local anesthesia showing the carina (a) and stenosed part of the trachea (b).

2.5 Airway endoscopy and trans-nasal tracheoscopy (TNT)

It is a form of indirectly visualizing the airway and larynx in which the clinician does not directly view the lower part of the airway or larynx [4]. Instead, it is visualized with fiber optic or digital laryngoscopes inserted trans-nasally.

The images from the scope can be displayed on a monitor for the clinician, patient and others to view at the time of the procedure; it can also be recorded. Experienced clinicians can also perform it on a wake tracheoscopy using local anesthesia on cooperative patients. They are an essential tool for identifying and planning strategies for management of difficult airway cases [5] (**Figure 4**).

3. Airway management for benign laryngeal surgery

3.1 Introduction

Working with our anesthesia colleagues at one place which is the upper airway passages is one of the most important (and often neglected) aspects of successful laryngeal operation. Lack of cooperation and pre-surgical planning with the anesthesiology team can make simple micro-laryngoscopy case into an airway crisis [1]. Benign laryngeal tumors are more common than the malignant one. Phono-surgery is used to excise most of those tumors whether is a vocal cord cyst, polyp, nodule, etc.

3.2 General important points should always be noticed

1. **Different plans + proper equipment's**: A good management plan for taking care of the patient's airway should be negotiated with the anesthetist before going to the surgery. An excellent plan (plan A), also another strategy (plans B and C) must be ready so that the airway management is algorithmic and automatic, as opposite to unplanned reaction. Before taking the patient into the operating theater, both the operating surgeon and the anesthesia team must have the right equipment in the room, opened, and "ready to use" if another plans become necessary.

2. **Positioning**: for optimal laryngoscopy exposure the patient put in the "sniffing positioning," head extended on the neck, and the neck flexed on the chest [6].

3. **In case of using surgical LASER:** a LASER-protected tube must be used. In case we use jet ventilation or apneic technique (both are safe for the LASER with some special FiO_2 settings).

4. **In case of the patient has a tracheostomy tube:** 5.5–6.0 mm Endo Tracheal Tube (ETT) inserted at the tracheal stoma into the trachea, **LASER** protected ETT should be used in case we use LASER. Using (apneic technique) if airway surgery is performed distal to the tracheal stoma site, applying frequent (reinsertion technique) of stomal ETT to give Oxygen in between the treatment.

5. Mask induction with anesthetic agents is the suitable method of airway management for endoscopic treatment of **subglottic/tracheal stenosis**, or using total intravenous anesthesia (TIVA) then using jet ventilation. Avoid using ETT intubation in those cases.

6. In case of scar formation because of **tracheostomy** was done in a patient with subglottic/tracheal stenosis, then the airway interning should be done at least 1 cm down to the level of the stenosis.

3.3 Anesthesia technique used in case of micro-laryngoscopy (MLS)

In general, lesions present at the anterior 2/3 (membranous vocal folds) of the larynx can be easily exposed and treated with size 5.5 mm or smaller micro laryngeal ETT. Lesions at the posterior 1/3 (vocal processes and posterior commissure/arytenoids region) of the larynx we can use one of those techniques (**Figure 5**):

A. **Oral intubation** using a small long ETT size: 5.0 mm or 5.5 mm micro-laryngoscopy tube (MLT) with a length (30 cm length) with adult tube's balloon that makes good airway sealing. Or using Tritube (**Figure 3**), an ultra-thin endotracheal tube (outer diameter 4.4 mm/inner diameter 2.4 mm).

B. **Jet Venturi ventilation:**

   1. Supra-glottic jet Venturi needle (**Figure 6**) Applied through port within laryngoscope or attached to laryngoscope.

   2. Tracheal Jet ventilation (where the tip of the jet is near the tip of the laryngoscope) or infra glottic jet ventilation.

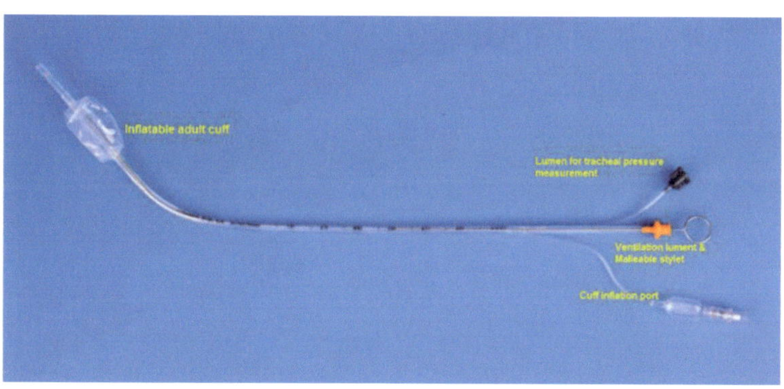

Figure 5.
Tritube: (Tritube, Ventinova medical, Eindhoven, the Netherlands).

Tracheal jet ventilation is better than supra-glottic jet ventilation [7], because tracheal jet ventilation helps the operating surgeon with less movement of the vocal cords. This is very important while performing phono-microsurgery. Also, it allows for better end-tidal CO_2 monitoring. On the other hand, Jet ventilation (supra-glottic, as opposed to subglottic) is safest when used proximally. However, movement of the vocal cords due to jet air will effect on the perfection of the surgical technique.

3. Tracheal Jet ventilation using plastic catheter inside the trachea: for example: Hunsaker Mon-Jet infra-glottic ventilation catheter (**Figure 7**) or tri-lumen catheter with Twin-stream jet ventilator.

C. **Apneic technique using high flow nasal cannula (HFNC)**

In our center we use this technique in 95% of the benign laryngeal lesion's surgery (**Figure 8**). High flow nasal cannula (HFNC) has been shown beneficial in pre-oxygenation, oxygenation after extubation & in the treatment of respiratory failure and heart failure. Recently HFNC proved to provide a very good oxygenation & ventilation for the patients who performing various upper airway surgeries without the need for the jet ventilation or endotracheal intubation. Delivery of O_2 via (HFNC) is an exciting & emerging therapy in acute adult medical practice. Humidified and worm O_2 is delivered at flow rate of up to 60–80 L/min.

D. **STRIV-Hi technique**

SponTaneous **R**espiration using **I**ntra **V**enous anesthesia & High flow nasal oxygenation. By using this way of anesthesia, we apply the concept of spontaneous ventilation according stepwise Target – Controlled Infusion (TCI Marsh technique) of Propofol applying the formula CP – Ce = 1.
Cp = the expected Propofol concentration at the plasma.
Ce = the predicted Propofol effect site concentration.

Benefits For all: (Patient, Surgeon, Anesthetist).

The use of STRIV-Hi technique decreases stress of endotracheal tube on cardio vascular system (CVS), respiratory system. Eventually it decreases post intubation complications. Because of the surgeon & the anesthetist are working at the same site there will be a high risk of affection on the ventilation, oxygenation and loss of airway.

It provides (wider field) for the surgeon & at the same time it can facilitate oxygenation during the induction of anesthesia in cases of severe laryngotracheal

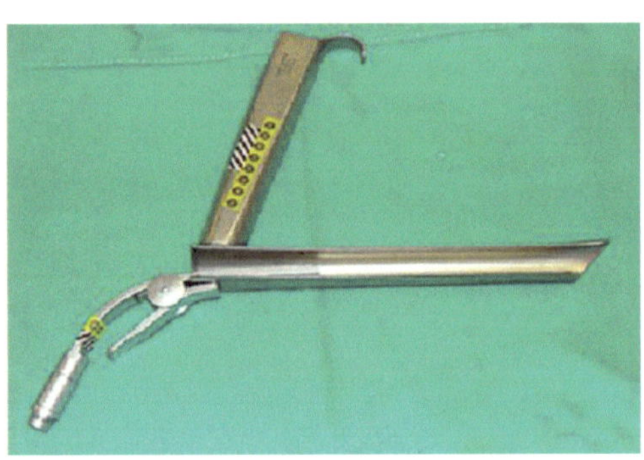

Figure 6.
Jet ventilation probe.

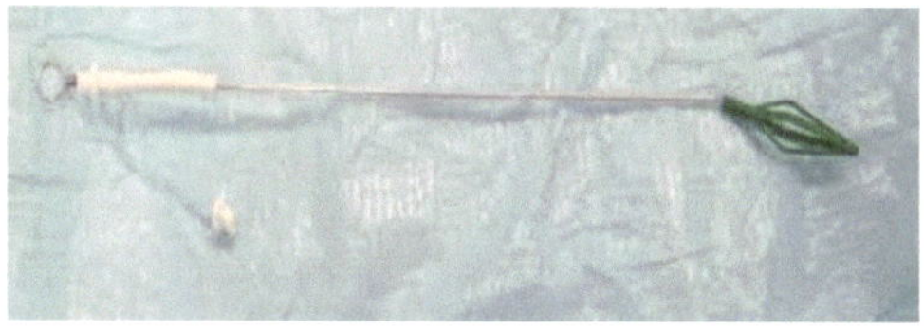

Figure 7.
Hunsaker Mon-Jet catheter.

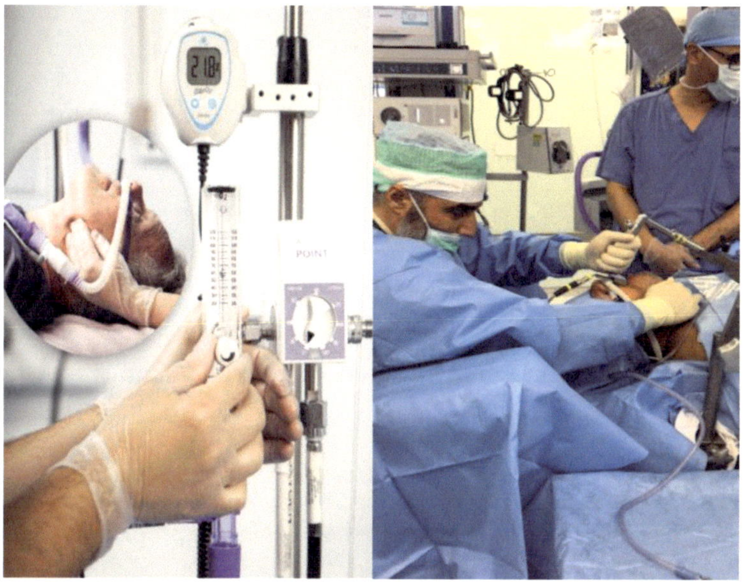

Figure 8.
HFNC in use.

stenosis which cannot be intubated conventionally. Also, it facilitates dynamic airway assessment & prevents risk of barotrauma (compared to jet ventilation).

3.4 Limitations of HFNC in MLS surgery

Duration of surgery: Operation less than 30 minutes so it is not suitable for junior staff both anesthetist and operating surgeon. It leads to CO_2 accumulation. It cannot be used in case of complete nasal obstruction, bleeding inside the airway & in case of Infection: opened abscess or COVID 19 patients. Also, not used in morbid obesity and predicted difficult airway.

3.5 In case of difficult exposure of the larynx

1. Difficult laryngeal exposure because of underlying anatomy which affect on the performance of micro-laryngoscope using rigid laryngoscopy/bronchoscopy. We may expect a "difficult exposure" per-orally in the following conditions:

A. Limited neck extension

B. Big tongue/difficult palatal visualization

C. Retrognathia

D. Short, thick neck

E. Trismus/reduced inter-incisor opening

3.6 Alternative techniques to get an airway in case of "difficult exposure"

A. Awake, flexible laryngoscopy with naso-tracheal intubation.

B. Tracheostomy done with local anesthesia.

C. Intubation by using specialized "anterior" laryngoscope.

D. Use of a curved ETT with stylet and Sliding Jackson laryngoscope.

E. Ossoff–Pilling laryngoscope.

F. Laryngeal Mask Airway (LMA).

G. Use of laryngoscopy and intubation without seeing of vocal cords.

4. Airway management techniques in head and neck cancer surgeries

4.1 Synopsis

Airway management for surgery of head and neck cancer (HNC) patients is a challenge for the otolaryngologist and anesthesiologist. Appropriate assessment and planning are mandatory for successful airway management. In this chapter, we will review the most common head and neck cancer imposing difficult airway and discuss the strategies of airway management in these patients undergoing head and neck cancer surgery.

4.2 Introduction

Head and neck tumors and malignancies are prominent and relatively frequent. Squamous cell carcinoma represents 90% of head and neck malignancies. (11).

Airway management for head and neck tumors surgery demands special consideration and high focus.

The difficulties and challenges in the airway management of surgical patients with head and neck malignancies are primarily secondary to distortion of normal anatomy (like mass effect) and alteration of the normal physiology (like trismus) of upper airways. In addition, any previous surgery or radiotherapy (neck stiffness and inadequate neck extension) add more difficulty to airway management in these patients. Also, head and neck malignancies resection surgeries are long and extensive procedures which usually lead to significant postoperative swelling and thus the risk of secondary iatrogenic upper airway compromise.

Detailed knowledge of tumor type and localization, size, and vascularity is essential for definitive planning of proper airway management and to avoid any complications during intubation or ventilation [8].

4.3 Recognition of the difficult airway

It is essential to identify any possible airway difficulty management preoperatively. During history taking, any obstructive symptoms should be noted.

Symptoms suggestive of airway obstruction:

- **Hoarseness:** an early symptom of glottic carcinoma; late with supra-glottic carcinomas.
- **Stridor**: biphasic one is suggestive of glottic narrowing, inspiratory one of a subglottic narrowing, and expiratory of a supra-glottic narrowing.
- **Dysphagia**: suggestive of a pharyngeal problem

There are other essential points to be checked as well:

Mouth opening: of at least 3 cm is necessary for successful laryngoscopy.

Mallampati classification can provide valuable and essential information about the size of the tongue in relation to the oral cavity and is a useful predictor of ease of intubation.

Size of the mandibular space: 2 fingerbreadths or more suggest easy intubation.

Can the patient assume the sniffing position? Ability to assume this position is predictive of a relatively straight axis to the glottis.

Endoscopic examination: to localize any narrowing and assess its significance.

CT scanning with 3D reconstruction and virtual bronchoscopy: is especially valuable in evaluating the size and extent of lesions. Three-dimensional reconstruction with virtual endoscopy improves the ability to more fully assess head and neck tumors and its extension and encroachment on the airway [9].

4.4 Common airway pathology that indicates difficult airway

Hypopharyngeal tumors:

The hypopharynx extends from the level of hyoid bone superiorly to the level of cricoid cartilage inferiorly and consists of three parts: pyriform sinus, post-cricoid area, and posterior pharyngeal wall. Tumors arising in the hypopharynx are most often localizing in the piriform sinus. Hypopharyngeal cancers are usually silent and grow to a significant size to cause symptoms; the central core can be necrotic.

Presentation: it is usually very late. Progressive dysphagia and late onset hoarseness.

Airway Management: given the potential for airway obstruction with apnea, a wake intubation is the most appropriate course.

- *A wake fiberoptic intubation* is the gold standard.
- *A wake oral laryngoscopy* is an acceptable alternative.
- Blind intubation techniques are relatively contraindicated because of the possibility of tumor disruption and significant bleeding (**Figure 9**).

Large goiters

Thyroid cancers or large goiters can be threatening to the upper airway by external airway compression, deviation, distortion, or even local invasion of the trachea. Long term compression may lead to softening of the trachea (tracheomalacia).

Involvement of the recurrent laryngeal nerve may jeopardize an already compromised airway by causing additional narrowing of the glottis. The status of the recurrent laryngeal nerve and glottis opening can be assessed by a routine preoperative flexible laryngoscopy.

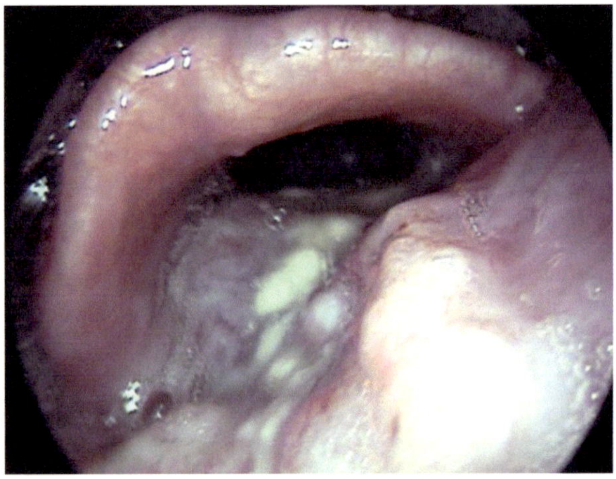

Figure 9.
Obstructive cancer of the hypopharynx.

Airway Management: Large extra-tracheal lesions should engender caution concerning airway management. In these cases, with a suspected difficult airway, a wake intubation is the most appropriate. The possible options: blind nasal, awake oral laryngoscopy, fiberoptic intubation or a wake tracheotomy.

- *Fiberoptic tracheoscopy provide perhaps the highest reliability*

- *A wake* oral *laryngoscopy* is unlikely to be successful in the presence of big goiter and significant airway distortion.

- *Blind nasal intubation* could be performed, but with the mass causing some compression and distortion of the airway, it may be unsuccessful (**Figures 10** and **11**).

Oropharyngeal cancers:

Airway Pathology: The oropharynx extends from the level of the hard palate superiorly to the level of the hyoid bone inferiorly. Laterally it houses the tonsils and faucial pillars.

Airway Management: The main concern is the conversion of a partially obstructed airway (by the tumor) to a completely obstructed (by swelling and/or bleeding) with upper airway or tumor manipulation. In cases of big oropharyngeal tumors, secure airway management requires the need to guarantee the airway before trying a definitive airway and avoidance of any instrumentation or manipulation of the pathology. Trans-tracheal puncture and block techniques are secure means to ventilate and oxygenate patients while more definitive maneuvers are performed (**Figures 12–14**).

Base of Tongue Lesion:

Airway Pathology: large midline tumors of base of the tongue can certainly present real difficulty for airway management. All of these patients should have preoperative fiberoptic nasal pharyngoscopy and CT scan. A CT scan shows the depth of tumor infiltration and involvement of epiglottis and pharynx.

Airway Management: Rigid tissue fixation and/or bleeding from the tumor often preclude successful oral laryngoscopy and intubation. Intubation with standard laryngoscopy in this situation is predictably difficult. A wake

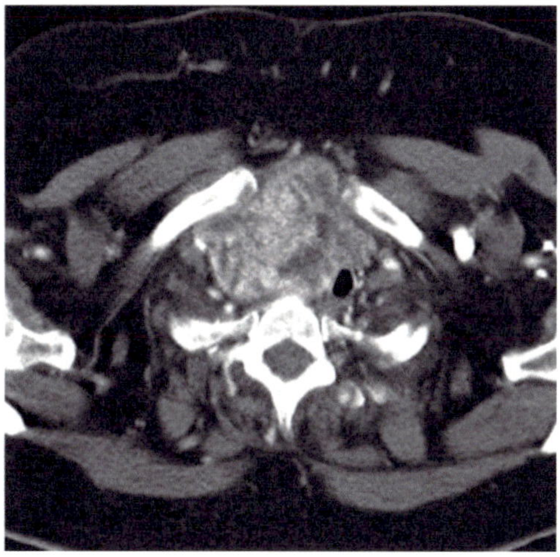

Figure 10.
Large thyroid goiter with tracheal compression and deviation.

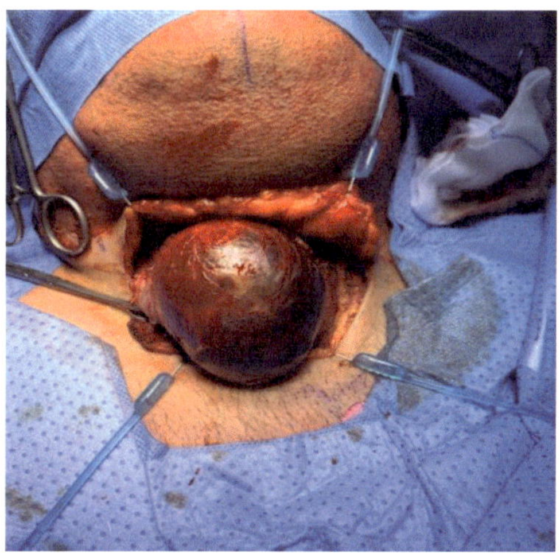

Figure 11.
Large goiter removal.

fiberoptic-trachesoscopy and intubation with the patient spontaneously ventilating is the most appropriate technique.

Vocal cord tumors for LASER cordectomy:

Symptoms range from mild dysphonia to marked stridor and severe respiratory distress. For T1 and T2 glottic cancers, **LASER** cordectomy is the standard treatment option. Inserting a laryngoscope and using **LASER** beam to resects the involved vocal cord with sufficient margin (**Figure 15**).

Airway management: Endoscopic excision of laryngeal vocal cord tumors requires adequate surgical exposure and thus special airway management, many options exist: Intubation with a special **LASER** tube, jet ventilation catheter, or spontaneous breathing with nasopharyngeal oxygen insufflations.

LASER use mandates that no combustible materials come in the field to avoid airway fires. *If fire occurs, the following urgent steps should be done immediately: stop ventilation, stop oxygen, remove the hot endotracheal tube, and wash with sterile saline to extinguish the fire.* Bronchoscopy should be next done to remove any debris and to determine the extent of the damage.

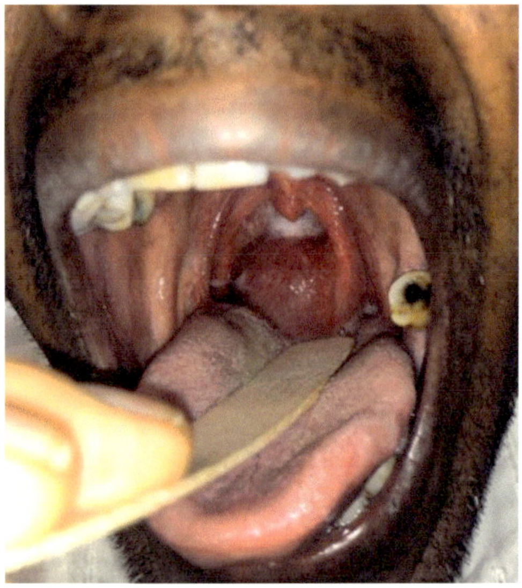

Figure 12.
Large oropharyngeal tumor with almost complete obstruction of the oropharynx.

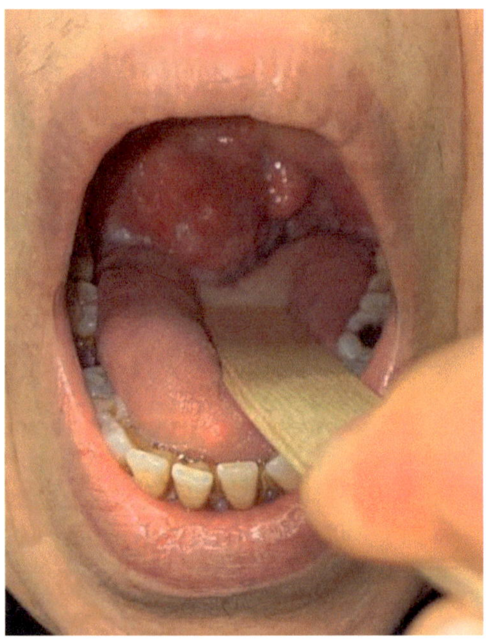

Figure 13.
Another example of a large oropharyngeal tumor arising from the right tonsil.

Supra-glottic Tumors

Airway Pathology: Laryngeal supra-glottic tumors present obvious and serious airway risk. In these tumors, with apnea airway obstruction may occur. In addition, these cancers are friable and can easily fragment and bleed with instrumentation which can convert partial obstruction into a complete obstruction. Therefore, a supra-glottic tumor presents definite intraoperative and postoperative airway risks.

Airway Management: *A wake oral fiberoptic laryngoscopy* is the gold standard.

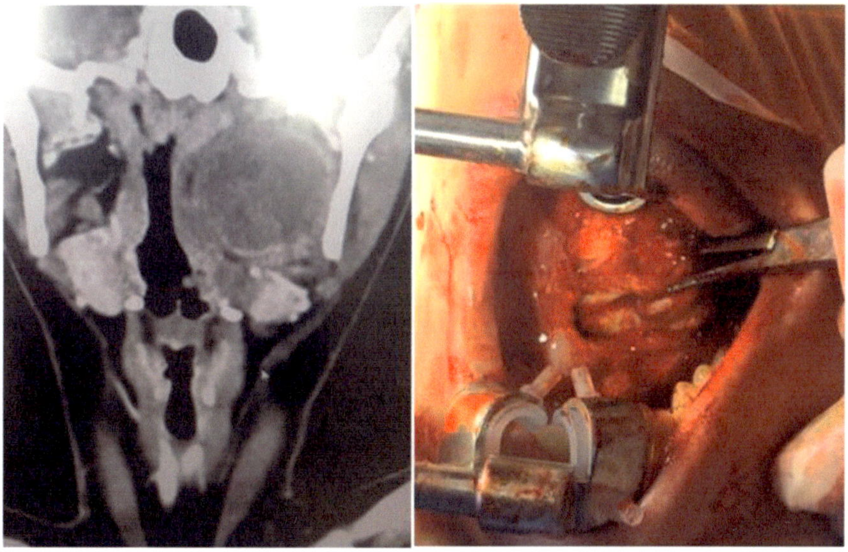

Figure 14.
Huge infra-temporal fossa encroaching on the oropharynx removed trans-orally.

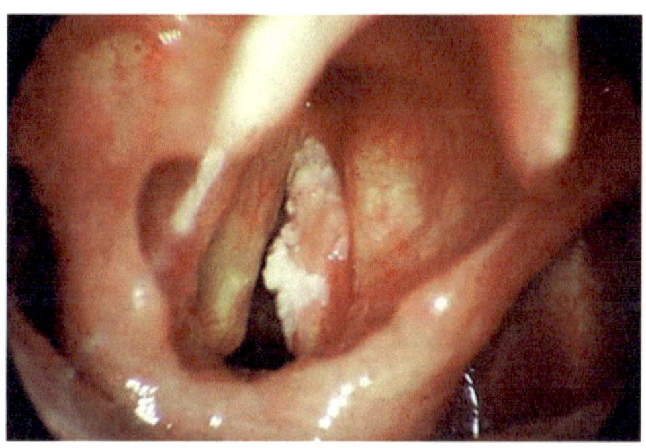

Figure 15.
Left vocal cord cancer for ***LASER*** *resection.*

The extent of postoperative edema should be properly assessed before extubation. In case extubation was decided, proper planning should be taken. These include the use of a fiberoptic bronchoscope, jet stylet catheter, or a tube changer (**Figure 16**).

4.5 Key points

- Patients with head and neck tumors usually present airway management challenges as difficult as any we confront.

- The situation cannot intubate/cannot ventilate episodes are best avoided because of the high associated morbidity.

- The history and physical examinations are essential in preoperative identification of the cases with a difficult **airway** that may need a wake intubation.

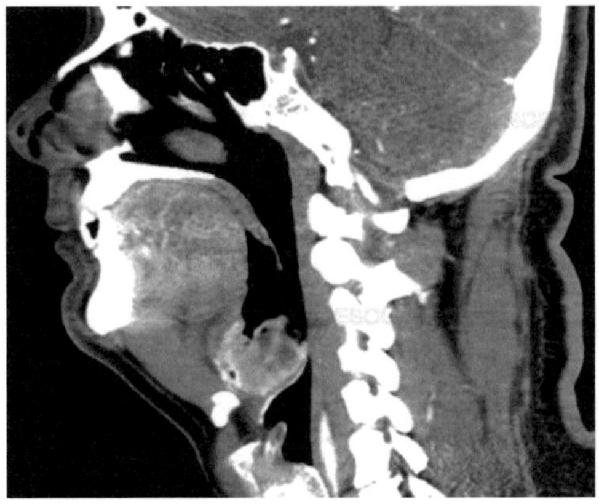

Figure 16.
Large supra-glottic cancer with airway obstruction.

- Symptoms of upper airway obstruction, findings on physical exam, and use of imaging enable us to properly evaluate head and neck tumors and alert us to the potential for airway management difficulty.

- A wake fiberoptic intubation is the most preferred technique in the management of a difficult airway.

5. Airway management post head and neck surgery

5.1 Introduction

There is a wide spectrum of head and neck surgeries ranging from major complex operations to simple minor day care surgical procedures [10].

It is not uncommon for head and neck surgery to affect the airway or to require changing the airway during the operation. For that reason, it is important to have a close and good cooperation between the theater teamwork (surgeons, anesthetists, anesthetic assistants, and nurses [10].

In the current practice now, there is wide range of diverse practice for post-operative airway management of head and neck patients. For example, some will do temporary tracheostomy for almost all head and neck free-flap reconstructions whereas others will manage the same case by overnight ventilation followed by extubation next day [11].

1. Laryngeal spasm	6. Haematoma of the neck
2. Oedema of the larynx	7. Bleeding in the airway
3. Paralysis of the vocal cord	8. Infection of the pharynx or larynx
4. Foreign body in the airway (as missed pharyngeal pack)	9. Reversal of neuromuscular blocking drug is inadequate
5. Obstructive sleep apnoea	10. Reduced venous drainage

Table 2.
Causes of postoperative airway obstruction.

5.2 Factors affecting the strategy of airway management

- A preoperative detailed history of the patient is very helpful to decide the best management of the airway post operatively. (Please refer to the pre-operative assessment).

- Careful preoperative examination of the face, mouth, pharynx, larynx and neck [12].

Causes of airway obstruction postoperatively are provided in **Table 2** [12].

5.3 How to predict postoperative airway difficulty

General factors:

1. If initial intubation is difficult then extubation may also be difficult.

2. Trauma to the airway will lead to oedema which may cause life-threatening airway obstruction postoperatively.

3. Obese patients and, or patient with obstructive sleep apnoea (OSA) are at high risk of postoperative airway obstruction.

4. Emergency patients or patient with gastro-esophageal reflux disease are at risk of aspiration postoperatively, a stomach decompression with nasogastric tube will be very useful [12].

5. Patients with unrelieved trismus (e.g. because of fibrosis) will need the use of an oropharyngeal airway or bite block (e.g. rolled gauze).

During induction:

If the mask ventilation at induction is difficult, this may predict difficulty during emergence [12]. The difficulty in mask ventilation at induction is mainly due to airway abnormality (tumor), OSA, facial asymmetry, Mallampati 3 or 4, receding mandible and age above 55 years old.

Surgical factors:

The airway in some of head and neck surgery can be changed from the preoperative state due to surgical intervention [11]. e.g. Operations on the tongue, pharyngoplasty, palatoplasty, tonsillectomy, operations on the cervical vertebrae, oedema following maxillofacial surgery and any major head and neck surgery.

5.4 Management strategy for difficult airway

General management:

Before safe extubation of the difficult airway we should consider number of requirements that are necessary and should be met.

The following techniques are suggested for a wake extubation of the difficult airway [12] (**Table 3**):

Excessive use of opioid and incomplete reversal of neuromuscular blocking agents may result in airway obstruction leading to hypoxia [12].

Therefore, quantitative neuromuscular monitoring is recommended.

1. Patient in sit up Position	8. Ensure giving adequate analgesia
2. Give Oxygen 100%	9. Ensure the patient is cardiovascular stabile
3. Ensure continuity of regular breathing and adequate gas exchange	10. Apply positive pressure, deflate cuff and remove tube
4. Insert bite block as rolled gauze	11. Ensure airway is patent
5. Airway suction	12. Continue giving oxygen
6. Ensure patient is awake, obeying commands with open eyes	13. Transfer the patient with high flow oxygen and with close observation and monitoring
7. Reversal of neuromuscular blocking	

Table 3.
Techniques to ease awake intubation in a difficult airway case.

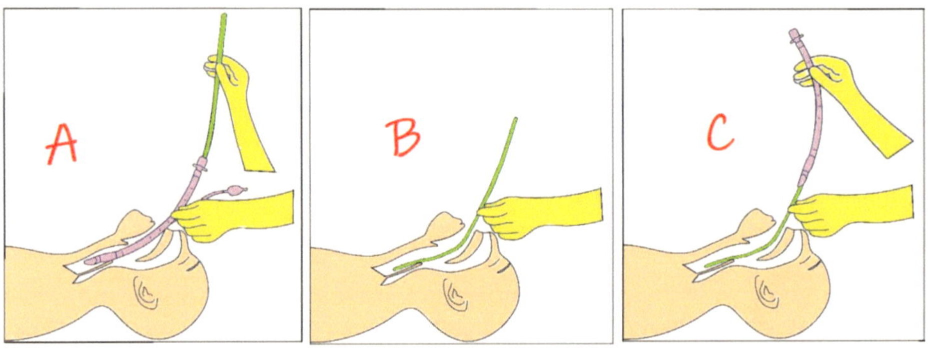

Figure 17.
(A) AEC introduced through the endotracheal tube. (B) AEC left inside trachea. (C) reintubation over the AEC.

Extubation:

Patient with expected difficult airway, extubation preferred to be on the operating table with all needed equipment are available. Patients with some degree of laryngeal oedema after extubation they will benefit from the use of humidified oxygen and nebulized Epinephrine [13].

But in case of total airway obstruction this treatment is not effective and there is a great possibility for re-intubation. Remifentanil used at the end of surgery to prevent coughing and facilitate a wake extubation.

Staged extubation with airway exchange catheters (AECs)

The AEC is usually used for patients known or suspected to have difficult airway, it is used to facilitate re-intubation if needed. The AEC (which is a long hollow boogie) introduced through the endotracheal tube (ETT) before extubation, and then the ETT can be safely removed (**Figure 17**).

In case the patient needs to be re-intubated, the AEC will be used as a guide for the ETT. The AEC can be left in place and tolerated for up to 72 H [14], but usually it is kept for few hours and removed after the patient is stable, fully awake and breathing normally.

Tracheostomy

Tracheostomy operation done within some of maxillofacial operations and in major head and neck operations where postoperatively the airway is expected to be compromised or the patient cannot protect his airway [15].

Usually the tracheostomy is temporary and patient can be weaned after healing of the wound, subsiding of the reactionary oedema and swelling and the patient is able to secure his airway.

Transferring the patient to intensive care unit (ICU)

If you are going to transfer the patient to the ICU with the endotracheal tube in, extra care to be taken to support the tube and avoid tube dislodgment [16].

5.5 Postoperative airway problems

Immediate stridor

Oedema from trauma to the airway is the most common cause for immediate stridor post extubation. This can be avoided by sitting the patient up, giving a dose of 8 mg Dexamethasone i.v. and also giving nebulized Epinephrine before extubation [17].

If the stridor persists and patient is deteriorating, you should examine the airway under anesthesia to rule out other causes as blood clot or retained throat pack.

Laryngeal compromise

This is due to oedema and malfunctions of the glottis and can lead to airway obstruction. It is usually happened after Ludwig's angina or dental abscesses drainage. It can start with postoperative sore throat and then progress to hoarseness of voice, weak cough, deep throat pain, and odynophagia, finally end with stridor, this situation usually will be associated with a difficult intubation. Close monitoring and early intervention are the key to early prediction and successful management of these patients [12].

Bleeding

In case of major bleeding as carotid blow out or rapidly expanding haematoma the patient requires urgent surgical and anesthetic intervention [12].

The removal of surgical skin clips may help to reduce airway deterioration. The patient should be immediately transferred to theater, and re-intubated with a small tracheal tube may be needed [12].

Obstruction or dislodgment of tracheal tube or tracheostomy tube

Usually the obstruction of either tube is due to thick secretion or clotted blood, regular suction and the use of humidified oxygen helps to prevent tube obstruction. Extra care to be taken to support the tube during moving or changing patient position. If there is a concern that the tube is obstructed or dislodged then immediate activation of documented action plan with early involvement of the surgical team if needed.

Post obstructive negative pressure pulmonary oedema

This commonly happened in the immediate postoperative time when the patient is trying to breathe while the airway is closed as he is biting on tracheal tube. This will create negative intrathoracic pressures, and this will lead to pulmonary oedema. Using bite blocks can reduce this risk. Deflating the cuff of the tube allowing the patient to breathe around it.

Using CPAP may help; but, if there is significant hypoxia, re-intubation should not be delayed.

Early management with re-intubation and ventilation will help for full recovery [12].

Laryngospasm

It usually happened due to stimulation during a light plane of anesthesia but may occur due to blood, secretions or foreign body in the larynx. The management is by clearing the oropharynx, applying CPAP with 100% oxygen, followed by deepening of anesthesia by an i.v. anesthetic agent. Also using short-acting muscle relaxant as Succinylcholine may be needed. But in case of significant laryngospasm, re-intubation will be the proper immediate action [12].

ICU Management of the difficult airway

Usually most of patients with head and neck pathology with high concern about the postoperative airway will be managed on the ICU. Suggestions for successful management includes good communication between all of the multidisciplinary team, handover to be written and verbal with clear description of the problem and how it was managed, the current state of the airway, what is the ongoing plane of management and whom to call in case of airway deterioration.

The decision to whether manage postoperative difficult airway interventions in ICU or in theater will depend on the clinical problem, availability of equipment, the urgency of the situation, and the relative proximity to theaters [12].

5.6 Key points

- Airway management continues from pre and peri-operative period to the postoperative period [11, 12].
- Postoperative airway obstruction usually leads to high incidence of morbidity if not managed in proper time.
- Close monitoring for patients with high risk of airway deterioration postoperatively is highly important.
- A plane of management of the difficult airway postoperatively should be agreed by the multidisciplinary team.
- Cooperation and harmony between anesthetists and surgeons are of extreme importance as both are working in the same field (shared airway).
- If expecting airway problem postoperatively, then the patient should be remained intubated or to do tracheostomy before extubation.
- Using the trans-nasal high-flow rapid insufflation ventilator exchange ("THRIVE") makes intubation and extubation less stressful and less traumatic.
- Staff dealing with patients either intubated or tracheostomized should receive proper training and to be aware of the relevant guidelines.
- A planned protocol should be developed for urgent airway management.

6. Airway management in obstructive sleep apnea (OSA) patients

6.1 Introduction

OSA is considered one of the important challenges in the peri-operative airway management. Obstructive apneas are defined as complete or near-complete cessation of airflow lasting for at least 10 sec. Obstructive hypopneas are characterized by at least 30% reduction in airflow for a minimum of 10 sec and are associated with a 4% oxygen desaturation [18].

The difficult airway in OSA patients is considered to be a main contributing factor to the higher rate of adverse respiratory and cardiovascular events, so to reduce the peri-operative complication [19], it is better to divide the management approach of OSA patients into: preoperative, intraoperative, and postoperative strategies.

6.2 Pre-operative assessment in suspected OSA patients

- A detailed history includes: loud snoring, observed apnea, daytime sleepiness, and morning headaches, with emphasis on airway examination and identifying comorbidities.

- Physical examination: characteristics predicting a difficult airway (highly modified Mallampati score, reduced thyromental distance) [19].

- OSA screening and diagnosis (results of screening tools/questionnaires such as those with STOP-BANG scores ≥5 with co-morbidities, full attended polysomnography (PSG) should be done prior to any major elective surgery and reviewed by sleep physician, while the other suspected OSA patients without co-morbidities and undergoing minor surgery, appropriate risk reduction steps can be taken [20].

- All patients after diagnosis of OSA has been established who use CPAP preoperatively (compliant and noncompliant) should be advised to bring the device to the hospital for use in the postoperative period, so that it is readily applicable whenever under the influence of narcotics or sedatives [21].

6.3 Intra-operative assessment and impact of anesthesia on OSA patients

During anesthesia; alteration of muscle activity results in upper airway collapse more at the level of retro-lingual. Such obstructive events require active intervention to arouse spontaneously, which is an important defense mechanism that occurs during natural sleep to overcome airway obstruction.

The administration of anesthetic agents exacerbates the upper airway collapse, alter the tone of the pharyngeal musculature, result in delay of the restoration of airway patency, therefore, in general the tendency for airway obstruction occurs out of proportion to the level of achieved sedation [22].

6.4 Post-operative assessment

Patients with OSA undergoing upper airway surgery are at high risk for difficult airway management and increased incidence of postoperative complications. These complications include higher re-intubation rates, hypercapnia, oxygen desaturations, cardiac arrhythmias, myocardial injury, delirium, unplanned ICU transfers, and longer hospitalization stays.

Several perioperative and anesthetic factors may contribute to these complications [22]:

1. *Medication*: drugs commonly used during general anesthesia (hypnotics, opioids and muscle relaxants).

2. The *patient's position* during anesthesia can negatively affect the traction forces in the trachea, leading to increased pharyngeal closing pressure and collapse of the upper airway.

3. Prolonged intubation may lead to pharyngeal edema and narrowing of the upper airway.

4. Decreased airway stability caused by prolonged postoperative patient's supine position.

5. Perioperative discontinuation of continuous positive airway pressure (CPAP) therapy.

6. Surgical stress and post-operative sedation may lead to disruption of sleep and apneic events at night affected by increased periods of rapid eye movement (REM) following surgery.

6.5 Highlights and pearls for upper airway mangament with elective surgery in adult OSA patients

1. Focused history, physical examination and implementing screening tool in the (pre-operative care) are crucial in studying high risk OSA cases to reduce post -operative complication [19].

2. In *mild OSA or low risk cases*, surgery can be proceeding with minimizing peri-operative complication risk.

3. In *high risk and diagnosed OSA* cases should have the following [23]:

6.6 In intra-operative care

- Consider minimal sedation or regional anesthesia if appropriate

- Prepare for difficult airway management, 25-degree head position, use short acting anesthetic drug.

- Consider invasive monitoring for respiratory & hemodynamic parameters.

- Extubate after the patient is completely awake

6.7 In recovery room

- Close observation for oxygen saturation and hemodynamic for at least 2 hours, with head position 30 degree.

- Consider use non-opioid anesthetic drug.

- Early use of positive airway pressure (PAP) in case of desaturation.

6.8 In-ward management

- Close monitoring and continuous supplemental oxygen therapy until they can maintain their oxygen saturation on room air.

- Continue PAP therapy in case needed.

- Discharged patient should follow with sleep physician for re-assessment.

7. Conclusion

- Patients who present with head and neck pathology are more likely to have difficult airways, are at increased risk of difficulties during airway management, and they are also more likely to require an emergency surgical airway when difficulties arise.

- Proper Preoperative assessment and Multidisciplinary planning is required for successful management.

- Virtual endoscopy can be used to supplement conventional airway endoscopy to help in planning the management of difficult airway cases

- Awake intubation is preferred in difficult airway cases where typical intubation may not be guaranteed.

- Using the trans-nasal high-flow rapid insufflation ventilator exchange ("THRIVE") makes intubation and extubation less stressful and less traumatic.

- OSA patients are becoming increasingly identified in the surgical population, therefore appropriate measures are needed in order to treat patients at the highest risk for OSA to reduce the perioperative complications.

- Obesity and obstructive sleep apnea increase the risk for anesthetic and sedative complications, including post -operative cardiorespiratory complications [20].

The lack of recognition of OSA cases pre-operatively poses significant challenges result from difficulties during airway management. To reduce encountered complication an appropriate anesthetic regimen including choice of medication, airway management and adequate postoperative monitoring should be optimized [24].

Author details

Muayad M. Radi Al-Khafaji[1,2]*, Hossam Makki[1,2], Hassan Haider[2], Furat Abbas[1,2] and Abhishek Menon[1]

1 Department of Otolaryngology - Head and Neck Surgery, Hamad Medical Corporation, Doha, Qatar

2 Clinical Otolaryngology - Head and Neck Surgery, Weill Cornell Medical College in Qatar, Doha, Qatar

*Address all correspondence to: mradi@hamad.com

References

[1] Sofferman RA, Johnson DL, Spencer RF (1997) Lost airway during anesthesia induction Alternatives for management, Laryngoscope 107:1476-1481

[2] Flint, Paul W, and Charles W. Cummings. Cummings Otolaryngology Head & Neck Surgery. 2010. Internet resource.

[3] Roth D, Pace NL, Lee A, Hovhannisyan K, Warenits AM, Arrich J, et al. Airway physical examination tests for detection of difficult airway management in apparently normal adult patients. Cochrane Database Syst Rev 2018; 5:CD008874.

[4] APA McAvoy, James MD; Ewing, Tyler MD; Nekhendzy, Vladimir MD The value of preoperative endoscopic airway examination in complex airway management of a patient with supraglottic cancer, Journal of Head & Neck Anesthesia: August 2019 - Volume 3 - Issue 3 - p e19 doi: 10.1097/HN9.0000000000000019

[5] Verma SP, Smith ME, Dailey SH. Transnasal tracheoscopy. Laryngoscope. 2012; 122(6):1326-1330. doi:10.1002/lary.23221

[6] Hochman II. Zeitels SM. Heaton JT (1999) Analysis of the forces and position required for direct laryngoscopic exposure of the anterior vocal folds. Ann Otol Rhinol Laryngol 108:715-724

[7] Hunsaker DH (1994) Anesthesia for micro-laryngeal surgery: the case for subglottic jet ventilation. Laryngoscope 104(Suppl.):1-30

[8] Management of the Difficult Airway: A Handbook for Surgeons. Francisco O M Vieira, Jerome W Thompson, and Michael Rutter)

[9] Imaging Tests for Predicting the Presence of Difficult Airway in Head and Neck Cancer Patients Undergoing Otorhinolaryngological Surgery By Juan Gutiérrez Franchi, S. Merino, P. de la Calle, C. Perrino, M. Represa and P. Moral)

[10] National Institute for Health and Care Excellence. Improving outcomes in head and neck cancers. NICE Cancer service guideline CSG6, 2004. https://www.nice.org.uk/guidance/csg6

[11] Anaesthesia for head and neck surgery: United Kingdom national multidisciplinary guidelines the Journal of Laryngology & Otology (2016), 130 (Suppl. S2), S23–S27.

[12] B Batuwitage, P Charters, I Ahmad, A Patel et al. Postoperative management of the difficult airway, BJA Education, 17 (7): 235-241 (2017)

[13] MacDonnell SP, Timmins AC, Watson JD. Adrenaline administered via a nebulizer in adult patients with upper airway obstruction. Anaesthesia 1995; 50: 35-36

[14] Biro P, Priebe HJ. Staged extubation strategy: is an airway exchange catheter the answer? Anesth Analg. 2007; 105(5):1182-1185. doi:10.1213/01.ane.0000286234.96551.67

[15] Biro P, Priebe HJ. Staged extubation strategy: is an airway exchange catheter the answer? Anesth Analg. 2007; 105(5):1182-1185.

[16] Mort TC. Continuous airway access for the difficult extubation: the efficacy of the airway exchange catheter. Anesth Analg 2007; 105: 1357-1362

[17] Lee CH, Peng MJ, Wu CL. Dexamethasone to prevent post extubation airway obstruction in adults:

a prospective, randomized, double-blind, placebo-controlled study. Crit Care 2007; 11: R72

[18] Adebola O. Adesanya, MD. Perioperative Management of Obstructive Sleep Apnea. CHEST/138/6/December 2010. DOI: 10.1378/chest.10-1108.

[19] De Raaff, Christel AL, et al. "Perioperative management of obstructive sleep apnea in bariatric surgery: a consensus guideline." Surgery for Obesity and Related Diseases 13.7 (2017): 1095-1109.

[20] Fauzia A Khan, Mohammad Ali. Perioperative Management of Patients with Obstructive Sleep Apnea - A Review. Indian Journal of Anesthesia 2008; 52 (2): 140-147.

[21] Hillman, et al. "Anesthesia, sleep, and upper airway collapsibility." Anesthesiology clinics 28.3 (2010): 443-455

[22] Victor Hoffstein, How and Why Should We Stabilize the Upper Airway?, Sleep, Volume 19, Issue suppl_9, November 1996, Pages S57–S60, https://doi.org/10.1093/sleep/19.suppl_9.S57

[23] ASMBS Clinical Issues Committee. "Peri-operative management of obstructive sleep apnea." Surgery for obesity and related diseases: official journal of the American Society for Bariatric Surgery 8.3 (2012): e27.

[24] Roesslein and Chung Obstructive sleep apnea in adults: peri-operative considerations. Eur J Anesthesiology (2018).; 35:245-255. DOI:10.1097/EJA.0000000000000765.

Chapter 9

An Approach to the Airway Management in Children with Craniofacial Anomalies

Brahim Boudjenah, Al Moataz Billah Adham, Surendra M. Chinnappa, Omed Assaf and Mashael Al-Khelaifi

Abstract

Managing the airways during anesthesia in pediatric patients with craniofacial abnormalities is a challenging and stressful situation for even experienced anesthesiologists. The prerequisites for a good management are a thorough understanding of the normal anatomy of the upper airway, its normal changes with growth, and the key features of congenital craniofacial abnormalities and their impact on the airways resulting in management difficulties. This chapter aims to provide an overview of various craniofacial anomalies and their airway management specificities. These include cleft lip and palate with or without Pierre Robin syndrome, craniofacial dysostosis (including Crouzon, Pfeiffer, and Apert syndromes), mandibulofacial dysostosis/Treacher Collins syndrome, hemifacial microsomia, Down's syndrome, and other anomalies.

Keywords: congenital syndrome, craniofacial anomalies, difficult airways, anesthesia, mandibulofacial dysostosis

1. Introduction

The incidence of difficult airway is higher in children with craniofacial syndromes than normal children, hence a thorough airway evaluation is crucial in order to anticipate difficult airway and to formulate a safe plan. Common challenges encountered upon examination of a child's airway include an uncooperative child and the unreliability of the Mallampati scoring for prediction of the difficult airway in children [1]. Airway assessment must focus on the general clinical systematic evaluation as well as the more specific airway issues of each syndrome and other associated organs involvement. The approach should include history taking, physical examination, and diagnostic tests.

2. Pediatric difficult airway evaluation

2.1 General airway assessment

General clinical history should focus on the presence of any problem affecting the airway or the respiratory system including history of snoring or apneas, upper respiratory tract infection (URTI), croup, stridor, voice hoarseness, recurrent aspirations, asthma, parental smoking, and most importantly a history of previous difficult airway management [2].

The general airway examination must include: a baseline oxygen saturation on room air, respiratory rate, preferred body position (prone position must be red-flagged as upper airway obstruction), mouth breathing, existence of any obstruction manifested by intercostal/suprasternal retractions, oral examination of the mouth opening, teeth, tongue size and Mallampati score, shape and position of the mandible, hyo-mental distance, and neck length/mobility.

Nevertheless, the airway examination in children may be difficult to perform in detail especially with an uncooperative child, thus it may be restricted to the general observation of the face, mandible, and breathing pattern in such situations.

The most critical step in airway examination of children pertains at taking a lateral "profile" look of the mandible which could spot a micrognathia or a retracted mandible that might be masked with the frontal look.

General diagnostic tests: they are seldom required especially when further details of the airway are needed. An X-ray of the head and neck can show the place and the level of upper airway obstruction; however, a CT scan/MRI can provide further details (especially in tumors and vascular malformations of the airway). CT virtual endoscopy (VE) is an excellent tool used to obtain an anatomically similar representation of the intraluminal geography of the airway, including supraglottic, glottic, and subglottic structures without the risk of exposure to ionizing radiation. Compared to conventional 3-D reconstructions, the images obtained through virtual endoscopy create the impression of a true endoscopic image allowing for a tailored approach toward the airway management. A flexible fiberoptic endoscopy maybe required in children with airway pathology especially children with an unexplained hoarse voice, suprasternal/intercostal retractions, and chronic aspirations.

2.2 Focused airway evaluation

The clinical evaluation should focus on risk factors which may potentially contribute to difficult airway management including (**Table 1**) [3]:

1. An extremely short thyro-mental distance with an overbite, with micro/retrognathia such as seen in Pierre Robin sequence and Treacher-Collins syndrome;

2. A fixed neck such as in Klippel-Feil syndrome;

3. A small oral opening and large tongue such as seen in Beckwith-Wiedemann syndrome;

4. Obstructive sleep apnea +/− secondary pulmonary hypertension;

5. Stiff subcutaneous tissues as seen in Mucopolysaccharidosis (high risk of difficult ventilation);

6. Midface hypoplasia as seen in Apert and Crouzon syndromes;

7. Obstruction of the airway when in supine position and the need to continuously maintain in prone positioning;

Anatomical malformation	Syndrome
Overbite	Pierre Robin-Treacher Collins-Goldenhar
Mandibular prognathism	Apert
Small mouth	Pierre-Robin, Treacher-Collins, Goldenhar, Down's syndrome
Large mouth	Mucopolysaccharidosis, Beckwith-Wiedemann
Palate (high arched)	Down, Crouzon, Apert, Pierre Robin, Treacher Collins, Mucopolysaccharidosis
Cleft Palate	Pierre Robin, Treacher Collins, Goldenhar, Down's, Apert, Crouzon
Tongue abnormality (Large or Glossoptosis)	Beckwith-Wiedemann, Mucopolysaccharidosis, Pierre Robin.
Short thyromental distance (less than 3 finger breadths used by the own child's fingers)	Pierre Robin, Treacher Collins, Goldenhar,
Subglottic narrowing	Down's syndrome
Tracheal abnormality (tortuosity)	Mucopolysaccharidosis
Cervical spine abnormalities	Down's syndrome, Klippel-Feil, Mucopolysaccharidosis, Goldenhar

Table 1.
Anatomical malformations related to difficult airway in craniofacial syndromes.

8. History of a previous failed airway;

9. Soft tissue tumors and vascular malformations with significant obstruction of the airway.

3. General airway management in patients with craniofacial syndromes

The airway management plan of the infants and children with difficult airway has many proposed algorithms but not unified as in the American Society of Anaesthesiologists (ASA) adult difficult airway algorithm [4–7]. The awake intubation is no more a popular option in pediatric intubations except for some emergency situations where the patient is in severe distress and obstruction, as it carries its own disadvantages (increase in intracranial pressure ICP and intracerebral hemorrhage ICH, gagging, uncooperative kid), hence induction of anesthesia with preservation of spontaneous breathing is the cornerstone for a safe airway management in patients with craniofacial syndromes with suspected difficult airway.

The airway provider should set a structured strategy for the management of the airway. Common practice is to have a "Plan A" as an initial approach with subsequent plan B and C in case of failure of the former.

An otolaryngologist attendance for emergency backup surgical access (Bronchoscopy/Tracheostomy) is recommended during the management of the potential difficult airway.

A secured peripheral IV line prior to induction is recommended in patients with cranio-facial anomalies.

Presence of two airway experts (pediatric anesthesiologists) during induction is advisable.

Plan A: Preserve spontaneous ventilation:

- Induction using IV sedative medication: propofol infusion or boluses (also dexmedetomidine, ketamine)

Or

- Inhalation induction with Sevoflurane

While patient is spontaneously breathing, a careful insertion of the laryngoscope blade may be attempted provided that the patient tolerates without bucking norcoughing.

A wide range of airway tools and techniques have been described for the intubation. However, it is crucial that the airway operator sticks with the tool that he is mostly familiar with. It is noteworthy to keep in mind that an airway tool is not a plan.

Techniques used for intubation of syndromic children with difficult airway include:

1. **Direct laryngoscopy**: a regular laryngoscope blade (a Macintosh curved or a Miller straight blade).
   The paraglossal approach with a straight blade is a well-described technique for intubation in children with difficult airway where conventional laryngoscopy technique fails. Using this technique may allow the operator to avoid the large tongue commonly encountered in cranio-facial syndromes via inserting the laryngoscope's straight blade through the trench between the tonsils and the base of the tongue. This technique allows a better exposure of an anterior larynx; however, it does not provide an adequate space for tube manipulation, hence it requires a high level of skills by the operator.
   Intubation with direct laryngoscopy may be facilitated with gum elastic bougie or a stylet.

2. **Video laryngoscopy**: video laryngoscopes such as the Storz video laryngoscope or the Glidescope have been successfully used for intubation in syndromic children with difficult airway. Despite the fact that the Glidescope provides an easy view, the intubation may be challenging due to the small "working" space and the curvature of the airway, especially in the smaller patients group.

3. **Fiberoptic bronchoscope intubation**: F.O.B intubation is a popular option as "first attempt" technique or as an alternative to a failed direct laryngoscopy and other techniques. It can be performed nasally, orally or through an LMA. However, its main disadvantage is that it might not be an option for neonates and smaller infants who require smaller endotracheal tubes that may barely accommodate the smallest F.O.B.
   It is also challenging to perform F.O.B intubation in neonates who have a small airway as the field of vision in the distal lens is very narrow and might get easily obstructed whenever touching any obstacle, hence it requires a high-level skill set and expertise.

4. **Fiber-optic bronchoscope intubation through LMA**: F.O.B intubation through LMA is a popular technique of intubation for children with difficult airway. The LMA can serve for ventilation/oxygenation during the process

of intubation which is a very favorable advantage especially in children with difficult bag-mask ventilation.

However, the removal of the LMA might get complicated with accidental ETT extubation, thus many techniques have been described for the removal; however, the safest strategy remains keeping both the LMA and the ETT in place after intubation and removing them together at extubation.

5. **Fiberoptic bronchoscope + GlideScope**: The fiberoptic bronchoscope can be used as a guiding bougie for intubation, while the view is provided by the Glidescope. This technique will require two personnel: with one handling the Glidescope while the other manipulating the F.O.B. It is called the video-assisted fiberoptic intubation (VAFI) technique.

Plan B: If Plan A fails and ventilation becomes problematic at any step of the airway management, then an LMA should be immediately inserted. If manual bag-mask ventilation gets possible after LMA insertion, then the operator has a choice whether to keep it if appropriate for the procedure, to proceed with F.O.B intubation through the LMA or to use other techniques for intubation.

If "Cannot ventilate" through LMA, then the operator should immediately move to plan C.

Plan C: If attempts at ventilating via "Bag-Mask" and LMA fail, one attempt at direct laryngoscopy can be performed aiming at intubating if possible.

If all the previous attempts fail, then an emergency surgical airway must imminently be resorted to by the otolaryngologist with either an emergent rigid bronchoscopy placement or an emergency tracheostomy.

Extubation and post-extubation strategies: Extubation of patients with craniofacial anomalies directly at the end of the procedure should only be performed in the following conditions:

1. An atraumatic intubation with minimal airway edema

2. A minor short surgery not involving the airway (excluding adeno-tonsillectomies)

3. Absence of a history of severe obstructive apnea

The extubation should be performed when the patient is fully awake with vigorous spontaneous breathing and resumption of airway reflexes. The anesthesiologist must be ready for a re-intubation with all the airway tools set up should the extubation trial fail.

Patients at risk of post-operative airway obstruction such as obstructive sleep apnea must be monitored overnight in a high dependency unit (Apnea monitoring).

Patients with significant obstructive apneas undergoing major airway surgeries (such as mandibular distraction osteogenesis surgery) in which intubation might have been difficult or traumatic should not be extubated at the end of the procedure as they are at high risk of obstruction post-op which may necessitate an intubation that would likely be extremely difficult as exacerbated by the airway edema. Such patients should be kept intubated, properly sedated, and transferred to the ICU for post-monitoring. Intravenous steroids regimen should be given to minimize airway edema.

4. Craniofacial anomalies and airway management

4.1 Down's syndrome

Overview: Down's syndrome is the leading chromosomal disorder associated with intellectual disability worldwide. It is characterized by a bundle of multisystemic morphologic features including cardiovascular, pulmonary, gastrointestinal, neurological, musculoskeletal, hematological, immunological, endocrine, ophthalmic, and hearing abnormalities. It was firstly described and published in the London Hospital Reports by a British doctor John Langdon Down in 1866 who called it "Mongolian type."

Genetics: Down's syndrome is a congenital autosomal disorder caused by the existence of a third copy, full or partial, of the chromosome 21 (HSA21), usually by nondisjunction [8].

Incidence: its average incidence is estimated to be about 1 in 800 live births and tends to increase with advanced maternal age.

Pathophysiology: This syndrome is caused by the existence of a third copy (either full or partial) of the chromosome 21 (HSA21) [8].

Clinical considerations: Down's syndrome is a multisystem disease associated with generalized growth retardation and varying degrees of mental impairment. Its clinical hallmarks encompass generalized neuromuscular hypotonia, atlantoaxial instability often associated with congenital cardiac anomalies (in particular an atrioventricular septal defect, a patent ductus arteriosus, or a tetralogy of Fallot) and gastrointestinal malformations (duodenal atresia and Hirschsprung disease) [4, 5, 9]. In addition, children with DS compared to healthy ones are more prone to multiple health issues, including obstructive sleep apnea, recurrent infections, hypothyroidism, epilepsy, audiovestibular and visual impairment, hematopoietic disorders (including leukemia), anxiety disorders, and early-onset Alzheimer disease. The physical appearance is pathognomonic with a chunky stature and a small round dysmorphic face.

In 1866, Dr. John Langdon Down, with few simple words, well described the main craniofacial features related to this disorder: a flat and broad face, narrow palpebral fissures, small nose, and long and thick tongue. These anomalies include a microcephaly, brachycephaly, a flattened occiput, a sloping forehead, midfacial hypoplasia, depressed nasal bridge, slanting eyes with epicanthic folds, hypotelorism, strabismus, and small ears with flat or absent helix. A cleft lip and/or palate may be present.

Airway and anesthetic implications: airway obstruction is common in children with Down's syndrome. A midface hypoplasia, narrow nasopharynx, choanal stenosis, high arched palate, pharyngeal muscle hypotonia, relative macroglossia, lingual tonsils, glossoptosis, adenotonsillar hypertrophy, micrognathia, short broad neck, and obesity, all these anatomical conditions combined together contribute to upper airway narrowing [6, 10]. In addition, various other structural airway anomalies may be present and diminish further the airway volume. They may be found isolated or combined together such as: laryngomalacia, subglottic stenosis, congenital tracheal, and bronchial anomalies [11]. They are highly suspected in children with Down's syndrome who have recurrent respiratory symptoms. Laryngomalacia and obstructive sleep apnea syndrome are the most common cause of upper airway obstruction below and above the age of 2 years old, respectively. Obstructive sleep apnea syndrome is reported with an incidence of approximately 30–55% of children with Down's syndrome and may be a potential indication of an adenotonsillectomy and/or home continuous positive airways pressure ventilation (BiPAP).

Collecting a detailed and accurate history from the parents is the first step in assessing the airways. Symptoms related to obstructive sleep apnea (snoring, choking, mouth breathing, sleep disturbances/restless sleep, diurnal drowsiness or fatigue) and a recent episode of upper respiratory tract infection should be noted. Any recent or active upper respiratory infection should prompt the physician to postpone any non-urgent surgery because of the high rate of postoperative respiratory complications. Examination of the oropharynx and head-neck is of utmost importance looking for any predictor of a difficult airway. A careful pulmonary examination is a must, and preoperative chest X-ray is not routinely required. An echocardiography is sometimes indicated to rule out any congenital heart defect or pulmonary hypertension [12].

The risk of upper airway obstruction at the induction of anesthesia for children with Down's syndrome is always present, hence a difficult airway management scenario must be anticipated. A difficult mask ventilation may necessitate insertion of an oropharyngeal or a nasopharyngeal airway. Tracheal intubation in children with Down's syndrome deserves special attention. The trachea is narrow and smaller than in healthy children, not only at the subglottic area but over its entire length and may be the site of numerous anatomical anomalies. When endotracheal intubation is indicated, a tracheal tube of 0.5 or 1 mm smaller than the expected one may be required due to the high risk of post-extubation stridor. It is recommended to monitor the ETT cuff pressure and keep it below 18 cm H_2O in order to lower the risk of post-extubation stridor, whereas a smooth and non-traumatic tracheal intubation should be the rule with cuffed ETT [1].

Craniocervical instability is reported to be common in children with DS with an incidence of about 15% of the cases, mostly secondary to a hyperlaxity of the transverse ligament. Nonetheless, a malformation of the craniovertebral junction bones may be associated. Atlanto-occipital and atlanto-axial joints are at high risk of subluxation during airway manipulation which may result in compression of the underlying spinal cord [13]. Thus, a gentle and cautious manipulation of the neck and the head is required during the airway management of children with DS especially those with potential risk of cervical spine instability causing neurological deficit or at risk of worsening while under anesthesia. A cervical spine manual in-line immobilization approach must always be provided by an assistant during mask ventilation and intubation.

After surgery, a "no touch technique" awake extubation with the child kept in lateral position is preferred. Down's syndrome children with a history of obstructive sleep apnea are hypersensitive to opioid effects and need to be admitted for post-operative apnea monitoring (with continuous SPO2 monitoring and a dedicated nurse) due to the high incidence of postoperative airway obstruction and hypoventilation. The use of non-invasive positive pressure support may be required for DS patients with severe OSA.

4.2 Pierre Robin sequence (PRS)

Overview: it is one of the congenital defects associated with abnormal anatomy of the airway imposing great challenges in its perioperative management. It was initially described by a French oral surgeon "Pierre-Robin" in 1923 as a clinical triad of: micrognathia (small mandible), glossoptosis (backward retraction of the tongue), and a subsequent airway obstruction [14]. The triad may be associated with a cleft palate in 50% of cases. PRS is classified as a sequence rather than a syndrome as it is representing succession of malformation events due to a sole cause, which is the failure in fetal mandibular development [15] (**Figure 1**).

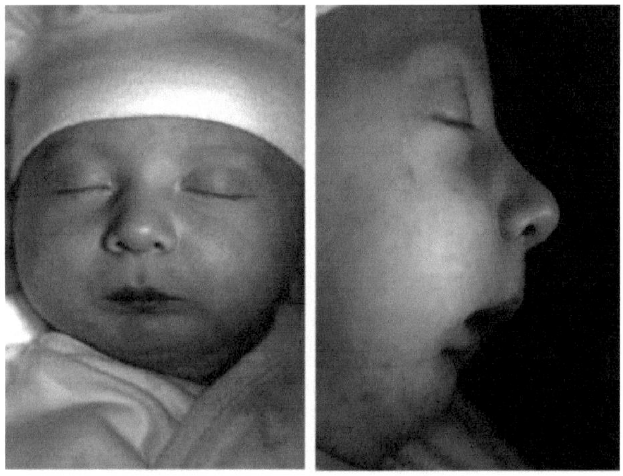

(a) (b)

Figure 1.
Pierre Robin sequence frontal (A) and lateral (B) facial [16].

Infants may present with airway obstruction (stridor) and respiratory distress and may require multiple surgeries (tongue adhesion, mandibular distraction osteogenesis, or tracheostomy).

The major challenge to the anesthesiologist is managing the airway of such patients who are infamous to be difficult to bag-mask-ventilate and extremely difficult to intubate.

Incidence: isolated PRS prevalence can range from 1/8500 to 1/14,000 of births [15]; however, around 40–60% of the PRS cases are associated with other facial syndromes including Stickler, Treacher Collins, Velocardial, and fetal alcohol syndromes [14].

Genetics: the genetic etiology of isolated PRS is still debatable as some authors attribute it to "in utero" compression secondary to oligohydramnios, and others suggest its association with SOX9 and KCNJ2 dysregulation on chromosome 17. However, syndromic PRS is associated with genetic mutations such as the 22q, 11.2 microdeletion in the Velocardial syndrome and the COL2A1 COL9A1 COL11A1 mutations associated with the Stickler syndrome.

Pathophysiology: in all cases, PRS is the consequence of primary failure of the development of the mandible, which leads to the backward and downward displacement of the tongue (the normal tongue has no place to be accommodated in the extremely small submandibular space), consequently resulting in airway obstruction. In 50% of cases, a superiorly displaced tongue may prevent the fusion of the palatal arches leading to a cleft palate. The resulting chronic airway obstruction leads to repeated episodes of hypoxemia and hypercapnia culminating in sleep apnea, pulmonary hypertension, poor feeding, gastroesophageal reflux, and failure to thrive and chronic ear diseases.

Preoperative considerations and airway evaluation: multiple procedures might be needed for the child with PRS such as tongue/lip adhesion, mandibular distraction osteogenesis, tracheostomy, bronchoscopies, MRI/CT imaging, gastrostomy tube insertion, and Nissen fundoplication.

The preoperative evaluation should focus on risk factors which may contribute to difficult airway management including:

1. An extremely short hyo-mental distance of less than 1 cm (or a maxillary to mandibular discrepancy of more than 1 cm)

2. Obstruction of the airway when in supine position and the need to continuously maintain in prone positioning

3. Frequent desaturations and the need to provide supplementary oxygenation

4. Presence of OSA (may indicate severe airway obstruction)

5. Presence of pulmonary hypertension

6. History of a previous failed airway

7. Co-existing pulmonary disease (secondary to reflux/recurrent aspirations, laryngo-tracheo-broncho malacia, chronic lung disease...)

8. Presence of reflux and feeding difficulties (nasogastric-tube dependent) [17]

The airway examination must focus on taking a lateral "profile" look of the mandible, assessing for the mandibulo-maxillary discrepancy and the degree of micrognathia. As well as examining the oral cavity for the degree of glossoptosis (size and position of the tongue) and for the presence of a co-existing "cleft palate."

The presence of any associated syndrome (Stickler, Velocardial, Treacher-Collins) or any heart murmur upon physical exam should prompt a request of a preoperative echocardiography as congenital heart anomalies are not uncommon in such patients.

Airway management in patients with PRS: the airway management plan of the infants and children with Pierre-Robin sequence must address the difficulties in bag-mask ventilation (BMV) and tracheal intubation [18]. The small chin may render the face mask difficult to provide a fit to seal the airway for BMV. With anesthetic induction, the backwardly placed tongue may adjoin the palate and subsequently completely block the airway rendering BMV more problematic. Insertion of a "Guedel" oropharyngeal airway (to overcome the obstruction) may not properly fit the patient because of the distorted airway anatomy, which adds further challenges to the BMV.

The glossoptosis and the micrognathia make the glottic opening more angled and further anteriorly displaced leading to a more anterior view with the laryngoscope. Also, the nearly absent submental space makes it impossible to accommodate the tongue during laryngoscopy which renders the view obstructed by the tongue as well as the difficulty to align the oro-pharyngo-laryngeal axes. The presence of a cleft palate may prevent proper position of the laryngoscope blade in the oropharynx hence further complicating the view.

Despite the subglottic anatomy is usually being normal in PRS, it should be remembered that the cricothyroid space is extremely small in infants which makes emergency crico-thyroitomy an impractical option in case of the need of an emergency airway access, thus the presence of an ENT surgeon as a backup for emergency tracheotomy is recommended as an integral part of the airway management in children with PRS.

The main aim during anesthetic induction is to preserve spontaneous ventilation by avoiding muscle relaxants as not to "burn your bridges." This could be achieved via a careful titration of IV propofol (infusion/boluses) or through inhalation induction.

Should the scenario of "Cannot Ventilate" occur at any moment of the airway management in children with PRS, a backup plan of alternative ventilation/oxygenation techniques must be imminently applied which includes first a two-handed ventilation technique with oropharyngeal/nasopharyngeal airway, and if failed, an immediate insertion of an LMA.

In case of failure of the above techniques, a laryngoscopy attempt may be tried once as to relief the obstruction done by the tongue and resumption of spontaneous breathing, or to possibly intubate. Should it fail, a prompt decision to establish an emergent surgical airway access (tracheostomy) by the otolaryngologist must be taken immediately.

If intubation was difficult and traumatic, then extubation should not be attempted at the end of the procedure, but rather the patient should be appropriately sedated/paralyzed and transferred to the ICU for post-operative care where extubation should be delayed until the patient is fully awake and has a positive leak test, along with the appropriate set up for a re-intubation in case of airway obstruction/respiratory distress.

4.3 Craniofacial dysostosis

4.3.1 Apert syndrome

Overview: also known as acrocephalosyndactyly Type I, this syndrome encompasses the following characteristics: premature closure of the cranial sutures, syndactyly of hands and feet, mid-facial hypoplasia, and midline calvarial defects from the glabella to the posterior fontanelle. Cervical spine fusion mainly at the level of C5-C6 is commonly involved, in addition to congenital cardiac defects. It was initially described by Eugene Charles Apert, a French pediatrician, in 1906 [4] (**Figure 2**).

Genetics: the genetic inheritance is of autosomal dominant nature, but mainly occurs through sporadic gene mutations of the FGFR-2 gene, mapped to 10q26.

Incidence: 1:65,000 to 1:160,000 of births. Males and females are equally affected. This syndrome represents 5% of all craniosynostoses.

Pathophysiology: Apert syndrome entails abnormal osseous development. The cranium and the extremities are most commonly implicated.

Clinical considerations: Characteristically, these patients have high forehead and flat facies, resulting mainly from coronal suture involvement. Abnormal facies have also been characterized by spheno-ethmoid-maxillary hypoplasia, a bulbous-tipped nose, a sunken nasal bridge, and a high arched palate and cleft. Frequently

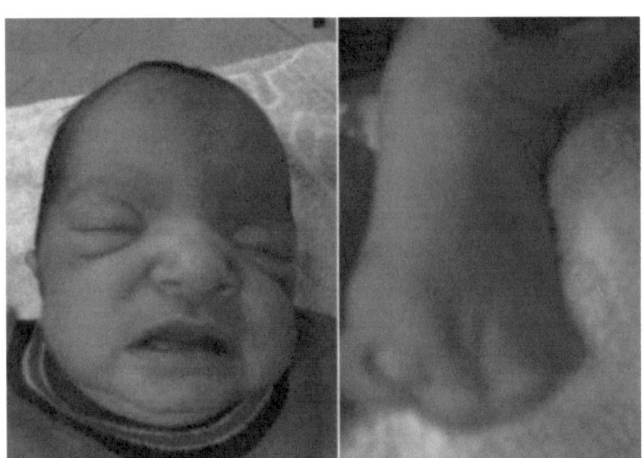

Figure 2.
Apert syndrome: prominent forehead, hypertelorism, proptosis, low set ears, open mouth, and feet with extensive syndactyly [19].

involved is choanal stenosis/atresia. In the context of the central nervous system, agenesis of the corpus callosum, hydrocephalus, an abnormal limbic system, and pyramidal tract have been portrayed. Early neurosurgical correction does not abate mental retardation in these patients. Seventy percent of these patients present with fusion of – more commonly – C5-C6 cervical vertebrae, although other levels may be involved. If limbs are involved, they often present with symmetric syndactyly (commonly the second, third, and fourth digits). Various joints (shoulders and hips) may be ankylotic or even aplastic. In the cardiac context, in 10% of the time, these anomalies involve patent ductus arteriosis (PDA), atrial septal defect (ASD), ventricular septal defect (VSD), Tetralogy of Fallot (TOF), pulmonary stenosis, or coarctation of the aorta. In the urologic context, 10% of these patients can present with polycystic kidneys, vaginal atresia, bicornuate uterus, hydronephrosis, and bladder neck stenosis. Airway/GI anomalies may occur in up to 2% of patients, including esophageal atresia, tracheoesophageal fistula, vertically fused tracheal rings, imperforate anus, biliary atresia, and pyloric stenosis [4, 7, 17].

Airway and anesthetic implications: thorough airway and head and neck evaluation is warranted prior to anesthesia administration in this condition. It would be important to ascertain whether there is any cervical spine fusion, abnormalities of the nasopharynx, palate, and/or trachea. Echocardiography is necessary to rule out congenital cardiac involvement. A chest radiograph may be indicated as many of these infants suffer respiratory complications during anesthesia. During anesthesia induction, one should prepare for likely difficult airway management. Maintenance of spontaneous ventilation until airway is secured is of vital importance. Alternate airway management techniques should be planned (video laryngoscope, fiberoptic intubation, and laryngeal mask airway). Depending on the type of the surgery, intravenous access and blood transfusion considerations are warranted accordingly [1, 20, 21].

4.3.2 Crouzon syndrome

Overview: this craniofacial dysostosis condition is very similar to Apert syndrome but does not necessarily involve extensive syndactyly. Crouzon syndrome is also known as acrocephalosyndactyly Type II. Clinical characters include hypertelorism (increased distance between the two orbits), exophthalmos, maxillary hypoplasia, and macrognathia. Initially designated by Octave Crouzon, a French neurologist, in 1912.

Genetics: autosomal dominant, but sporadic mutations occur in up to 50% of the cases. Genetically mapped to 10q26, encoding for the FGFR-2.

Incidence: 1:25,000 of births, with both males and females being equally affected, accounting for 4.5% of all cases of craniosynostoses.

Pathophysiology: the genetic mutation in this condition leads to accelerated maturation of osteoblastic cells, such that during fetal development, there is premature ossification of the calvaria leading to craniosynostosis (mainly involving the coronal, sagittal and at times the lambdoidal sutures).

Clinical considerations: maxillary hypoplasia associated with mandibular prognathism is commonly seen. Hypertelorism and proptosis are common ophthalmologic findings. It is common to find a high arched palate with a cleft and a bifid uvula. Choanal atresia has been demonstrated in Crouzon syndrome. Central nervous system findings include mental retardation, progressive hydrocephalus with associated intracranial hypertension, and very commonly an associated chronic herniation of the cerebellar tonsils. Twenty five percent of these patients present with cervical spine fusion most commonly at the level of C2-C3. Syndactyly is considered much less severe as compared to Apert syndrome [6, 7, 17].

Airway and anesthetic implications: Serious airway examination is necessary in this condition. Maxillary hypoplasia may lead to poor mask fit, and visualization of the vocal cords can be difficult with standard laryngoscopy. Choanal atresia must be assessed prior to anesthesia induction. Cervical spine fusion must be evaluated pre-operatively, as it can lead to difficulty with neck extension. One must also be mindful of intracranial pressure in the setting of progressive hydrocephalus and chronic tonsillar herniation. Depending on the degree of mental retardation, separation from family may pose a challenge. Difficult airway management is to be expected. Maintenance of spontaneous ventilation and oxygenation is necessary until the airway is secured. Alternate airway management techniques must be planned and pre-arranged (video laryngoscope, fiberoptic intubation, and laryngeal mask airway). A pre-operative echocardiograph is necessary, along with certain intraoperative management measures depending on the cardiac anomaly involved. Special consideration must include eyes protection in the setting of proptosis. Large bore intravenous access must be considered for major surgeries. In case of cranial vault reconstruction for craniosynostosis repair, the anesthesiologist must be mindful of the possibility of venous air embolism [1, 21, 22].

4.3.3 Pfeiffer syndrome

Overview: also known as acrocephalosyndactyly Type V, Pfeiffer syndrome involves sagittal craniosynostosis, maxillary retrusion of variable degrees, and soft tissue syndactyly. Mental retardation and congenital heart disease are commonly associated (**Figure 3**).

Genetics: it is autosomal recessive, with some cases presenting as de novo/sporadic mutations.

Incidence: extremely rare.

Pathophysiology: the genetic mutation involves the FGFR-1 and FGFR-1 genes involved in fetal mesenchymal integrity of the tissue that forms the bones, resulting in premature bony maturation and closure of the sutures, along with accelerated ossification of the calvaria.

Clinical considerations: much like Crouzon syndrome, Pfeiffer syndrome is commonly characterized by maxillary hypoplasia and flat facies, along with proptosis and hypertelorism. Strabismus is commonly present. This condition is linked to mild craniosynostosis and mainly involving the coronal and sagittal sutures. Limb findings are associated with broad thumb, great toe, and polysyndactyly. These

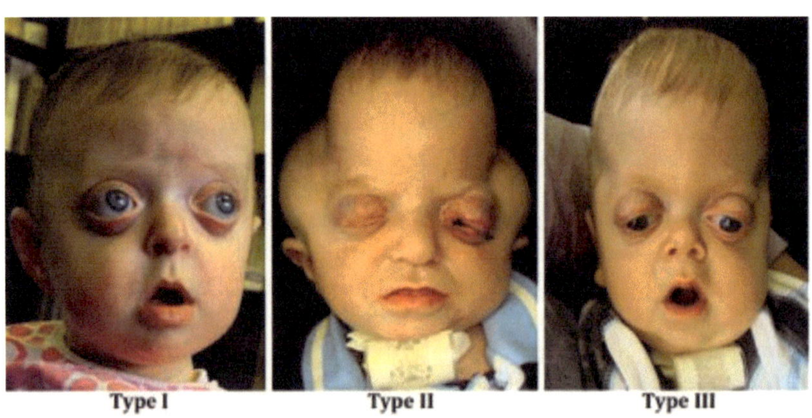

Figure 3.
Images of children with type 1,2,3 Pfeiffer syndrome [23].

patients also present with unpredictable degrees of hearing loss, mainly moderate to severe in most patients. Also, common findings are choanal atresia and cleft palate. Occasional associations include laryngomalacia, tracheomalacia, and bronchomalacia, along with fused cervical spine at varying levels in 30% of Pfeiffer syndrome patients. Other less common associations include Arnold-Chiari malformation, imperforate anus, and congenital heart disease [6, 7, 17].

Airway and anesthetic implications: the degree of mental retardation will dictate the difficulty of parental separation when shifting the patient to the operating room. Special consideration must include protecting the eyes in the presence of proptosis. Difficulty in airway management is to be expected and anticipated. Maintenance of spontaneous ventilation and oxygenation until the airway is secured is of vital importance. Alternate airway management techniques must be prepared and available (video laryngoscope, fiberoptic intubation, and laryngeal mask airway). Depending on the degree of congenital cardiac anomalies present, special considerations are to be undertaken. A large bore intravenous or central venous access is to be considered for more involved procedures, along with readiness for blood transfusion. In the setting of increased intracranial pressure, special consideration includes the maintenance of cerebral perfusion pressure intraoperatively, with a keen eye on mean arterial blood pressure [1, 24, 25].

4.4 Treacher Collins syndrome (TCS)

Overview: also known as mandibulofacial dysostosis or Franceschetti-Zwahlen-Klein syndrome, Treacher Collins syndrome (TCS) is recognized as being one of the most severe craniofacial malformation disorders and one of the most challenging airways encountered by an anesthesiologist [26]. Hallmark features include malar and mandibular hypoplasia, bilateral anotia or microtia often associated with bilateral conductive hearing loss, antimongoloid slanting of the eyelid fissures and lower lid colobomas. Although this syndrome was firstly described in 1846 by Thompson, and reported as a congenital disease with coloboma of the lower eyelids by George Andreas berry in 1889, its name is associated to a British ophthalmologist Edward Treacher Collins, who, in 1990 published a case report of two patients with these ocular and periorbital sequelae (**Figure 4**).

Genetics: known to be a very rare genetic disease, TCS results from a mutation on the TCOF1 gene in most individuals but rare cases were reported secondary to mutation of the POLR1C or POLR1D gene. It is an autosomal dominant inherited disorder. Only about 1% of cases are inherited in an autosomal recessive pattern [28].

Incidence: it has a prevalence of about 1 in 50,000 live births, without predisposition for sex or race.

Pathophysiology: this is a defect of the neural crest formation which affects the first and second branchial arches, grooves, and pouches during the second month of intrauterine life resulting in an oto-mandibular dysplasia associated with other craniofacial anomalies [28].

Clinical considerations: the clinical features associated with Treacher Collins syndrome involve the head and neck and appear to be bilateral with relatively symmetrical distribution. They are variable in severity, mainly including zygomatic, mandibular and maxillary hypoplasia, micrognathia, external ear malformations, hearing loss, high arched palate, antimongoloid slanting of the eyelid fissures, colobomas, total or partial absence of lower eyelashes, and midface bones hypoplasia resulting in a pathognomonic bird-like face appearance with a protruded nose and small rounded face. It may also impact the oral cavity with dental malocclusion and anterior open bite. The hypoplasia of the mandible is more severe at the condyle than at the ramus and the body, which could be potentially responsible for temporomandibular joint

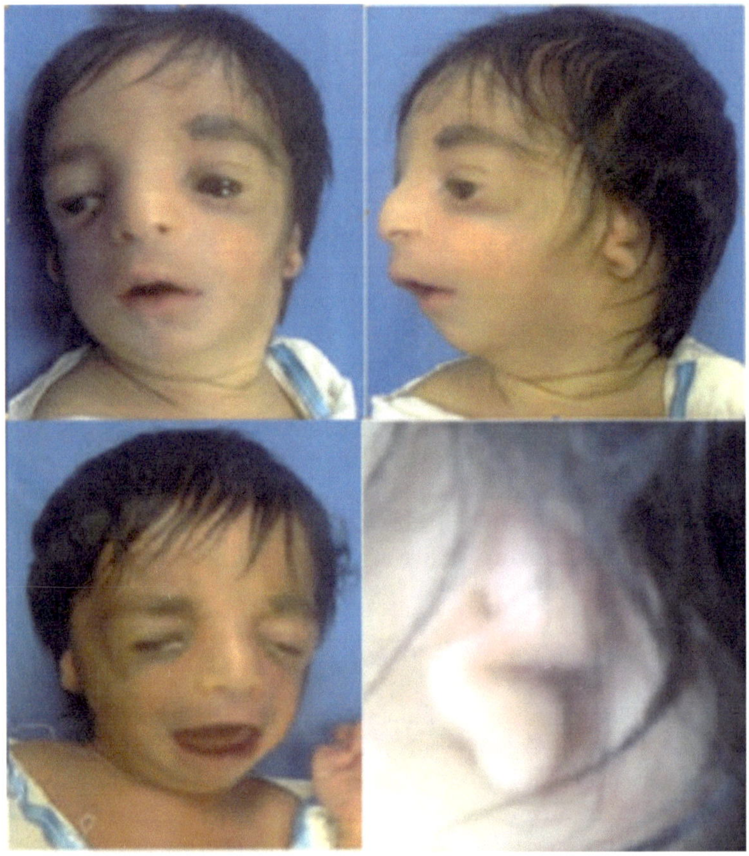

Figure 4.
Treacher Collins syndrome with characteristic facial features including downward and laterally slanting palpebral fissures, paucity of lashes and lack of naso-frontal angle, bird like appearance, micrognathia, microtia (deformed pinna), macrostomia, and large tongue [27].

dysfunction and mouth opening limitation. TCS is associated with Cleft Palate in 30% of the cases, and pharyngeal hypoplasia is commonly associated as well. All these anomalies can disrupt several functions like breathing, swallowing, chewing, and speech. Systemic manifestations, namely cardiac, renal, and skeletal, especially cervical vertebral defects, may also be observed [1, 4, 6, 7, 17].

Airway and anesthetic implications: Treacher Collins syndrome (TCS) was firstly reported as a hazard for general anesthesia in 1963 by Edward Ross due to the difficulty in maintaining a free and adequate airway. Several associated mechanisms are the cause, namely mandibular hypoplasia, micrognathia, retrognathia, posterior displacement of the bulky tongue, and the pharyngeal hypoplasia, resulting in a small and narrow retromandibular space [29, 30]. The presence of a temporomandibular joint abnormality or a small mouth aperture may further worsen the case. Thus, upper airway obstruction is common at induction of anesthesia and may require an airway manual maneuver (a two-hand mask ventilation, chin lift, and jaw thrust) and insertion of an oropharyngeal/nasopharyngeal airway. If unsuccessful, insertion of a supraglottic airway device such as a laryngeal mask airway before intubation is indicated. In addition, the failure rate of direct intubation is extremely high owing to the difficulty in alignment of the three axes (oral, pharyngeal, and laryngeal axes), which complicates further the visualization of the glottis. The degree of severity worsens with increasing age mainly because of the decreased mandibular growth.

A rigorous and warily planned algorithm is the success key in the management of the airways in children with Treacher Collins syndrome. Consultation of previous anesthesia records is of valuable aid, and a meticulous airway reassessment is required. A preoperative 3D tomographic images help assess anatomical features of the upper airway and guide the choice of the best airway management plan.

A laryngeal mask airway (LMA) is indicated for short and superficial procedures. But, whenever tracheal intubation is required, the spontaneous ventilation during anesthetic induction must be maintained until securing the airways. Fiberoptic intubation represents the preferred technique. It is facilitated by application of traction on the tongue, and a jaw thrust with a backward-upward-rightward pressure ("BURP") maneuver. Awake fiberoptic intubation is challenging in the pediatric population owing to the lack of cooperation. Other several techniques have been successfully used for tracheal intubation, namely fiberoptic intubation through LMA, fiberoptic-assisted laryngoscopy, blind nasal intubation, retrograde intubation, Shikani Optical Stylet (SOS), indirect videolaryngoscopy with GlideScope Ranger, Airtraq optical laryngoscope, Airway Scope or C-MAC videolaryngoscope with D-Blade, and tracheostomy as the last option. The use of TruView EVO2 laryngoscope for reintubation after accidental extubation in a neonate with TCS was also reported [26, 31].

TCS patients undergoing major surgical procedures involving the airway should be kept intubated and sedated in the intensive care unit (PICU) until subsidization of the edema. For short surgical superficial procedures not involving the airway, extubation may be attempted based on the clinical judgment of the anesthesiologist and the hospital set up. Before extubation, a nasopharyngeal airway must be inserted and maintained during the postoperative period in order to prevent upper airway obstruction.

4.5 Goldenhar's syndrome (GS)

Overview: Goldenhar's syndrome, also called Facio-auriculo-vertebral syndrome or Oculo-Auriculo-Vertebral syndrome, is a variant of hemifacial microsomia disorders that affect the eye, ear, nose, lip, soft palate, and mandible, and often associated with vertebral and cardiac anomalies. It was initially reported in 1952 by a Belgian-American ophthalmologist Maurice Goldenhar. In 1963, Gorlin introduced the term "Oculo-Auriculo-Vertebral syndrome" due to the presence of associated vertebral anomalies (**Figure 5**).

Genetics: the exact etiology remains unclear. Most cases are sporadic, but some rare familial cases were reported suggesting autosomal dominant or recessive inheritance [33].

Incidence: Goldenhar's syndrome occurs in about 1 in 3000 to 1 in 5000 live births, affecting males predominantly. Male to female ratio is 2:1.

Pathophysiology: this hemifacial microsomia is caused by the underdevelopment of the first and second branchial arches during the 4th week of gestation resulting in craniofacial anomalies, ocular anomalies, vertebral anomalies, and cardiac defects.

Clinical considerations: Goldenhar's syndrome (GS) is a multisystem syndrome with a wide spectrum of clinical features. Craniofacial anomalies are unilateral in 90% of the cases and include mandibular hypoplasia, hypoplastic zygomatic arch, micrognathia, macrostomia, external and middle ear malformations (microtia, preauricular appendages, and atresia) often with sensorineural hearing loss, and eye anomalies (epibulbar dermoids, lipodermoids, microphthalmos, and coloboma). Nevertheless, in 10% of cases both facial sides may be affected with one side typically more affected than the other. Oral cavity anomalies like palate anomalies

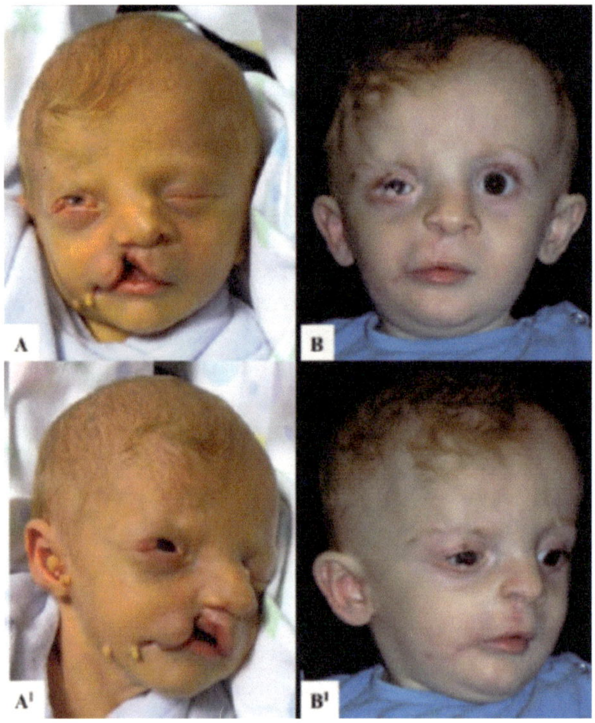

Figure 5.
Goldenhar's syndrome before and after surgical procedure for lip and palatoplasty, correction of macrostomia and nasal septum deformity, excision of pre-auricular tags: (A) preoperative; (B) postoperative [32].

(high arch or cleft) and tongue anomalies are often associated. Additionally, almost 50% of children with Goldenhar's syndrome may have vertebral defects, especially at the cervical level, such as hemivertebrae or hypoplasia, along with a potential risk of subluxation at the atlanto-occipital joint. Neck movements are limited during flexion and extension, increasing the rate of difficult or failed tracheal intubation procedure. Congenital cardiac structural malformations (Tetralogy of Fallot and septal defects) are present in about one third of the cases. In rare cases, some degrees of mental retardation and other systemic anomalies, mainly genitourinary, pulmonary, and vascular are reported [4, 6, 7, 17].

Airway and anesthetic implications: anesthesia or sedation may be provided for children with Goldenhar's syndrome for various procedures (ear reconstruction, distraction osteogenesis, soft tissue reconstruction, skin graft, cardiac, etc.).

The anesthetic management is risky because of the difficult airway. The degree of difficulties depends directly on the severity of craniofacial anomalies and associated vertebral defects and tends to worsen progressively with increasing age. Detecting patients at risk in the preoperative setting may anticipate challenging airway situations. Consultation of previous anesthesia records is of a valuable help; however, the airway must be reassessed before any new airway manipulation. The degree of severity of mandibular hypoplasia correlates with difficult tracheal intubation. Virtual imaging using 3D CT or cone-beam computed tomography may be indicated for selected patients to assess the airway anatomy looking for anomalies [34].

Facemask ventilation is challenging in children with Goldenhar's syndrome due to a poor mask seal, often requiring the use of a gauze with self-adhesive tape to provide an adequate seal. The reason for this poor mask fit is the facial asymmetry and the presence of a soft tissue slit extended from the side of the mouth to the middle of the cheek on the abnormal hemi-face.

Tracheal intubation is usually more difficult to achieve than maintaining airway patency, especially in the case right-sided hemifacial microsomia. Several combined conditions may contribute to difficult intubation, including retrognathia, micrognathia, asymmetrical hypoplasia of the mandible, limited mouth opening, palatal anomalies, potentially associated vertebral defects, and limited neck motion. The hypoplastic mandible reduces the retromandibular space. The relatively bulky tongue is displaced posteriorly overhanging the larynx, thus making visualization of the vocal inlets difficult, even nearly impossible during conventional laryngoscopy.

Although fiberoptic intubation (FOB) technique is one of the popular options for securing difficult airways of patients with GS, various strategies can be adopted successfully to perform tracheal intubation; however, it is recommended that the airway operator sticks with the tool and technique that is the most familiar to his practice. These include: FOB through LMA (video-assisted fiberoptic intubation (VAFI)), GlideScope, Air-Q, Airtraq, C-MAC D-blade or C-MAC Miller-blade videolaryngoscopy, Pentax-AWS Airwayscope with tracheal introducer, Laryngeal Mask Airway helped by Pediatric Boussignac Bougie or retrograde tracheal intubation. The Truview PCD® laryngoscopy has proven its effectiveness and offers the advantage of continuously supplying oxygen via its oxygenation side port during the procedure. When the intubation is not required, LMA or nasopharyngeal airway constitutes a possible alternative [1, 35, 36].

4.6 Klippel-Feil syndrome (KFS)

Overview: it was initially described by Klippel and Feil in 1912 as a clinical triad of an extremely short "compressed" neck, a low hairline at the rear end of the skull, and a limited mobility of the neck caused by fusion of two or more cervical vertebrae. Despite being discovered as a triad, it is not uncommon for patients with KFS to meet just one clinical criterion of the above. It may be associated with other anomalies (**Figure 6**).

Genetics: Klippel-Feil syndrome is an inherited autosomal dominant condition. It is the result of an anomalous partition of the cervical somites during embryogenesis between the third and eighth week of gestation.

Incidence: KFS has a prevalence of 1:40000 to 1:42000 of live births.

Clinical considerations: KFS is classified into three classes according to the level and severity of the spine fusion, with type 1 representing a considerable fusion of numerous cervical vertebrae, type 2 representing fusions of one or two cervical vertebrae, and type 3 representing cervical vertebrae fusions combined with thoracic and/or lumbar vertebral fusions.

KPS may be related to other anomalies such as cranio-facial deformities including craniosynostosis, cleft lip, micrognathia, and laryngeal defects. Thoracic deformities such as scoliosis may be present in addition to other skeletal deformities like scapular elevation (Sprengel's). Uro-genital malformations are commonly present as well as congenital heart defects most commonly the VSD.

Neurological deficits with hyperlaxed cervical spines and neuro-degeneration with fused spines are commonly associated with KPS [17].

Airway and anesthetic implications: KFS is often associated with difficult intubation, evidently because of the fixed neck which does not allow proper extension of the atlanto-axial joint during laryngoscopy and the subsequent advanced Cormack-Lehane view. Many reports describe a grade 4 view with a conventional laryngoscope.

Screening patients at risk for cervical spine instability is a crucial step before airway management in order to avoid spinal injury, especially those with

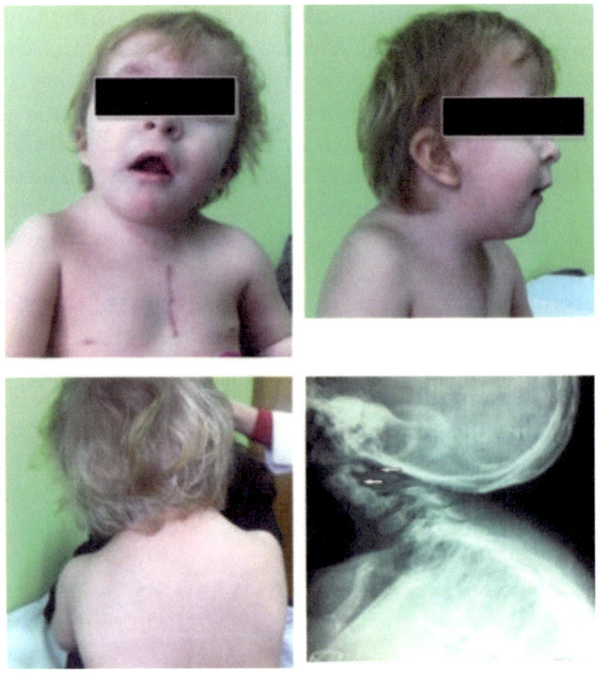

Figure 6.
Child with Klippel-Feil syndrome and anomaly of the Occipito-cervical junction. The images show an elevated left shoulder due to a Sprengel anomaly, a short, webbed neck, and a low hairline (scar on the thorax after surgical repair of nonrestrictive atrial septal defect) [37].

hyperlaxed spines who may require C-spine precautions with in-line-stabilization during intubation. This is performed via a lateral neck X-ray in flexion and extension positions [1, 4–7].

Obstructive sleep apnea (OSA) is not uncommonly encountered in patients with KFS, hence a preoperative sleep study may be indicated along with postoperative apnea monitor. A preoperative echocardiography must be considered especially in patients with pulmonary hypertension secondary to OSA and scoliosis.

A history of previous smooth intubation in KPS patient does not implicate a future favorable outcome due to the progressive nature of the disease. Hence, a careful preoperative assessment and planning is critical for safe airway management.

Bag-mask ventilation is likely difficult in those patients as well as direct laryngoscopy owing to the fixed neck or the in-line neck stabilization.

Should the older child be cooperative enough to sustain an awake fiberoptic intubation (with light sedation) that would be the approach of choice avoiding both the risks of difficult ventilation and neck injury secondary to airway manipulation.

Otherwise, a plan to preserve spontaneous ventilation during anesthetic induction should be performed with either total intravenous anesthesia (TIVA) or inhaled Sevoflurane (IV Dexmedetomidine and IV Ketamine can be used as well) avoiding the use of neuro-muscular blockers.

A trial of manual bag-mask to assess for ventilation is used by some practitioners before airway manipulation. The various arrays of airway tools including videoscopes (Glidescope/C-MAC etc.) as well as the fiberoptic bronchoscope have been used successfully for intubation in patients with KFS. They are preferred as first line intubation technique due to the lower incidence of cervical spine mobilization when used.

It is important to keep in mind that the option of an emergency surgical airway such as cricothyrotomy/tracheostomy is very limited in patients with KFS due to the extremely short neck, thus the airway approach must be very carefully planned.

Extubation must only be attempted when the patient is fully awake and in the presence of protective airway reflexes. An opioid-sparing anesthetic technique is recommended (regional anesthesia whenever possible) as the presence of OSA may increase narcotic-sensitivity. KFS patients should preferably be monitored in the post-operative setting in a high dependency unit or an intensive care unit according to the severity of their cardio-pulmonary and airway pathology.

If the patient is on a home BIPAP, it will be required after extubation.

4.7 Beckwith-Wiedemann syndrome

Overview: it was initially reported by J Bruce Beckwith and Hans-Rudolf Wiedemann. It is one of the syndromes associated with a huge tongue that may impose challenges to airway management (**Figure 7**).

Genetics: it is caused by genetic alterations on chromosome 11p15 region.

Incidence: 1 per 13,700–15,000 of live births.

Clinical considerations: Beckwith-Wiedemann syndrome is characterized by a clinical tetrad of macroglossia (Most common), omphalocele, umbilical hernia, and neonatal hypoglycemia.

These children are associated with exomphalos, macroglossia, gigantism, macrosomia, visceromegaly, horizontal earlobe creases, renal medullary dysplasia, cardiac malformations, hypoglycemia, hypothyroidism, hyperlipidemia, polycythemia, hypercalciuria, and embryonal tumors. The presence of three features out of the above will confirm the clinical diagnosis of BWS after ruling out the clinical features of overgrowth syndromes. The risk for embryonal tumor development especially hepatoblastoma, neuroblastoma, rhabdomyosarcoma, gonadoblastoma, and adrenal carcinoma has been observed [6, 7, 17].

Airway and anesthetic implications: the main anesthetic considerations in BWS are abnormal airway anatomy, hypoglycemia, and cardiac anomalies (cardiomegaly and other cardiac structural defects). A detailed pre-operative assessment of the airway, the cardiac, and the urinary system is mandatory. Visceromegaly may shift the diaphragm upward reducing functional residual capacity. Associated congenital malformations, prematurity, and interventions early in life may complicate anesthetic management. These children frequently require corrective surgical

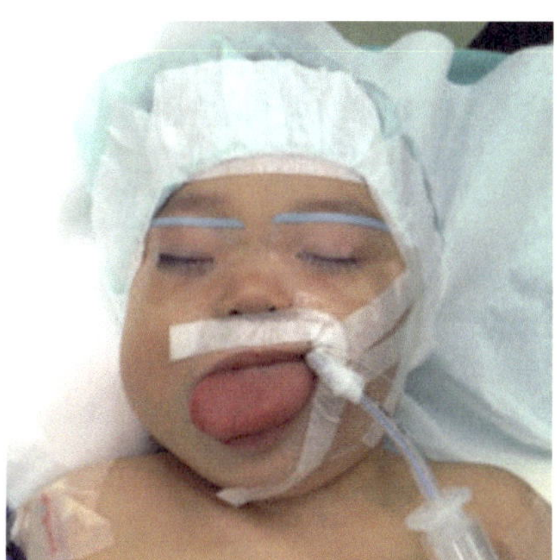

Figure 7.
Macroglossia in the patient with Beckwith-Wiedemann syndrome after intubation [38].

interventions in infancy such as tongue reduction surgeries, hernia repair, exomphalos repair or hepatectomy.

Preoperative assessment should include a careful evaluation of the airway focusing on the mouth opening, tongue size, and preoperative head and neck imaging if required. It should focus also on other systems involvement such as the heart, hence an echocardiography is recommended. The genito-urinary system and the liver must be evaluated in addition to the preoperative glucose homeostasis.

The major challenge during airway management of a patient with Beckwith-Wiedemann syndrome pertains to the huge tongue which might completely obstruct the airway with anesthetic induction rendering the bag-mask ventilation and intubation difficult to perform [39, 40].

Hence a careful plan A, with a backup plan B and a plan C must be organized beforehand. An intravenous line is recommended to be secured before induction. Keeping spontaneous ventilation is considered to be the safest approach to the airway that can be achieved with intravenous anesthetics or inhalational Sevoflurane and by avoiding non-depolarizing neuro-muscular blockers. Some practices may use muscle relaxants after making sure of the ability to ventilate by a trial of ventilation after induction. Sugammadex muscle (rocuronium antidote) has allowed more confidence for anesthesiologists to give muscle relaxants in order to facilitate intubation.

A variety of tools can be used for intubation ranging from the direct laryngoscopes aided by a Gum elastic Bougie or a stylet, to the Videoscopes including the C-MAC and the Glidescope, to the fiberoptic bronchoscope.

A plan B consists of inserting a laryngeal mask airway should ventilation become problematic, and in case of the latter's failure, a plan C with a surgical airway must be immediately implemented.

Extubation must only occur when patient is fully awake and may be helped with a nasopharyngeal airway "in-situ" to help overcoming the tongue's obstruction in the immediate post-operative period. Patients with BWS must have a post-operative monitoring after surgery in the high dependency area or the intensive care unit.

4.8 Mucopolysaccharidosis (MPS)

Overview: the mucopolysaccharidoses (MPS) are a set of storage diseases caused by a disordered or absent lysosomal hydroxylase enzyme leading to the build-up of muco-polysaccharides (glycosaminoglycans (GAG)) in the connective tissues, the musculo-skeletal system and the visceral organs. They are classified as seven syndromes with each involving a mix of 11 enzymatic disorders [41]. Mucopolysaccharidoses patients are associated with a high incidence of difficult bag-mask ventilation which represents the "nightmare" for the anesthesiologist or the airway operator.

Incidence: as a rare set of conditions, MPS accounts for less than 0.1% of all genetic but have been reported throughout the world in various forms. Region and ethnic background may affect the phenotype of MPS.

Genetic: inheritance autosomal recessive.

Pathophysiology: the mutation in lysosomal hydroxylase enzyme leads to an impaired metabolism of mucopolysaccharides (GAG) which will accumulate in multiple body tissues leading to macroglossia, adenotonsillar hypertrophy, and laryngeal/tracheal tissue distortion and narrowing.

Some types of MPS (Type1: Hurler, Type 4: Morquio, and Type 6: Maroteaux-Lamy) may be associated with atlantoaxial subluxation and odontoid hypoplasia which may lead to spinal cord compression with subsequent neurological deficit. Accumulation in the cervical spines may lead to a short and fixed neck. The temporo-mandibular joint may get affected with restricted mobility. Deposition of mucopolysaccharides in the heart and vascular tissues may lead to cardiomyopathies, arrhythmias, and pulmonary hypertension [5].

Clinical considerations and airway management: difficult ventilation and intubation are common concerns in patients with mucopolysaccharidoses as the thick and uncompliant infiltrated tissues (skin, tongue, and mucous membranes of the airway, bones, and joints) may render the natural airway narrow and not distensible by the positive pressure ventilation applied by the bag-mask. Laryngoscopy is often challenging due to difficult manipulation of the laryngoscope as a result of the stiff and thick tissues. The large tongue, the hypertrophied tonsils, and the limited mouth opening are caused by the immobile temporo-mandibular joints [40]. This effect is compounded if there is a subluxation of the atlanto-axial joint or cervical-spine affection which mandates an in-line-stabilization during airway management.

A narrow/distorted trachea may prevent an appropriately sized endotracheal tube from passing throughout the vocal cords.

Fortunately, the enzymatic replacement therapy may hinder the progression of the disease, hence an adequately treated mucopolysaccharidosis patient may have a lesser risk of difficult airway than the untreated patient.

Preoperatively, the MPS patient must be well assessed for the extent of the disease as well as a focused airway assessment including the mouth opening, tongue and tonsillar size, presence of obstructive sleep apnea (which is very common in MPS), and pulmonary hypertension. A preoperative echocardiography is essential to rule out any associated cardiomyopathy. Patients with MPS type 1 (Hurler), 4 (Morquio), and 6 must be checked for any cervical spine or atlanto-axial instability [42].

Intravenous cannulation in MPS patients may be challenging due to the thick infiltrated skin, hence a preoperatively inserted intravenous line before anesthetic induction is preferable.

Spontaneous ventilation must be maintained during induction of anesthesia due to the high risk of difficult ventilation in case of apnea. This could be achieved with either intravenous or inhalational induction agents and by avoiding neuro-muscular blockers.

An LMA must be used as a second plan whenever encountering difficulties in ventilation; it can also be used to facilitate fiberoptic intubation.

Video-laryngoscopies are other favorable options for intubation in MPS patients especially those with unstable cervical spine owing to the lesser risk of neck mobilization when used. Establishment of a surgical airway access such as tracheostomy may be difficult due to the thick tissues and the associated tracheal deformities.

5. Craniofacial vascular malformations (VMs)

Vascular anomalies are disorders of abnormal vasculogenesis or lymphogenesis. They can involve any part of body and can present in any phase of development. They include different types according to histopathology and anatomical site.

VMs may be with other syndromic malformations such as Parkes-Weber, Sturge-Weber, Klippel-Trenaunay Servelle-Martorell, PHACE and LUMBAR syndromes.

5.1 Subglottic hemangiomas

Overview: infantile hemangioma (IH) is the most prevalent vascular anomaly of the head and neck. It may cause a life-threatening airway obstruction if located in the glottic/subglottic area.

Incidence: its prevalence is approximately 4–5% mainly in fair-skinned kids. It is more common in girls and commonly associated with cutaneous hemangiomas.

Pathophysiology: the infantile hemangioma is a benign proliferative disorder of the vascular endothelial-like cells. It is believed to be due to a dysregulated angiogenesis resulting in neovascularization caused by the disordered differentiation of the embryonic mesenchymal cells. It has two phases, a proliferative one which starts as early as the first few weeks of life and continues progression and growth in size until late childhood, and an involution phase where the tumor begins shrinking in size until complete disappearance which is eventually due to the replacement of the endothelial cells with fibroblasts and fat cells. IH may occur at any place in the head and neck, starting as a small lump and then enlarging in size. Patients with IH are usually asymptomatic unless the tumor is present in the airway and reaches considerable size to cause obstructive symptoms. Hemangiomas of the airway may cause snoring, hemoptysis, hoarseness, stridor, and respiratory distress, which requires early intervention. Propranolol therapy plays a great role in its shrinkage [43].

Airway evaluation and management: history, imaging (MRI), and endoscopic studies are essential in the preoperative evaluation. Patients with glottic/subglottic lesions may easily get airway obstruction upon anesthetic induction. An LMA/supraglottic for rescue ventilation may not be an option if the obstruction is infraglottic. Laryngoscopy and intubation may be complicated by bleeding if the tumor is traumatized which may completely impede the view and render airway management more challenging. Preserving spontaneous breathing with either inhalational or intravenous anesthetic and avoiding muscle relaxants is a safe approach until the airway is secured. Postoperative extubation should not be attempted until resolution of the airway edema. Intensive care (PICU) and postoperative steroids are indicated after major airway lesions endoscopic excision.

5.2 Lymphatic/lymphaticovenous malformations (cystic hygroma)

Overview: also called cavernous hemangioma. It is a multi-loculated benign congenital tumor affecting preferably the head and neck. It can present as a neck mass on prenatal ultrasound [5]. Airway compromise can be the sequelae of direct compression from the mass and/or bony changes following mandibulomaxillary hypertrophy (**Figure 8**).

Incidence: approximately 1 in 6000 live births, 70–80% occur in the neck, usually in the post cervical triangle.

Pathophysiology: it is a combination of lymphatic and venous cells. They may present at different sizes and progress in growth after birth. It might get complicated with bleeding or infection which may considerably increase their size. The clinical presentations are related to its size and the anatomy involved.

Clinical evaluation and airway management: large masses involving the airway can cause potential airway compromise according to the location and the size of the tumor. Tracheal compressions can be present with neck and mediastinal lesions. Tongue, pharyngeal or laryngeal involvement may present with significant airway obstruction. The treatment is often LASER or surgical excision and always requires a pre-inserted tracheostomy or an "in place" endotracheal tube prior to the procedure. Imaging is required in all cases, and tumors located in the mediastinum require further investigation. Sedatives should be used with caution because of their potential to aggravate the airway obstruction. Maintaining spontaneous ventilation via inhalational or intravenous induction is the cornerstone of a safe anesthetic approach when managing the airway of patients with CH. In case of complex and high-risk lesions, a tracheostomy under local anesthesia may be indicated prior to the procedure. Aspirating the cyst to shrink its size prior to

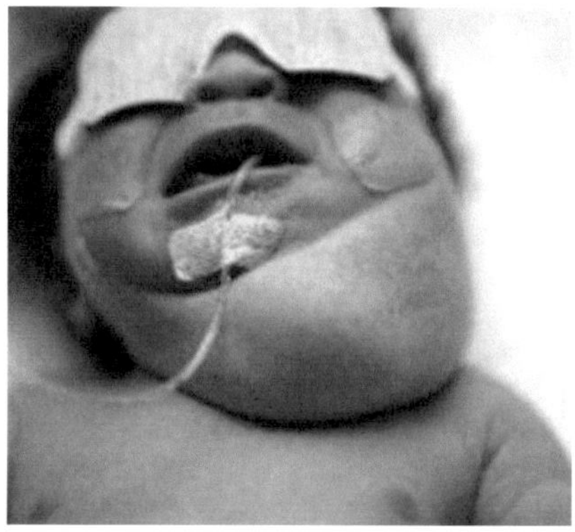

Figure 8.
Huge movable mass is found out on the left neck [44].

facilitate intubation has been reported but at the expense of complicating further the surgery. Post-operative intensive care (PICU) monitoring is indicated for high-risk lesions [45, 46].

5.3 Arterio-venous malformations

Arterio-venous malformations (AVM) involving the face and the airway are rare to occur. The main issue with airway management is the risk of massive bleeding that can occur if the AVM has been traumatized when managing the airway.

Clinical evaluation and airway management of children with vascular malformations involving the airway: a thorough preoperative history and physical exam are of utmost importance in anticipating a potentially difficult airway in children with vascular malformations. Clinical imaging (CT, MRI and 3-D reconstruction) and endoscopic evaluation may be necessary to establish the diagnosis and identify the size and location of the pathology. Even with a meticulous airway evaluation, an unanticipated difficult airway can still occur, hence an effective preparation before airway evaluation is crucial. An airway management strategy should be tailored according to each patient's airway pathology including a back-up approach should the initial one fails and an emergency rescue plan [47].

General anesthesia with an inhaled agent such as Sevoflurane or an intravenous agent (such as propofol, ketamine or dexmedetomidine) while maintaining spontaneous ventilation is the technique of choice. Video laryngoscopy, FOB-guided endotracheal intubation, and endotracheal intubation through an LMA are the most popular strategies for intubation.

A pre-procedure tracheostomy inserted under local anesthesia may be indicated for high risk malformations with severe airway obstruction [48].

6. Conclusion

The airway management of children with craniofacial abnormalities imposes great challenges owing to the difficulties in ventilation and intubation potentially encountered in most of the syndromes as well as the other systems involvement. A careful anticipation, preparation, and planning are key elements for a safe and successful airway management. The approach to each patient should be tailored according to the extent of the relevant abnormalities following a strategy of a simple clear plan A with a backup plan B and C. Preserving spontaneous breathing is one of the safe practices when patients are at risk of difficult ventilation. The use of the most familiar airway tools is pivotal in achieving favorable results. Extubation is an integral part of the airway management and should only be performed when the child meets its criteria and in a controlled environment. Post-extubation monitoring in a critical care or an observation area must be carried out for patients at risk of airway obstruction.

Acknowledgements

Special thanks for Dr. Habib El Bechouti, senior anesthesia consultant in Sidra Medicine, Qatar and Dr. Yasser Hammad, senior anesthesia consultant in Hamad Medical Corporation, Qatar for their valuable comments, chapter editing, and reviewing.

Conflict of interest

The authors declare no conflict of interest.

Author details

Brahim Boudjenah[1*], Al Moataz Billah Adham[2], Surendra M. Chinnappa[1], Omed Assaf[1] and Mashael Al-Khelaifi[1]

1 Hamad Medical Corporation, Doha, Qatar

2 Sidra Medicine, Doha, Qatar

*Address all correspondence to: bboudjenah@hamad.qa

References

[1] Raj D, Luginbuehl I. Managing the difficult airway in the syndromic child. Continuing Education in Anaesthesia, Critical Care & Pain. 2015;**15**(1):7-13. DOI: 10.1093/bjaceaccp/mku004

[2] Waisel DB, Truog RD, Todres ID. Ethical issues in pediatric anesthesiology. In: Cote CJ, Lerman J, Todres ID, editors. The Pediatric Airway. 4th ed. Vol. 8. Philadelphia, PA: Saunders Elsevier; 2009. pp. 71-87

[3] Krishna SG, Bryant JF, Tobias JD. Management of the difficult airway in the pediatric patient. Journal of Pediatric Intensive Care. 2018;**7**(3): 115-125. DOI: 10.1055/s-0038-1624576

[4] Mann D, Garcia PJ, Andropoulos DB. Anesthesia for the patient with a genetic syndrome. In: Andropoulos DB, Gregory GA, editors. Gregory's Pediatric Anesthesia. 6th ed. Wiley-Blackwell; 2020. pp. 1085-1105. DOI: 10.1002/9781444345186.ch38

[5] Oliveira CRD. Pediatric syndromes with noncraniofacial anomalies impacting the airways. Paediatric Anaesthesia. 2020;**30**(3):304-310. DOI: 10.1111/pan.13810

[6] Garcia-Marcinkiewicz AG, Stricker PA. Craniofacial surgery and specific airway problems. Pediatric Anesthesia. 2020;**30**:296-303. DOI: 10.1111/pan.13790

[7] Nargozian C. The airway in patients with craniofacial abnormalities. Paediatric Anaesthesia. 2004;**14**(1):53-59. DOI: 10.1046/j.1460-9592.2003.01200.x

[8] Antonarakis SE, Skotko BG, Rafii MS, et al. Down syndrome. Nature Reviews. Disease Primers. 2020;**6**(1):9. DOI: 10.1038/s41572-019-0143-7

[9] Stoll C, Dott B, Alembik Y, Roth MP. Associated congenital anomalies among cases with Down syndrome. European Journal of Medical Genetics. 2015;**58**(12):674-680. DOI: 10.1016/j.ejmg.2015.11.003

[10] Korayem M, Nuha MA, Waleed B, Eman A, Wafa A, Reem A. Craniofacial manifestations of Down syndrome: A review of literature. Academia Journal of Scientific Research. 2019;**7**(3):176-181

[11] De Lausnay M, Verhulst S, Boel L, Wojciechowski M, Boudewyns A, Van Hoorenbeeck K. The prevalence of lower airway anomalies in children with Down syndrome compared to controls. Pediatric Pulmonology. 2020;**55**(5):1259-1263. DOI: 10.1002/ppul.24741

[12] Lewanda AF, Matisoff A, Revenis M, et al. Preoperative evaluation and comprehensive risk assessment for children with Down syndrome. Paediatric Anaesthesia. 2016;**26**(4): 356-362. DOI: 10.1111/pan.12841

[13] Rodrigues M, Nunes J, Figueiredo S. Neuroimaging assessment in Down syndrome: A pictorial review. Insights into Imaging. 2019;**10**:52. DOI: 10.1186/s13244-019-0729-3

[14] Cladis F, Kumar A, Grunwaldt L, Otteson T, Ford M, Losee JE. Pierre Robin sequence: A perioperative review. Anesthesia and Analgesia. 2014;**119**(2):400-412. DOI: 10.1213/ANE.0000000000000301

[15] Izumi K, Konczal LL, Mitchell AL, Jones MC. Underlying genetic diagnosis of Pierre Robin sequence: Retrospective chart review at two children's hospitals and a systematic literature review. The Journal of Pediatrics. 2012;**160**(4):645-650.e2. DOI: 10.1016/j.jpeds.2011.09.021

[16] Kılıç SC, Kılıç N, Oktay H, Kiki A. Pierre Robin sequence from orthodontic and surgical perspective. World Journal

of Stomatology. 2014;**3**(4):30-37. DOI: 10.5321/wjs.v3.i4.30

[17] Bissonnette B, Luginbuehl I, Marciniak B, Dalens B. Syndromes: Rapid Recognition and Perioperative Implications. New York: McGraw-Hill Education; 2006. Available from: https://accessanesthesiology.mhmedical.com/book.aspx?bookid=852

[18] Elmatite W, Haykal N, Upadhyay S, Pizzuto M, Watt S. Airway management in neonates with Pierre Robin syndrome along with Mobius syndrome and platoglossal fusion. Journal of Anesthesia and Clinical Research. 2017;**8**:1000757. DOI: 10.4172/2155-6148.1000757

[19] Panigrahi I. Craniosynostosis genetics: The mystery unfolds. Indian Journal of Human Genetics. 2011;**17**(2):48-53. DOI: 10.4103/0971-6866.86171

[20] Nargozian C. Apert syndrome. Anesthetic management. Clinics in Plastic Surgery. 1991;**18**:227

[21] Cinalli G, Renier D, Sebag G, et al. Chronic tonsillar herniation in Crouzon's and Apert's syndromes: The role of premature synostosis of the lamboid sutures. Journal of Neurosurgery. 1995;**83**:575

[22] Sculerati N, Gottlieb MD, Zimbler MS. Airway management in children with major craniofacial anomalies. Laryngoscope. 1998;**108**:1806

[23] Amjadi H. The role of genetic mutations in genes FGFR1 & FGFR2 in Pfeiffer syndrome. Journal of Pediatrics and Neonatal Medicine. 2019;**1**(2):110

[24] Digilio MC, Marino B, Borzaga U, Giannotti A, Dallapiccola B. Intrafamilial variability of Pfieffer-type cardiocranial syndrome. American Journal of Medical Genetics. 1997;**73**:480

[25] Meyer P, Renier D, Blanot S, Orliaguet G, Arnaud E, Lajeunie E. Anesthesia and intensive care of craniostenosis and craniofacial dysmorphism in children. Ann Fr Anesth Reanim. 1997;**16**:152

[26] Hosking J, Zoanetti D, Carlyle A, Anderson P, Costi D. Anesthesia for Treacher Collins syndrome: A review of airway management in 240 pediatric cases. Pediatric Anesthesia. 2012;**22**:752-758

[27] Al-Mosawi AJ. Genetic and hereditary disorders in Iraqi children. Annals of Medical & Surgical Case Reports: AMSCR-1000011; 2019

[28] Duque C, Lopes Cardoso I. Treacher Collins syndrome and implications in the oral cavity. Clinical Research and Trials. 2019;**5**:1-5. DOI: 10.15761/CRT.1000278

[29] Ribeiro A d A, Smith FJ, Nary Filho H, Trindade IEK, Tonello C, Trindade-Suedam IK. Three-dimensional upper airway assessment in Treacher Collins syndrome. The Cleft Palate-Craniofacial Journal. 2020;**57**(3):371-377. DOI: 10.1177/1055665619885555

[30] Ma X, Forte AJ, Berlin NL, Alonso N, Persing JA, Steinbacher DM. Reduced three-dimensional nasal airway volume in Treacher Collins syndrome and its association with craniofacial morphology. Plastic and Reconstructive Surgery. 2015;**135**(5):885e-894e. DOI: 10.1097/PRS.0000000000001160

[31] Ratnamma V, Navaratnarajah J. 141 Treacher Collins syndrome – Retrospective review of airway management techniques. Archives of Disease in Childhood. 2018;**103**:A56-A57. DOI: 10.1136/goshabs.141

[32] Villani R, Michelina VV, Fabbri E, Zarabini AG, Morselli PG. Goldenhar

syndrome: Surgical planning in a severe case with cleft lip and palate, coloboma and macrostomia. JSM Head and Face Medicine. 2017;**2**(1):1003

[33] Bogusiak K, Puch A, Arkuszewski P. Goldenhar syndrome: Current perspectives. World Journal of Pediatrics. 2017;**13**(5):405-415. DOI: 10.1007/s12519-017-0048-z

[34] Molins G, Valls A, Guijarro R, Hernández-Alfaro F. Mandibular hypoplasia and narrow airway in Goldenhar syndrome: Anticipation of difficult intubation with cone-beam computed tomography. Journal of Clinical Anesthesia. 2016;**34**:1-2. DOI: 10.1016/j.jclinane.2016.03.031

[35] Orozco ST, Latorre JLR, Saldarriaga CA. Infant with Goldenhar syndrome: Failed intubation and rescue using fiberoptic and i-gel laryngeal mask. Trends in Anaesthesia and Critical Care. 2020;**30**:e30. DOI: 10.1016/j.tacc.2019.12.077

[36] Sinha R, Pangasa N, Nethaji R, Maitra S. Successful use of C-MAC Miller blade in neonate with Goldenhar syndrome and cleft lip with cleft palate: A case report. Acta Anaesthesiologica Belgica. 2019;**70**:39-41

[37] Bejiqi R, Retkoceri R, Maloku A, Bejiqi R, Mustafa A, et al. How often is Klippel-Feil syndrome associated with congential heart disease presentation of five cases and a review of the literature. Journal of Cardiology and Cardiovascular Medicine. 2019;**4**:110-116. DOI: 10.29328/journal.jccm.1001050

[38] Tsukamoto M, Hitosugi T, Yokoyama T. Perioperative airway management of a patient with Beckwith-Wiedemann syndrome. Journal of Dental Anesthesia and Pain Medicine. 2016;**16, 4**:313-316. DOI: 10.17245/jdapm.2016.16.4.313

[39] Batra M, Valecha UK. Anesthetic management of tongue reduction in a case of Beckwith-Wiedemann syndrome. Journal of Anaesthesiology Clinical Pharmacology. 2014;**30**:562-564

[40] Channabasapa SM, Pradeep SH, Dharmapa S, Sarji D. Anesthetic management of a neonate with Beckwith-Wiedemann syndrome posted for repair of exomphalos. Saudi Journal of Anaesthesia. 2016;**10**:249-250

[41] Kloesel B, Holzman RS. Anesthetic management of patients with inborn errors of metabolism. Anesthesia and Analgesia. 2017;**125**:822-836

[42] Walker R, Belani KG, Braunlin EA, Bruce IA, Hack H, Harmatz PR, et al. Anaesthesia and airway management in mucopolysaccharidosis. Journal of Inherited Metabolic Disease. 2013;**36**:211-219

[43] Shayan YR, Prendiville JS, Goldman RD. Use of propranolol in treating hemangiomas. Canadian Family Physician. 2011;**57**(3):302-303

[44] Hyunzu K, Hyuk-Soo K, Jung-Tak O, Jeong RL. Anesthetic management for neonate with giant cystic hygroma involved upper airway – A case report. Korean Journal of Anesthesiology. 2011;**60**(3):209-213. DOI: 10.4097/kjae.2011.60.3.209

[45] Rao KS, Shenoy T. Anesthetic management of a large cystic hygroma in a newborn. Anesthesia, Essays and Researches. 2015;**9**(2):270-272

[46] Braga AFA, Frias JAF, Braga FSS, et al. Anestesia para tratamento intraparto extra-útero em feto com diagnóstico pré-natal de higroma na região cervical. Revista Brasileira de Anestesiologia. 2006;**56**(3):278-286

[47] Clarke C, Lee EI, Edmonds J Jr. Vascular anomalies and airway concerns. Seminars in Plastic

Surgery. 2014;**28**(2):104-110. DOI: 10.1055/s-0034-1376265

[48] Jacobs IN, Cahill AM. Special considerations in vascular anomalies: Airway management. Clinics in Plastic Surgery. 2011;**38**(1):121-131. DOI: 10.1016/j.cps.2010.08.008

Chapter 10

Airway Management during Pregnancy and Labor

Kemal Tolga Saracoglu, Gul Cakmak and Ayten Saracoglu

Abstract

Pregnant women undergo non-obstetric surgeries as well as cesarean operations. Airway management can be complicated due to physiological changes which occur in the respiratory system of labors. The most common causes of pregnancy-specific hypoxic respiratory failure are eclampsia, preeclampsia, and pulmonary edema that develops secondary to tocolytics. Approximately 10–15% of pregnant women undergo emergency cesarean section. Regional anesthesia is a preferred technique worldwide most commonly, and general anesthesia is applied with rapid sequence induction for the rest of the patients. Difficult Airway Society Master Algorithm for Obstetric Patients is a useful method to manage the airway in labors.

Keywords: airway management, respiratory failure, tracheal intubation, pregnancy, labor

1. Introduction

1.1 Pregnancy and physiological changes in the airway

Several physiological changes develop in the systems during pregnancy. Airway management can be complicated due to these changes that occur in the respiratory system (**Table 1**). Capillary dilatation that occurs during pregnancy due to the gestational hormones including progesterone and estrogen. This causes congestion in the nasopharynx, larynx, trachea, and bronchi. On the other hand, as the uterus expands, the diaphragm elevates approximately 4 centimeters. The decrease in the abdominal muscles' tonus and activity allows the diaphragm to take on more respiratory function. The rise of the diaphragm decreases total lung capacity and functional residual capacity. Relaxation in the airway muscles increases the dead-space capacity. Expiratory reserve and residual volume are reduced. Increased alveolar ventilation and decreased functional residual capacity (FRC) increase the maternal uptake and elimination of inhalation anesthetics. However, decreased FRC and increased metabolic rate predispose to apnea or hypoxemia during hypoventilation periods which can precipitated by airway obstruction and prolonged tracheal intubation attempts.

The changing position of the stomach during pregnancy shifts the intra-abdominal segment of the esophagus towards the thorax in many pregnant women. This leads to a decrease in the tone of the lower esophageal high pressure area, which normally prevents reflux of stomach contents. Hence, pulmonary aspiration risk occurs. The risk is higher during anesthesia induction and tracheal intubation. Therefore, rapid sequence induction is recommended.

Volume	
Tidal Volume	**Increases by 45%**
Inspiratory Reserve Volume	Increases by 5%
Expiratory Reserve Volume	Decreases by 25%
Residual Volume	Decreases by 15%
Capacity	
Total Lung Capacity	Decreases by 5%
Vital Capacity	Does not change
Inspiratory Capacity	Increases by 15%
Functional Capacity	Decreases by 20%

Table 1.
Changes in lung volume and capacity during pregnancy.

2. Anatomic changes in pregnant women

The main changes occur by the consequences of growing uterus. The diaphragm is placed upwards. Hence, a shortening of the ribcage and an increase in the anteroposterior and right–left planes take place. Expansion from the ligamentous attachment areas of the ribs facilitates adaptation to these anatomical changes. With the effect of the increasing weight in the pregnant, the obscurity of the anatomical signs on the face and the enlargement of the breasts are among the reasons that cause the difficulty of tracheal intubation. As the uterus continues growing during pregnancy, the intraabdominal part of the stomach and esophagus are displaced to the left of the diaphragm. With this physiological change, progesterone and estrogen cause a decrease in esophageal lower sphincter pressure.

3. Aspiration prophylaxis and fasting in obstetric patients

Four main drugs are used for aspiration prophylaxis:

1. Sodium citrate: is a non-particulate antacid and increases gastric pH

2. H2-antagonists: Famotidine, cimetidine. They block histamine on the gastric parietal cells.

3. Proton pump inhibitors: Pantoprazole, omeprazole. They block H^+K^+ATPase enzyme system in the parietal cells of stomach.

4. Metoclopramide: stimulates upper gastrointestinal motility, and the lower esophageal sphincter tone rises.

Clear liquids are recommended up to two hours before general anesthesia induction. The fasting period for solids is six to eight hours.

4. Pregnancy and respiratory failure

The most common causes of pregnancy-specific hypoxic respiratory failure are eclampsia, preeclampsia, and pulmonary edema that develops secondary to tocolytics. Cardiogenic pulmonary edema due to peripartum cardiomyopathy is another cause. Also, placental abruption, chorioamnionitis, obstetric hemorrhage, or endometritis are among emergencies that cause Adult Respiratory Distress Syndrome (ARDS) [1]. On the other hand, non-pregnancy specific causes include aspiration pneumonia, pulmonary embolism, venous air embolism, pneumothorax, atelectasis, pulmonary contusion, trauma, burns, and sepsis.

In pregnancy the chest wall compliance is reduced. The functional residual capacity decreases. This lead to rapid oxygen desaturation during airway management. Upper airway edema becomes another problem. Besides, pulmonary aspiration, viral pneumonitis or thromboembolism risk increases in pregnant patients. Pregnancy carries a risk of increased susceptibility of some pulmonary. Pneumonia is a significant risk factor for maternal morbidity.

5. Preoperative preparation

Approximately 10–15% of pregnant women undergo emergency cesarean section [2]. Regional anesthesia is preferred worldwide most commonly, and general anesthesia is applied with rapid sequence induction (RSI) for the rest of the patients. Some tests and examinations are required to evaluate the airway before anesthesia applications. The ideal test should be simple, fast, and cost-effective in the preoperative evaluation. Most bedside testa are affected with anatomical and physiological changes of pregnancy [3]. It should also have high sensitivity, high specificity, and positive predictive value. According to the American Society of Anesthesiologists (ASA) difficult intubation guidelines, the difficult airway definition can be described as an experienced anesthesiologist experiencing difficulties in ventilation, tracheal intubation, or both [4]. Difficult laryngoscopy is defined as an experienced anesthesiologist's inability to perform intubation in more than three attempts with a conventional laryngoscope. Difficult mask ventilation is defined as the anesthesiologist's inability to maintain oxygenation without assistance, the inability to increase the peripheral oxygen saturation above 90% despite using 100% oxygen, or the inability to correct improper ventilation findings. Gas leakage from the face mask, decreased chest movements and auscultation findings, dilatation of the stomach with air, hypoxemia, cyanosis, or hypercarbia indicate improper ventilation. One of the most commonly used preoperative evaluation tests is the Modified Mallampati score. Mallampati score of 3 and 4, BMI of >26 kg. m^2, mandibular protrusion defect, snoring history, abnormal facial anatomy, and high thyromental distance are among the markers of difficult mask ventilation in pregnant women. Obstructive sleep apnea is another marker of difficult mask ventilation. In the preoperative period, difficult laryngeal mask placement can also be evaluated. Components of the shortening of RODS are listed in **Table 2**.

Protruding maxillary incisors, receding mandible, short interincisor distance, and increased neck circumference are among other difficult airway markers in pregnant women. Other potential risk factors include obesity, short neck, receding

Restricted mouth opening
Obstruction or obesity
Distorted anatomy
Stiffness

Table 2.
Difficult laryngeal mask ventilation markers: RODS.

Difficult intubation story
Interincisor distance < 4 cm
Tiromental distance < 6 cm
Sternomental distance < 12 cm
Head and neck extension < 30°
Mallampati 3–4
Mandibular protrusion (defect or prognathism)
Neck circumference > 40 cm
Submental compliance defect

Table 3.
Preoperative examination findings for direct laryngoscopy and intubation difficulty.

mandible, swollen tongue, and facial edema. The distances that should be measured in the preoperative examination and examination findings that are predictive for direct laryngoscopy and intubation difficulty are given in **Table 3**. In pregnant patients the physiological and the anatomical changes constitute the difficulty for airway management. The susceptibility to hypoxaemia, friability and mucosal engorgement are main causes of failed airway management [2].

6. Preoxygenation and apneic oxygenation in obstetric patients

As obstetric patients are prone to have airway management difficulties, preoxygenation is essential to increase the oxygen reserve before anesthesia induction. The ideal way to determine the sufficiency of preoxygenation is to monitor end tidal oxygen (FeO_2) concentration. $FeO_2 < 90\%$ shows inadequate preoxygenation. We have a critical level the oxygen consumption about 250 mL/min. This rate increases during pregnancy. As oxygen is removed from lungs the alveolar partial oxygen pressure decreases during airway interventions. Therefore apneic oxygenation is recommended. Oxygen delivery systems include nasal canula, simple face mask, Ventury mask, non-rebreather mask, insufflation by transtracheal or endobronchial catheters, dual bladed laryngoscopes. High flow nasal cannula is also commonly used for this purpose today. During apneic oxygenation, carbon dioxide levels continue to rise, which can lead to a decrease in pH and respiratory acidosis. However, the use of higher flow more than 15 L/min oxygen during apnea provides better gas washout.

7. Awake intubation

When it is thought that oxygenation and manual ventilation cannot be guaranteed after anesthesia induction in a pregnant woman with difficult intubation, awake intubation is recommended. Expecting a high rate of leakage between the face mask and the face, upper airway collapse as a result of general anesthesia are among the conditions that require awake intubation. Awake intubation can be performed using a video-laryngoscope or flexible bronchoscope [5, 6]. During the procedure, low or, if possible, high flow oxygen applications are recommended to extend the apneic window. If the patient will be intubated under general anesthesia or if it is understood that there is a difficult airway following induction, the use of a video-laryngoscope is often recommended [7]. Different types of video-laryngoscopes have been presented in studies and case reports. Kariya et al. [8] reported that awake tracheal intubation with Airway Scope is safe in pregnant women with hemodynamic instability.

Topicalization can be performed in different ways. N. Glossopharyngeus nerve block can be performed in palatoglossal arc. It provides the blockade of gag reflex. N. Laryngealis recurrens and superior can be blocked in cervical level. Another technique is to apply local anesthetic infiltration at the oropharyngeal area. Mucosal atomization devices, inhalational lidocaine or lidocaine lolipops are aother alternatives. EMLA contains 2.5% lidocaine and 2.5% prilocaine and is another option for topicalization. The disadvantages include uncooperated patients, oversedation risk and failure due to inexperienced operator.

8. Surgical cricothyroidotomy

The frequency of obesity is increasing in pregnant women. Although regional anesthesia is recommended, surgical intervention may be required under general anesthesia. It is important to identify neck landmarks while performing surgical cricothyroidotomy. Cricothyroidotomy complications vary from 6.1% to 54.5% [9, 10]. Ultrasonography can provide advantages over traditional digital palpation in obese pregnant women by improving the image and increasing the accuracy of cricothyroid membrane identification [11].

9. Difficult airway guide in obstetrics

The incidence of failed tracheal intubation in obstetric patients is 1/390 [12]. In 2015, the Obstetric Anesthetists' Association and Difficult Airway Society in the UK came together and published the Guideline for difficult intubation in obstetrics [13] (**Figure 1**). Three algorithms are defined according to this guide. These consist of safe obstetric general anesthesia, obstetric failed tracheal intubation, and cannot intubate cannot oxygenate (CICO) steps. The first step is the Pre-induction planning and preparation and planning should be done with a team discussion. RSI is the recommended technique. However, mask ventilation can be performed so that the intraabdominal pressure does not exceed 20 cmH20. The practitioner can attempt at most two times in the presence of difficult tracheal intubation. The third attempt should only be performed by an experienced anesthesiologist. If there is a failure, a failed intubation declaration is made, and help is sought. Continuity of oxygenation is essential. 2 ventilation attempts can be made with a laryngeal mask. Ventilation should be continued with a face mask in case of failure. The 3rd algorithm is initiated if oxygenation fails with the mask. CICO is declared. 100% oxygen is continued to be given. Laryngospasm and insufficient muscle relaxation are excluded. If necessary, neuromuscular blockade is repeated. If oxygenation still fails, the front-of-neck access procedure is applied. If oxygenation of the patient can be achieved before starting the surgical airway, the team should decide according to the clinical condition of the pregnant woman. The patient can be awakened or a decision to continue can be given by evaluating the clinical situation of the pregnant woman and the experience of the operator. Maternal and fetal condition, obesity, surgical factors, aspiration risk, and airway require hazards consideration. Obstetric airway may provide a stressful environment because of failure risk of tracheal intubation and difficult mask ventilation. This may cause a risk of

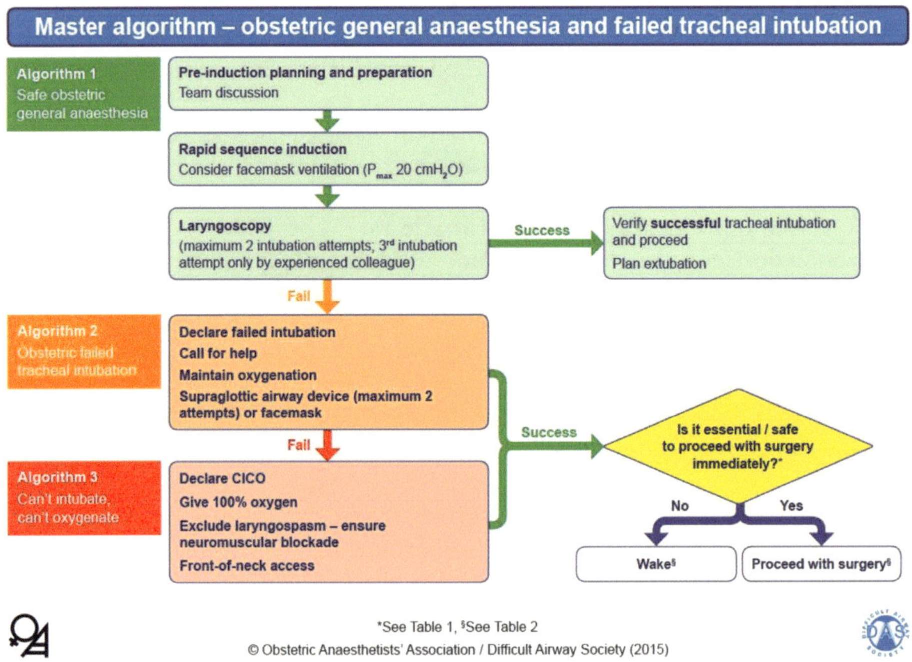

Figure 1.
Difficult airway society master algorithm for obstetric patients.

hypoxaemia, and trauma. Besides, team working should be managed carefully and the team leader should overcome possible errors related with decision-making or time management.

10. Video-laryngoscopes

It is widely available in obstetric units and is often used as a routine tracheal intubation device. It has been reported that it is available in 90% of obstetric units in the UK [2]. Aziz et al. [14] analyzed the data of 180 obstetric patients over 3 years. The first attempt success rate was found to be 100% with video-laryngoscopes. In case of failure in direct laryngoscopy, VL is also used as the rescue device.

Video-laryngoscopes can be classified as unchanneled, channeled, disposible, reusable, standart, angulated, and with tube channels. The selection criteria contains information about experience and competency, training purposes, shape, portability and cost. Necessity of stylet, angle of view, trauma incidence and blade types are among other reasons. For training purposes Macintosh shaped blade with monitor is recommended. In bloody or soiled airway, both Macintosh shaped blade and an extra-curved blade are useful.

11. Supraglottic airway devices

Supraglottic airway can be defined as medical devices that provide ventilation, oxygenation and delivery of anesthetic gases without tracheal intubation. Supraglottic airway devices are less invasive than tracheal tubes. They provide a better airway than a face mask. In DAS Difficult Airway Algorithm, these devices are recommended as resque techniques after failed tracheal intubation. The main

Elective surgeries should be postponed until after birth.
Non-emergency non-obstetric surgical procedures should be postponed as much as possible to the 2nd trimester with the lowest risk of preterm contractions and spontaneous abortion.
An obstetric care provider should be ready in the operating room ready during surgery.
Surgery should be planned in units with neonatal and pediatric services.
It should be decided to remove the fetus or maternal positioning by applying fetal heart rate monitoring.

Table 4.
Tips for anesthesia for non-obstetric surgery in pregnancy.

advantages are providing hemodynamic stability, the protection of mucociliary clearance, easy and fast insertion, less laryngeal trauma, and being easy to learn.

Supraglottic airway devices are also used for flexible bronchoscopic intubation. The success rate ranges from 76% to 100%. Aintree catheter is often used as an indirect method.

12. Training

Studies have reported inexperience as an important cause of failed airway management [15]. Creating checklists and teaching assistants this way is an important educational tool. Simsek et al. [16] reported that the checklist with video-based feedback can be placed in clinical practice permanently. Simulation-based training is among the most frequently used training techniques. However, knowledge and skills acquired through simulation should be able to be transferred to the clinical environment [17].

13. Non-obstetric anesthesia during pregnancy

Approximately 2% of pregnant women require non-obstetric surgery in any trimester [18]. Negative results occur after non-obstetric surgery during pregnancy. Maternal death was reported in 1/12.542 cases (0.006%), and the risk of miscarriage or fetal loss was reported to be 10.5% in the first trimester before the 20th week [19]. This rate was found to be 5.8% when all trimesters were evaluated. The practices to be followed by the ACOG Committee regarding non-obstetric surgeries are summarized in **Table 4** [20].

Airway management can be challenging because of breast engorgement, and weight gain. Edema and bleeding may occur during tracheal intubation or supraglottic airway device insertion. Reduced functional residual capacity and high oxygen consumption should be balanced with apneic oxygenation and preoxygenation. Preparations should be made according to difficult airway management guidelines.

14. Airway management in obstetric patient during COVID-19 pandemic

On admission, COVID-19 test should be performed for the obstetric patients. The testing is vital to protect the hospital staff and to prevent the vertical transfer to the neonate [21]. A checklist should be used for pre-anesthesia evaluation. Patients with COVID-19 may be presented with respiratory symptoms including pneumonia, Acute Respiratory Distress Syndrome (ARDS), lung effusion, and hypoxemia. As a physiological arrangement, functional residual capacity (FRC) reduces in pregnancy. However these pulmonary conditions increase oxygen consumption, deplete the oxygen stores and cause a deeper decrease in FRC. Besides FRC may be lower than closing capacity when the patient lies in supine position for sugery. Therefore effective preoxygenation with left uterus dislocation is required. The operator should take cautions against fluid overload as the patients are sensitive. The delivery or the cesarean section should be performed in an isolation delivery room or negative pressure operating room [22]. Multi-disciplinary based team work isessential with detailed plans. Rapid sequence induction is recommended. A clamp is also recommended during the preparation period. Following tracheal intubation, lung-protective strategies should be followed including low tidal volume and PEEP titration. The risk of droplet and aerosol transmission of COVID-19 is a potential problem during mask ventilation and tracheal intubation. Personal protective equipment is recommended [23]. The use of barrier-enclosure devices were used in small case series or small-sample simulation studies. The ability to perform airway manuplations is a major concern for these devices. Therefore there is lack of evidence in this regard [24].

15. Extubation of obstetric patients

Stimulation of laryngeal reflexes, oxygen depletion, suppression, airway edema, loss of protective reflexes, an increase in sympathetic adrenergic tonus are main problems related with obstetric patients during extubation. Difficult Airway Society recommends awake extubation in patients with associated risk factors [25]. Bailey maneuver, remifentanil technique, staged extubation set, and tube exchange catheters are among advanced techniques [26]. Bailey maneuver is a technique for laryngeal mask exchange. Behind the tracheal tube a supraglottic airway device is inserted. By this way the operator can both ventilate the patient and extubate through the guidance of fiberoptic visualization. Thus, laryngospasm, bleeding, or edema can be treated early. In remifentanil technique, the patient receives low dose remifentanil infusion in order to prevent cough and postoperative pain. Airway exchange catheters are frequently used during extubation. Awake patients can tolerate these aduncts and oxygenation is possible. If reintubation is indicated the operator can advance the tracheal tube.

16. Postoperative monitoring

Awake extubation should be preferred. Muscle relaxant agents should be reversed. Sugammadex is recommended in cases with rocuronium. The patient can deteriorate and the airway may become obstructed. Therefore monitoring and supervision by experienced personnel are essential. A backup plan should be created and the team should be ready for reintubation. Ventilation, oxygen and carbon dioxide levels should be monitored. Severe preeclampsia, volume overload or existing co-morbidities may complicate the postoperative period.

17. Conclusion

Pregnant women come to the operating room for non-obstetric surgeries as well as cesarean operations. Pregnancy is characterized by significant physiologic changes in the respiratory system and airway. Reduced functional residual capacity, airway edema, and increased oxygen consumption are main factors. These changes cause airway management to be complicated and difficult. Therefore effective pre-oxygenation is essential. Besides, apneic oxygenation is recommended in obstetric patients by using low and high flow oxygen delivery systems.

Regional anesthesia is preferred over general anesthesia because of its high risk of complications. Guidelines specific to pregnant women have been published and difficult airway management steps should be followed in patients undergoing general anesthesia. Patients with Covid 19 disease may present with Acute Respiratory Distress Syndrome (ARDS), lung effusion, and hypoxemia. Postoperative care should be planned. Extubation of pregnant patients should be considered awake and advanced techniques should be ready.

Author details

Kemal Tolga Saracoglu[1]*, Gul Cakmak[2] and Ayten Saracoglu[2]

1 Department of Anesthesiology and Intensive Care, Health Sciences University Kartal Dr. Lutfi Kirdar Training and Research Hospital Istanbul, Turkey

2 Department of Anesthesiology and Intensive Care, Marmara University Medical School Istanbul, Turkey

*Address all correspondence to: saracoglukt@gmail.com

References

[1] Ende H, Varelmann D. Respiratory Considerations Including Airway and Ventilation Issues in Critical Care Obstetric Patients. Obstet Gynecol Clin North Am. 2016 Dec;43(4):699-708. doi: 10.1016/j.ogc.2016.07.002.

[2] Mushambi MC, Athanassoglou V, Kinsella SM. Anticipated difficult airway during obstetric general anaesthesia: narrative literature review and management recommendations. Anaesthesia. 2020 Jul;75(7):945-961. doi: 10.1111/anae.15007.

[3] Pilkington S, Carli F, Dakin MJ, Romney M, De Witt KA, Doré CJ, Cormack RS. Increase in Mallampati score during pregnancy. Br J Anaesth. 1995 Jun;74(6):638-42.

[4] Apfelbaum JL, Hagberg CA, Caplan RA, Blitt CD, Connis RT, Nickinovich DG, Hagberg CA, Caplan RA, Benumof JL, Berry FA, Blitt CD, Bode RH, Cheney FW, Connis RT, Guidry OF, Nickinovich DG, Ovassapian A; American Society of Anesthesiologists Task Force on Management of the Difficult Airway. Practice guidelines for management of the difficult airway: an updated report by the American Society of Anesthesiologists Task Force on Management of the Difficult Airway. Anesthesiology. 2013 Feb;118(2):251-70. doi: 10.1097/ALN.0b013e31827773b2.

[5] Kariya N, Kimura K, Iwasaki R, Ueki R, Tatara T, Tashiro C. Intraoperative awake tracheal intubation using the Airway Scope™ in caesarean section. Anaesth Intensive Care. 2013 May;41(3):390-2. doi: 10.1177/0310057X1304100319.

[6] Goldszmidt E, Brimacombe J, Keller C. Awake intubation is indicated in pregnant women with difficult airways. Anesth Analg. 2004 Nov;99(5):1577-8; author reply 1578. doi: 10.1213/01.ANE.0000137446.94850.9A.

[7] Zaouter C, Calderon J, Hemmerling TM. Videolaryngoscopy as a new standard of care. British Journal of Anaesthesia 2015; 114: 181-3.

[8] Kariya N, Kimura K, Iwasaki R, Ueki R, Tatara T, Tashiro C. Intraoperative awake tracheal intubation using the Airway Scope™ in caesarean section. Anaesth Intensive Care. 2013 May;41(3):390-2. doi: 10.1177/0310057X1304100319.

[9] Hamaekers AE, Henderson JJ. Equipment and strategies for emergency tracheal access in the adult patient. Anaesthesia 2011; 66: 65-80.

[10] Cook TM, Woodall N, Frerk C; Fourth National Audit Project. Major complications of airway management in the UK: results of the Fourth National Audit Project of the Royal College of Anaesthetists and the Difficult Airway Society. Part 1: anaesthesia. British Journal of Anaesthesia 2011; 106: 617-31.

[11] You-Ten KE, Desai D, Postonogova T, Siddiqui N. Accuracy of conventional digital palpation and ultrasound of the cricothyroid membrane in obese women in labour. Anaesthesia. 2015 Nov;70(11):1230-4. doi: 10.1111/anae.13167.

[12] Kinsella SM, Winton AL, Mushambi MC, Ramaswamy K, Swales H, Quinn AC, Popat M. Failed tracheal intubation during obstetric general anaesthesia: a literature review. Int J Obstet Anesth. 2015 Nov;24(4):356-74.

[13] Mushambi MC, Kinsella SM, Popat M, Swales H, Ramaswamy KK, Winton AL, Quinn AC; Obstetric Anaesthetists' Association; Difficult Airway Society. Obstetric Anaesthetists'

Association and Difficult Airway Society guidelines for the management of difficult and failed tracheal intubation in obstetrics. Anaesthesia. 2015 Nov;70(11):1286-306. doi: 10.1111/anae.13260.

[14] Aziz MF, Kim D, Mako J, Hand K, Brambrink AM. A retrospective study of the performance of video laryngoscopy in an obstetric unit. Anesth Analg. 2012 Oct;115(4):904-6. doi: 10.1213/ANE.0b013e3182642130.

[15] Asai T. Airway management in patients undergoing emergency Cesarean section. J Anesth. 2015 Dec;29(6):927-33. doi: 10.1007/s00540-015-2037-5.

[16] Simsek T, Yilmaz M, Saracoglu A, Saracoglu KT. Preoperative airway management checklist: the transfer of knowledge into clinical practice by video based feedback. South Clin Ist Euras 2020;31(1):26-30.

[17] Saracoglu KT, Saracoglu A. Airway management education: an update. Acta Anaesth Belg 2017;68:175-186.

[18] Heesen M, Klimek M. Nonobstetric anesthesia during pregnancy. Curr Opin Anaesthesiol. 2016 Jun;29(3):297-303. doi: 10.1097/ACO.0000000000000311.

[19] Cohen-Kerem R, Railton C, Oren D, et al. Pregnancy outcome following nonobstetric surgical intervention. Am J Surg 2005; 190:467-473.

[20] ACOG Committee on Obstetric Practice. ACOG Committee Opinion No. 474: nonobstetric surgery during pregnancy. Obstet Gynecol 2011; 117:420-421.

[21] Bauer ME, Bernstein K, Dinges E, Delgado C, El-Sharawi N, Sultan P, Mhyre JM, Landau R. Obstetric Anesthesia During the COVID-19 Pandemic. Anesth Analg. 2020 Jul;131(1):7-15.

[22] Wang Y, Yang M, Wang L, Dong H, Lu Z. Pregnancy and COVID-19: what anesthesiologists should know? Minerva Anestesiol. 2020 Nov 24. doi: 10.23736/S0375-9393.20.14647-9. Epub ahead of print.

[23] Saracoglu KT, Dalkilinc Hokenek U, Saracoglu A, Sorbello M, Demirhan R. COVID-19 patients in the operating room: a concise review of existing literature. Minerva Anestesiol. 2020 Dec 17.

[24] Sorbello M, Rosenblatt W, Hofmeyr R, Greif R, Urdaneta F. Aerosol boxes and barrier enclosures for airway management in COVID-19 patients: a scoping review and narrative synthesis. Br J Anaesth. 2020 Dec;125(6):880-894.

[25] Popat M, Mitchell V, Dravid R, Patel A, Swampillai C, Higgs A. Difficult airway society guidelines for the management of tracheal extubation. Anaesthesia 2012;67:318-40.

[26] Saracoglu KT, Yilmaz M, Duzyol IY, Turan AZ, Okuyucu KA, Yurt E. Advanced techniques in extubation: Bailey maneuver, tube exchange catheter and staged extubation set. J Clin Anesth. 2018 Aug;48:28-29.

Chapter 11

Challenges to Airway Management in Space

Preethi Reddy

Abstract

Human interest in space exploration is boundless. We are driven to investigate the unknown and push the limits of our understanding of our universe. Given that space flights are for extended periods of time—in the hazardous environments of space and the growth of the space tourism industry is credibly anticipated; the incidence of medical and surgical events is bound to increase during space travel. Airway management becomes an essential skill in such situations. Microgravity, shortage of medical personnel, inability of the crew to return to earth expeditiously or access real time assistance from earth are some of the reasons that warrant training and preparation of the crew, towards this end. The purpose of this chapter would be to explore the challenges and the various recourses available for airway management during space travel.

Keywords: space travel, airway management, space medicine, space flight, anaesthesia

1. Introduction

There is expanded access to space. Government agencies and private companies alike have planned manned missions to the moon and to Mars, for the coming years. Currently, we are also witnessing a meaningful growth in the space tourism sector.

It is now more important than ever to increase our understanding of human physiology and pathology in space. Furthermore, it is of prime importance that astronauts can manage medical and surgical emergencies, that may arise especially given that a space tourist—as against the typical astronaut—is unprepared for the rigours of space travel and therefore exposed to a higher risk of medical complications [1].

Man's tryst with space began in 1961. The International Space Station (ISS), which has been in orbit for almost 20 years now, has enabled humans to stay in space for long durations. This has provided a swifter and a more profound bioastronautics development.

The environment of space is harsh and challenging, with a prolonged exposure to multiple stressful stimuli, radiation, weightlessness, isolation, and confinement to tight enclosed spaces for long periods of time. Microgravity, which affects all organ systems, has the most profound effect on human physiology [2].

Travelling to Mars will require transitioning between three different gravitational fields: being weightless during a six month interplanetary flight, being at about one third of the Earth's gravity on Mars, and re-acclimatising to Earth's gravity upon return [3].

2. Airway management in space

With increasing flight durations, there is an increased prospect that a medical emergency will entail airway management. It is currently estimated that the probability of a medical intervention requiring general anaesthesia, over the course of a 950 day mission to Mars and with six crew members is 2.6%. This speaks to the importance of how even the unlikeliest of events could imperil the mission and lead to loss of life [1]. Airway management is an important skill that is required to manage a great many medical emergencies. Some of the possible scenarios necessitating airway management in space are listed in **Table 1** [1, 4, 5].

Seventeen medical emergencies were documented during spaceflight between the periods of 1961–1999 [1]. In one instance, in 1962, on the Mercury 7 flight, Scott Carpenter, an American astronaut, aspirated food crumbs in orbit and in 1975 several astronauts on the Apollo-Soyuz mission developed a mild form of chemical pneumonitis after accidentally inhaling propellent fluid during re-entry [4]. Incidentally, none of the seventeen cases have required intubation. Also, no one has required GA in space to date [1].

Medical evacuation is not an option, in case of an airway emergency, owing to the distance as well as the absolute need to maintain oxygenation to avoid brain death. It is therefore necessary that immediate care is provided, while on board [6]. This warrants a crew equipped with emergency care skills as well as continuous training, to prevent skill erosion [1, 6, 7]. Furthermore, communication delays prohibit real time telemedicine support. For example, the communication delay between Earth and Mars is about twenty minutes—one way [1]. Airway management skills are thus critical to the mission of exploring space safely.

In the first half of this chapter, we will deal with the physiology of airway management and the physiological adaptations of the human body in space. This would provide the essential foundation to understand the challenges associated with airway management in space.

The term 'Airway Management' refers to the maintenance of airway patency and ensuring adequate ventilation and oxygenation. Successful airway management entails that the practitioner anticipates and predicts difficult airway and at the same time devises an airway management plan. The practitioner should also be adequately skilled to execute that plan, with the available resources. In order to enable this plan, anaesthesia is typically required—to provide patient comfort, limit airway reflexes, and to moderate the hemodynamic response to airway instrumentation [8].

3. Physiology of airway management

3.1 Pre-oxygenation

Hypoxaemia can occur on induction of anaesthesia and muscle paralysis on account of hypoventilation and apnea. Pre-oxygenation or denitrogenation helps to replace the nitrogen in the lungs with oxygen. This, consequently, extends the apnea time and allows the anaesthesiologist to secure the airway and resume ventilation.

Pre-oxygenation is achieved by providing 100% oxygen via a face mask, at a flow rate of 10-12 L/min to prevent rebreathing. This can be achieved by asking the patient to breathe for 3 min using tidal volume ventilation; or by taking 8 vital capacity breaths over 60 seconds. During this process, it must be ensured that there are no leaks around the face mask [8].

1. Hypoxic cardiopulmonary arrest
2. Airway obstruction
3. Foreign body aspiration
4. Burns or smoke inhalation
5. Coma
6. General Anaesthesia (GA)

Table 1.
Indications for airway management in space.

3.2 Pulmonary aspiration of gastric contents

Patients are required to have an empty stomach to reduce the risk of regurgitation and pulmonary aspiration of acidic gastric contents. The American Society of Anaesthesiologists task force recommends 4 hours of fasting from breast milk, 6 hours of fasting from infant formula, non-human milk and solid foods; and up to 8 hours or more from fried or fatty food. Clear fluids may be allowed up to 2 hours prior to anaesthesia [9].

Prophylactic drugs may be beneficial in patients with specific risk factors for aspiration. They help in decreasing gastric volume and increasing the gastric fluid pH. The commonly used drugs (alone or in combination) are—non-particulate antacids, promotility drugs and H2-receptor antagonists. These drugs may be used alone or in combination [8].

3.3 Airway reflexes and the physiological response to intubation of the trachea

One of the main functions of the larynx is protection of the airway. Sensory receptors in the glottic and subglottic mucosa are triggered—on airway instrumentation—leading to the adduction of the vocal cords and laryngospasm. Furthermore, foreign body irritation of the lower airway can result in bronchospasm [8].

Airway instrumentation causes an intense noxious stimulus via the vagal and glossopharyngeal afferents. This results in a reflex autonomic activation, manifesting as hypertension and tachycardia. Although this response lasts only for a short duration, it may have serious consequences in patients with significant cardiac disease. Also, CNS activation can occur leading to an increase in the electroencephalographic activity, cerebral metabolic rate and blood flow, which may result in an increased intracranial pressure [8].

3.4 Anaesthesia for airway management

General anaesthesia is the most common technique employed in airway management. A rapid acting intravenous anaesthetic agent is most commonly used for induction of anaesthesia, followed by a neuromuscular blocking agent to provide muscle relaxation [8, 10].

Rapid sequence induction is used when there is an appreciable risk for gastric regurgitation and pulmonary aspiration of gastric contents. In this technique, after pre-oxygenation, cricoid pressure is applied. This is followed by an induction dose of an intravenous anaesthetic and 1–1.5 mg/kg of intravenous succinylcholine. The trachea is then intubated without any attempts at positive pressure ventilation. The cricoid pressure is applied constantly until the airway is secured.

Inhalation induction of anaesthesia with volatile anaesthetics is commonly used in paediatric patients—to provide a needle free experience—and in adults where intravenous access is difficult or when this technique is desirable [8].

Intravenous induction without neuromuscular blocking drugs is used for LMA (laryngeal mask airway) placement. Propofol is the drug of choice for this technique due to its distinct ability to suppress airway reflexes and produce apnea [11, 12].

Awake airway management is indicated, but not limited to, difficult mask ventilation and difficult intubation [13]. In such a case, the pharyngeal muscle tone and patency of the upper airway is maintained. This allows for spontaneous ventilation and acts as a safeguard against aspiration. It also provides an opportunity for a quick neurological examination, if indicated. Awake airway management is achieved by topicalisation of the airway with local anaesthetics [8].

3.5 Equipment for airway management

Equipment for basic airway management includes face masks for pre-oxygenation and delivery of inhalational anaesthetic agents, supraglottic airways are devices that are inserted blindly into the pharynx to provide a conduit for ventilation without requiring tracheal intubation, and endotracheal tubes, that provide maximum protection against the risk of aspirating gastric contents while establishing a definitive airway and at the same time, allowing positive pressure ventilation with higher airway pressures.

In patients with known or predicted difficult airway, videolaryngoscopy, rather than direct laryngoscopy is indicated since videolaryngoscopy inherently provides better glottic visualisation as well as effortlessly employed by non-experts [8].

3.6 Laryngoscopy and endotracheal intubation

Endotracheal intubation is established as the gold standard for airway management. It is typically achieved by direct laryngoscopy with patients placed in the sniffing position. A line of sight must be established from the mouth to the larynx. Direct laryngoscopy displaces the hyoid, tongue and epiglottis anterior to a line running from the upper teeth to the glottis.

In this technique, the mouth is opened, the laryngoscope blade is inserted and the tip is positioned to apply a lifting force exposing the glottis. The endotracheal tube is then inserted through the vocal cords into the trachea [8, 14].

4. The human body in space

The Earth's constant gravitational force is an important factor in the evolution of life on this planet. It has determined the development of all forms of life. All biological adaptations on land and water have been influenced by its interactions with gravity forming complex systems for stability, fluid regulation, gravity sensing, and locomotion.

The human body responds to microgravity in the same manner that it responds to senescence (ageing): Both ageing and microgravity produce a decline of biological function [15]. Also, like ageing, microgravity causes a negative calcium balance leading to a loss of bone density, muscle atrophy, cardiovascular and haematic changes, and metabolic, endocrine, and sleep disturbances. In microgravity, astronauts undergo rapid senescence. However, they subside over time on returning to Earth, departing from the typical path of the ageing process. This correspondence of symptoms combined with a prolonged stationing in space requires that we are alive to the issue of accelerated ageing in space [15].

4.1 Cardiovascular system

Changes in the cardiovascular system because of microgravity are paramount from the standpoint of the anaesthesiologist. Gravity influences the equilibrium of the various functional fluid compartments of the vascular system and in particular that of the venous capacitance vessels [16]. In the upright posture, there is higher arterial pressure in the feet (200 mmHg) and lower pressure in the head (70 mmHg) relative to the heart (100 mmHg). In space, this gradient is absent, leading to redistribution of body fluids toward the head [2, 15, 17]. This phenomenon is referred to as "fluid shift". As a result of this, astronauts develop facial puffiness coupled with reduced volume in the lower limbs [2, 16].

Also, due to this 'fluid shift', there is engorgement of the central circulation. Mechanoreceptors sense this blood redistribution activating autonomic offloading and volume regulating reflexes leading to vasodilation and pooling of blood in the viscera and tissues, and initial renal fluid and salt loss. Most of these adaptations occur within 6–10 hours of spaceflight. After one week in space, the plasma volume reduces and the intracellular volume increases [15, 16]. In the same period, the RBC mass drops by about 10%. This "space anaemia" can again be attributed to the fluid shift toward the upper body, which is associated with an increase in kidney tissue oxygen partial pressure leading to the inhibition of erythropoiesis. A second hypothesis explains this as being due to haemolysis of recently formed RBCs [2, 16, 18].

Despite the headward fluid shift, paradoxically the central venous pressure is not increased. Further, a reduction in the intrathoracic pressure and the loss of gravitational force on the cardiac muscle may even reduce it [15, 16].

Microgravity affects the heart rate and blood pressure minimally [16, 19]. The initial headward fluid shift increases the stroke volume and cardiac output. Subsequently, after a few days of adaptation, the resulting hypovolemia and cardiac atrophy, increase the ejection fraction and decrease the stroke volume. The left ventricle mass reduces by 8% due to reduced myocardial load in microgravity [16, 20–22]. The left ventricular systolic function is minimally affected even though diastolic dysfunction has been identified in astronauts [16].

The nitric oxide release as a result of endothelial cell adaptation to microgravity and the loss of tone due to smooth muscle cell deconditioning causes vasodilation. Systemic vascular resistance reduces after 1 week of weightlessness due to this vasodilation [15, 16].

The baroreflex response is weakened by 50% after just 24 hours of being in space. It is constrained after long-duration spaceflight and these changes linger on for up to 2 weeks after returning to Earth. There are changes in adrenergic-receptor sensitivity in microgravity: beta-adrenergic receptors sensitivity is increased and alpha-adrenergic receptors sensitivity is decreased. There is also an increased risk of arrhythmias in space due to catecholamine discharge [16].

In space, aerobic capacity may be either maintained or increased. On return to Earth, there is an orthostatic challenge due to readaptation to gravity. As a result of this, astronauts experience reduced stroke volume and cardiac output which leads to landing-day orthostatic stress [2].

4.2 Endothelial changes

Microgravity and reduced motor activity produces endothelial changes by altering the regional blood flow and vascular transmural pressure, which in turn, produces an adaptation of vasomotor tone and long term vascular remodelling mainly in the endothelium and smooth muscular cells [16].

This microvascular endothelial dysfunction in astronauts, plays a material role in osteoporosis, muscle atrophy and cardiovascular deconditioning considering that the endothelial cells of the microvasculature cover a surface area that is fifty times larger than that of all the large vessels put together [15].

4.3 Space motion sickness

Space motion sickness is a result of neurovestibular disturbance that happens to about two-thirds of astronauts. It occurs within a few minutes of being in space and gradually resolves over a period of 48–72 hours. Nevertheless, it can last up to a few days and can reappear after landing. Some causes that are suggested as a possible hypothesis include: an increase in cerebrospinal fluid and intracranial pressure due to the headward fluid shift, a lowered threshold for vestibular stimulation due to central volume expansion and the absence of gravity triggering an abnormal vestibular activity leading to a parasympathetic overstimulation [15, 23].

Space motion sickness is characterised by an imbalance in spatial orientation, balance, gaze control and autonomous vestibular function. Symptoms include facial pallor, cold sweating, stomach awareness, anorexia, vomiting, nausea, headache and malaise [2, 15, 16].

4.4 Eye

On Earth, venous return from the head, neck and upper trunk is supported by gravity. Unlike the lower half of the body, the veins draining this region do not have valves and lack muscular contraction. In space, there is reduced arterial blood supply and venous flow from the eye. This increases the venous pressure and filtration at the capillaries causing an increase in both intracranial pressure and IOP [15].

4.5 Effects on the musculoskeletal system

Extended exposure to microgravity leads to a loss of bone and muscle mass due to its reduced use and perfusion changes. Inadequate nutrition and stress are additional reasons that lead to muscle atrophy [2]. Weight bearing bones: lumbar spine, pelvis, femoral neck and trochanter, and calcaneus and postural muscles: back, abdominal wall, lower limbs are most commonly affected [2, 24].

In addition to absence of gravitational loading, decreased Vitamin D production—partly due to low levels of sunlight—leads to decreased calcium fixation in bones and reabsorption in kidneys. Higher ambient levels of carbon dioxide, leading to respiratory acidosis also contribute to bone loss [2, 15] Increase in urinary calcium coupled with a reduction in diuresis and decreased fluid intake increases the risk of kidney stones [25–27].

4.6 Effects on the respiratory system

Microgravity induced changes in the lungs have been the subject of much interest for decades. The ventilation to perfusion ratio attains equilibrium in the absence of gravity [15, 16]. There is an increase in the total alveolocapillary surface which in turn improves the lung diffusing capacity [16]. Gas exchange in space does not undergo a substantial change but there is reduced oxygen consumption and carbon dioxide production. This is attributed to a reduced physical activity in space and change in the ventilation to perfusion ratios between the upper and lower lung regions. These factors lead to an overall reduction in the metabolic rate [15].

Changes in the thoracoabdominal compliance is advantageous to the pulmonary function [16].

Microgravity can cause weakening of the respiratory muscles leading to a reduced rib cage expansion. Thus, there is an increased contribution of the abdomen to tidal volume [28]. Intra-abdominal pathology and subsequent intra-abdominal hypertension is important to providing life support and mechanical ventilation. However, it has been demonstrated that intra-abdominal gas insufflation during laparoscopic surgery in space and the subsequent intra-abdominal hypertension is made better by the absence of gravity [15, 16].

It has been suggested that changes in the respiratory system are similar to those that occur to individuals on prolonged bed rest and are anatomical in nature [15]. These typically occur over several weeks. There is a significant reduction in tidal volume [15, 16] and residual volume [29]. Vital capacity and forced vital capacity reduce initially followed by subsequent recovery. Functional residual capacity (FRC) reduces by 500 ml and remains at that level for the remainder of the period in space [29, 30]. Peak inspiratory and expiratory flows are also not significantly altered. However maximum inspiratory pressure significantly reduces, while the maximum expiratory pressure (MEP) at total lung volume initially reduces at month 2 and month 4, but recovers by month 6 of being in microgravity. The MEP at FRC however is not affected [15].

4.7 Immune system

Immune system dysregulation occurs in space. High levels of physical and psychological stress—immediately before and after space flight— physiological stress, isolation, confinement, disrupted circadian rhythms are some of the contributing factors to immune system dysregulation [2]. Additionally, increase in levels of glucocorticoids and catecholamines, may also contribute to change in the immune system [3, 31]. Various studies have demonstrated that lack of gravity impairs the signalling pathways that are necessary for early T-cell activation. This leads to changes in the organisation of the cytoskeleton and microtubule organising centres [2].

Immune system dysregulation can lead to an increased incidence of hypersensitivities, autoimmunity, allergies, infectious diseases, latent viral reactivation and even malignancies [3].

Microbes undergo several changes in their characteristics in space. Notably, bacteria cultured on board have increased pathogenicity [32]. The microorganisms present in the human body, are transmitted easily between persons, in such confined habitats [3].

4.8 Gastrointestinal motility

Gastrointestinal motility is reduced in space especially in the first 72 hours. It has also been observed that the gastric content pH decreases [16].

4.9 Weight loss

Astronauts experience a weight loss of up to 5% after a 6 month stay on the International Space Station (ISS). This is explained by a mismatch between caloric intake and caloric expenditure [16, 33, 34].

4.10 Psychological effects

Confinement and isolation in constrained spaces, for extended periods of time, affects one's psychological health. Even with screening, training, and support; behavioural issues, cognitive conditions, and psychiatric disorders among crew members, is to be expected. Decline in mood, cognition and morale can occur. Sleep disorders due to changes in their circadian rhythms is also quite common [2, 3].

Extended exposure to stress, isolation and changes in circadian rhythm can have a psychological impact on astronauts. Cognitive impairment, sleep disorders, psychosomatic symptoms, anxiety and even depression can occur [7].

Personnel skills like team coordination, communication, logistics, etc. and technical skills like troubleshooting equipment, use of safety equipment, orientation, etc. contribute to the health and safety of astronauts. Selection of suitable crew, training and maintenance of skills during the mission, is important. Therefore, medical and psychological benchmarks for crew-member selection ought to be very high [7].

4.11 Exposure to radiation

Space travel presents the additional risk of exposure to harmful radiation. On Earth, we are shielded from cosmic radiation by the Earth's magnetic field and its atmosphere. However, on a space station astronauts are exposed to up to ten times the radiation they are exposed to while on Earth. Radiation in space can cause radiation sickness and degenerative tissue disease, among many other serious issues [3].

5. Challenges to anaesthesia delivery and airway management in space

Anaesthesia is important for airway management. Blunting airway reflexes and hemodynamic response to airway instrumentation is a chief consideration. This can be achieved by anaesthesia.

Delivery of anaesthesia in space is highly demanding and complicated, and the reasons can be grouped into three main categories: physiological, technical and human as shown in **Table 2** [16, 17, 35].

5.1 Physiological considerations

5.1.1 Challenges related to cardiovascular changes in space

In weightlessness, a new physiological equilibrium is established, adapted to the reduced loading conditions. However, this equilibrium is delicate as is the tolerance to any additional event or even an interventional procedure. Reaction of the human body to blood loss, anaphylaxis or any event that reduces cardiac function, may be further compromised. General anaesthesia and mechanical ventilation may also adversely affect this physiological equilibrium [16].

On landing in gravity environments different from Earth, cardiovascular changes and hypovolemia causes orthostatic intolerance. The aerobic capacity is also impaired as a result of hypovolemia, anaemia and orthostatic intolerance [16, 36]. These factors combined with space motion sickness, limits the crew's ability to perform tasks effectively.

Preloading with intravenous (IV) fluids before the induction of general anaesthesia is important to prevent cardiovascular collapse [37]. Any significant

1. Physiological
    - Cardiovascular changes
    - Fluid shift
    - Gastrointestinal System
    - Pharmacology in Space environment
    - Choice of anaesthetic technique
2. Technical
    - Fluid generation and handling
    - Vascular access
    - Closed cabin pressures
    - Medical equipment
    - Use of restraints
    - Telemedicine and information technology
3. Human
    - Crew Skills
    - Psychological effects on crew

Table 2.
Factors complicating delivery of medical care in space.

hypovolemia should be treated concomitantly with IV fluids and vasopressors. Alpha agonists such as phenylephrine, metaraminol, midodrine, norepinephrine should be at hand; higher doses than usual may be required. Beta-agonists and beta-antagonists should be used with care [16]. For induction of anaesthesia, drugs that preserve cardiovascular stability, such as ketamine, are preferred [37].

5.1.2 Fluid shift

Although not documented, headward fluid shift and facial oedema can complicate the intubating conditions [16]. Drug distribution during spinal anaesthesia may also be altered due to the cephalad fluid shift and is therefore not recommended, in microgravity [38].

5.1.3 Gastrointestinal system

Space motion sickness accompanies gastroesophageal reflux in astronauts, sometimes lasting the entire mission. It may even persist after their return to Earth. The gastroesophageal reflux along with decreased gastrointestinal motility puts the crew at a risk for pulmonary aspiration, both during and after flight [16, 17].

5.1.4 Pharmacology in the space environment

Both the pharmacokinetics and pharmacodynamics of drugs are altered in weightlessness [39].

Cardiovascular changes, weight changes, changes in hormonal, electrolyte and immunoglobulin levels, decrease in the amount of microsomal P-450 as well as its dependent enzymes are some of the factors that cause changes to the pharmacokinetic and pharmacodynamic properties of drugs in space [16, 40]. As a result, the corresponding drug dosages need to be altered as well [39].

Also, long term storage of drugs may render them ineffective or even toxic [16].

A notable mention: the depolarising muscle relaxant succinylcholine is contraindicated due to disuse atrophy of muscles and changes in the neuromuscular junction, and the increased risk of hyperkalemia after prolonged exposure to microgravity [17, 39]. Instead, rocuronium is recommended to be used as an alternative [16, 41].

5.1.5 Choice of anaesthetic technique

One of the limiting aspects of the anaesthesia protocol for microgravity is that it should be carried out by a small crew of non-medical personnel, with limited training. In several low-income countries, anaesthetic procedures are regularly performed by non-medical personnel, with relatively low complications. Simplified versions of the protocols—one which can easily be followed by non-physicians—must be developed.

The worst case scenario approach should be the basis for making the choice of the anaesthetic technique. It must be borne in mind that astronauts who may require anaesthesia in space may have to be managed by nonmedical personnel with limited training, in case the crew medical officer (CMO) is incapacitated or deceased. In addition, they maybe hypovolemic, deconditioned, at a risk for rhythm disturbances and gastric aspiration, and intolerant to succinylcholine [16].

Although ultrasound guided regional anaesthesia may be used safely and successfully, it requires considerable training [16, 38, 42, 43]. Spinal anaesthesia is not feasible in microgravity, its safety and efficacy is unpredictable because the heavy local anaesthetic solutions used depend on gravity. Epidural anaesthesia may be used, but it also requires considerable training and absolute asepsis, and therefore carries significant risks [16].

General anaesthesia with endotracheal intubation is suitable for all types of surgical conditions and is the recommended choice of anaesthetic technique.

Intubation, in general, is facilitated by use of general anaesthesia and muscle relaxants [16]. Furthermore, use of video laryngoscopy also increases the intubation success rate especially among new users [44, 45].

5.2 Technical considerations

5.2.1 Fluid generation and handling

Intravenous (IV) fluids have a limited shelf life and usually remain unused during that period. Shipping and storing them is expensive due to the added weight and the wastage of valuable storage volume. It is however expedient, and necessary to be able to generate IV fluids on demand using drinking water. This process was successfully tested on the ISS (project IVGEN) [16, 46].

Fluids and gases do not separate in space, owing to their different densities, which complicates fluid handling and drug preparation. Hence most drugs and intravenous fluids exist as a foamy liquid [16, 17].

It is advisable that injectable drugs be carried in prefilled syringes. Needleless vial adapters that allow direct drug aspiration into the syringe without the need for a needle to pierce the vial septum are also preferred. Experiments have been successfully conducted by NASA Scientific and Technical Information Program for removal of air bubbles [16, 17, 47].

Another important concern is that many medical devices such as anaesthetic vaporisers and suction equipment, that depend on gravity induced separation of fluids and gases, do not function properly in microgravity [17, 37].

5.2.2 Vascular access

During a medical emergency, vascular access may be difficult to obtain. In space, securing the body of the IV administrator as well as mastering fine motor skills to perform the required task can be a challenge. Also, microgravity causes small objects to float away. Sharp objects such as IV cannulae can present a potential hazard to the crew [47].

Using ultrasound to obtain central venous access either autonomously or robotically is currently under development. An intraosseous access kit has also been included in the ISS medical gear [16].

5.2.3 Closed cabin atmospheres

A spacecraft offers a tightly sealed environment. Medical procedures requiring the use of oxygen would risk oxygen enrichment in the closed cabin atmosphere, increasing the risk of explosion and fire. Use of a closed ventilation circuit limits the dumping of oxygen in the cabin. Volatile anaesthetics cannot be used in such an environment, as a gas leak can contaminate the on-board closed loop environment and therefore general anaesthesia must be provided by the technique of total intravenous anaesthesia (TIVA) [16, 17, 38]. Xenon may find utility as an anaesthetic gas in such space operations [17].

5.2.4 Medical equipment

Advanced medical care requires equipment such as a monitor, ventilator, suction equipment, and oxygen concentrator. Equipment carried to space must comply with specific spaceflight standards. There are a number of stipulations in terms of weight, size, and power consumption. For perspective: It costs about US$ 22,000 USD to transport one kilogramme of material into low Earth orbit. Drugs that do not need refrigeration and that which have a long shelf life are preferable, in this regard [16, 17].

5.2.5 Use of restraints

Airway management is made possible during spaceflight using restraints, allowing the operator's hands to be free to hold and guide the endotracheal tube into the airway [38]. Use of restraints are absolutely necessary to hold instruments, patients and personnel in place. For surgical procedures, it has been demonstrated that it is possible to restrain instruments in microgravity using various supplies ensuring sterility, operator accessibility, safe waste disposal, while maintaining ergonomic capability [48, 49].

5.2.6 Telemedicine and information technology

Telemedicine, as a medium for healthcare delivery, has tremendously improved and finds great many applications, in the current healthcare setting. Today, availing a virtual opinion, of an expert, at a remote location, is fairly uncomplicated. This becomes very useful during spaceflight operations. However, a delay of about 20 minutes to receive one way communication is to be expected during a journey to Mars [4]. Since anaesthetic procedures and airway management require prompt and expedient responses, telemedicine—with its inherent latency issues—may not prove to be the most optimal solution. Hence, other advanced on-board information systems will need to supplement telemedicine technology in space [17].

5.3 Human factors

5.3.1 Medical skills and training

It must be borne in mind that the crew is unlikely to have a trained physician on board. Therefore anaesthetic procedures and airway management may have to be carried out by non-anaesthetists and non-physicians [35]. At present the Crew Medical Officer in each mission receives a training of about 80 hours [17]. Fading of skills during flight is an important concern and continuous training of the crew members is essential [1]. Fatigue and sleep debt during long duration space flight [2] can further affect performance of the medical officer during emergencies.

5.3.2 Incomplete knowledge about human physiology in partial gravity

At present we have very little information about human physiology in partial gravity. This knowledge is important in helping to plan the mission as well as preparing for medical contingencies. The moon has about one-sixth the Earth's gravity and Mars has about one-third. The Apollo moon missions did not include extensive physiological experiments unfortunately.

We have information about short term changes from transitioning from 1G to partial gravity levels. This has been obtained during parabolic flight, head-up tilt, lower body unweighting experiments. However, physiological impact of prolonged stay in reduced gravity is not available [16].

6. Airway management in space

An integrated space surgery research found that most procedures performed on Earth can be performed in microgravity with the right equipment and with the operator, subject and tools sufficiently restrained [38].

6.1 Training of crew

The medical team identified for the space exploration mission can be as lean as a single crew medical officer (CMO)—who is not necessarily a medical doctor [35].

On Earth, anaesthesia techniques, in high income countries, are performed only by experienced practitioners. In space, however, sophisticated medical expertise may be absent, or the CMO may have become injured, incapacitated or seriously ill, even requiring anaesthesia [35]. Since real-time telemedical support is not immediately forthcoming, the crew will have to be self-reliant. It may be imperative that lifesaving procedures may then have to be performed by personnel with limited training. Until now, neither an anaesthetic technique nor human surgery has been performed in space, except for local infiltration [50].

Simulation and ground research are important programmes in framing protocols since there is a poor knowledge base about managing medical events in space. Simulation tools and techniques are routinely used in the medical field for continuous training of doctors [51–53]. The benefits of such training on their performance has been well documented [51, 54]. Needless to say, the simulation setup must resemble the target environment as closely as possible [54, 55].

In low income countries, especially ones facing a shortage of trained medical professionals, non-physician medical professionals regularly provide anaesthesia and perform surgical procedures. Many of them have a modest medical background [7]. They are trained mostly on the job and often work alone, even lacking recommended equipment and safety levels [35, 56–60] Ketamine based anaesthesia combined with the considerable skills that the providers acquire in a limited time could explain the perioperative mortality rate in these countries—which is "only" about two to three times more— when compared to high resource ones [35]. However, a crucial difference between anaesthesia providers in these low income countries and future space exploration missions is that the former treat a high number of patients and therefore skill redundancy is not a factor [7].

Personnel with modest medical training may be able to perform invasive procedures safely which is being witnessed in austere environments in different parts of the world. Astronauts are perhaps best positioned to respond to such a challenge [35]. Apart from their multitude of skills, astronauts are also selected for their ability to tolerate extreme stress. They are unquestionably among the best candidates, besides healthcare providers, to be able to perform advanced and invasive medical procedures, in the remotest of settings [35].

Currently, the International Space Station (ISS) has an on-board crew medical officer (CMO), who is not necessarily a trained medical doctor [7]. Given the uniqueness of future long distance space missions, the ideal profile of a crew physician is a subject for discussion [61, 62].

The CMO will need to possess a broad spectrum of knowledge, be competent in basic surgical skills and in the management of the critically ill [61–63]. He/She will have to be resourceful and flexible in his/her thinking and approach, and have the ability to improvise for unanticipated medical scenarios [62]. A single physician is required to manage both surgery and anaesthesia. If the CMO herself becomes ill, injured, incapacitated or dies, it is imperative that non-physicians take over. It is therefore prudent to train several of the crew members to manage at least the most common emergencies [7].

Recently, progress has been made in the field of artificial intelligence, especially in its application in medicine. It is now possible to achieve better monitoring, improve disease detection and bring in more efficient clinical decision support systems. Safety of crew members could be improved by autonomous diagnostic systems, closed-loop automated anaesthesia or other clinical decision support systems. Furthermore, these measures could also simplify the training programme [7].

6.2 Equipment

Devices for airway management that are brought on board the space shuttles, comprise of: a face mask, a pressure-cycled ventilator, a single-bladed laryngoscope, tracheal tubes, an introducer, a capnograph, and a tracheostomy kit [64].

Care has to be taken to ensure that the airway equipment carried on board is adequately restrained and made conveniently accessible to the person performing the procedure.

Cuffed endotracheal tube is the recommended device in view of the changes in gastric motility and reflux. However several studies have shown that non-anaesthesiologists can secure the airway more easily with supraglottic airways than with endotracheal intubation [65–67]. A laryngoscope is not required to be used in order to insert these devices and hence one hand is now available to stabilise the head as well as the neck [64]. The second generation supraglottic airways provides a better seal and also allow gastric drainage making it a good fit for emergencies, in microgravity [1].

Videolaryngoscopy may also be used with increased success in these scenarios since they have better glottic visualisation and a higher success rate with less experienced clinicians [68–70].

6.3 Technique

Airway management in space, with all its challenges, is amplified for non-medical personnel. Checklists and other such simple and minimal protocols will immensely help to streamline the process [7].

A mandatory pre-anaesthetic evaluation of all space travellers, before their departure from Earth, is recommended. A thorough airway assessment and detailed clinical documentation for every space traveller would prove to be valuable in case of emergencies. Clinical documentation may include details like the size of the endotracheal tube, requirement of additional intubation equipment, etc. Checklists for airway management and anaesthesia may include details of that equipment that must be available conveniently with the corresponding drug doses calculated and made available.

Conventional laryngoscopy and intubation with the patient placed in the sniffing position, without the use of restraints, is likely to have a high failure rate in microgravity. The head and neck move out of the field of vision during direct laryngoscopy, due to the anterior force exerted. It is not possible for the hand—the one not holding the laryngoscope—to stabilise the head–neck as well as direct the endotracheal tube toward the glottic opening simultaneously [64]. Anaesthesiologists exert a force of about 40 N, lasting for about 10–20 s during direct laryngoscopy. This force is sufficient for a 70 kg human to move about 0.3 m in 1 second in microgravity. Use of a restraint (**Figure 1**) will allow the stabilisation of the head and neck, so that the hand not holding the laryngoscope is free to direct the endotracheal tube toward the glottic opening [64]. However, there are some limitations in applying them during a medical emergency. Data indicates that it takes 5 to 10 seconds for strap application [71].

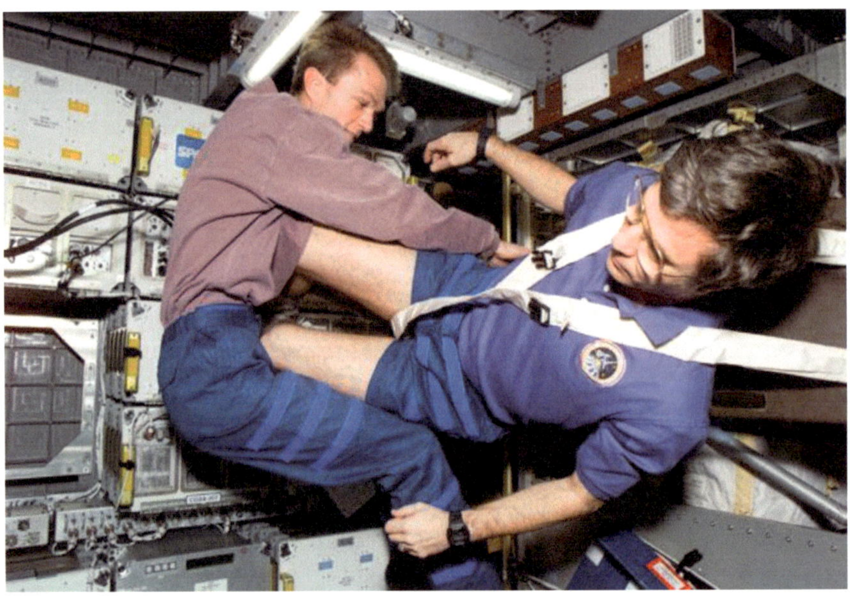

Figure 1.
*Crew medical restraint system used during the space shuttle missions. Restraints hold the patient in place and allow the operator's hands to be free. Source: Photograph S81E5933 - STS-081 - RME 1327 - Crew Medical Restraint System (**CMRS**); "STS-81 pilot Brent Jett straps mission specialist John Blaha into the Crew Medical Restraint System (**CMRS**) in the Spacehab module." January 1997; File Unit: STS-81, 4/12/1981 - 7/21/2011; Series: Mission photographs taken during the space shuttle program, 4/12/1981–7/21/2011; Record Group 255: Records of the National Aeronautics and Space Administration, 1903–2006; National archives at College Park, Adelphi road College Park (MD). Accessed on 30th April, 2021.*

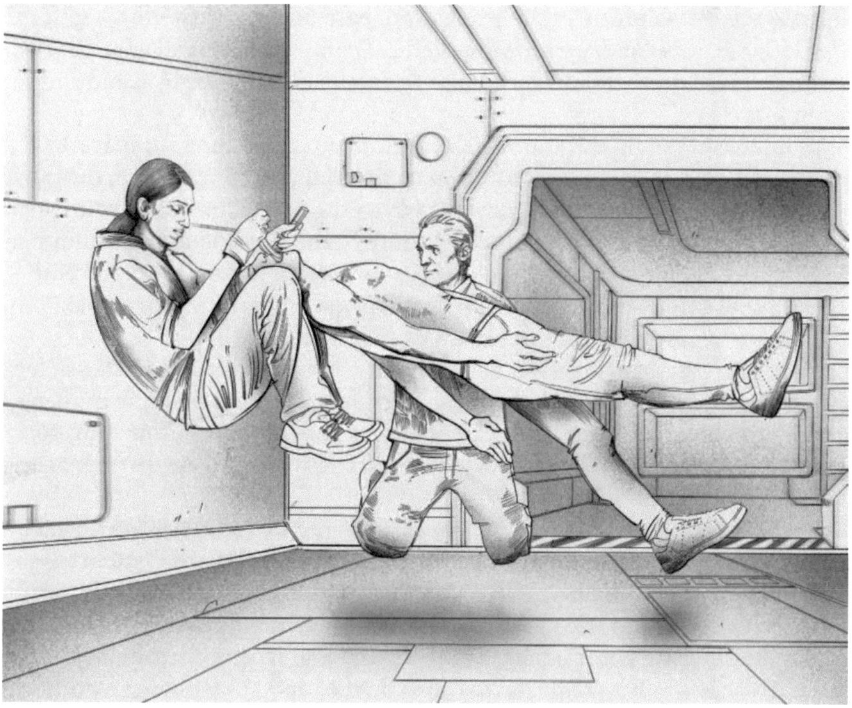

Figure 2.
An artist's representation of the sit down-lean back technique. (Image provided by the author.)

A self-retaining, bivalved laryngoscope may allow the hand that is holding the laryngoscope to be free in order to help stabilise the head and neck. The head and neck of the patient may also be stabilised between the knees of the person intubating the patient [64, 71].

During cardiopulmonary resuscitation, stabilising the head by gripping it between the knees (**Figure 2**) is recommended [71]. Even though this technique provides a distant view of the glottic inlet, it is stable and saves time. This technique may be compared to the "sit down–lean back technique" used by paramedics to stabilise the victim's head [72].

In the case of elective procedures, it is advisable to use restraints. If exercise of restraints is not feasible then extra tracheal airway devices may prove to be useful. It is not essential to position oneself at the head end of the patient for use of the extra-tracheal airway devices, in the interest of saving time [64].

Restraints are not necessary for either the patient, the equipment or the operator—on Mars—since its gravity is approximately one-third of Earth's gravity. In microgravity, however, restraining is recommended [35].

Robotic intubation may not find an application, at least in the foreseeable future, as far as space is concerned, in view of the undue up-mass they constitute and given that the chances of using this technique is remote [1].

7. Conclusion

Recent technological advances and scientific discoveries will lead mankind to realise its aspirations as a spacefaring species. If we are to support an enduring human exploration of space, we would have to rapidly update our understanding of human physiology, as well as find better ways to manage medical and surgical events in space. Persons other than professional astronauts are unprepared for the rigours of space travel and are prone to medical complications and emergencies. In this regard, it is of great importance that astronauts manage medical and surgical events in space.

With increasing flight durations, as a result of advances made in spaceflight enabling technologies that would afford deeper exploration into space, the prospect of a medical emergency entailing airway management is increased. Medical evacuation is not an option in such cases and therefore becomes imperative that immediate care is provided, while on board. Such situations call for a crew equipped with emergency care skills and training. Airway management is an important skill that is required to manage a great many medical emergencies.

This chapter briefly overviews the physiology of the airway, anaesthesia delivery and airway management, on Earth, to compare with and highlight the challenges to human physiology in space given the unique nature of the environment, so as to understand the specific challenges to anaesthesia delivery and airway management, in space.

The enabling technology for space travel, powered by Artificial Intelligence and Machine Learning algorithms, is advancing exponentially. Medical science typically tends to follow a more measured trajectory and tends to trail relative to the strides made by technology. We will also likely travel to Mars in the near future and this particular mission will come under more scrutiny than any other previous space missions. The crew will be required to travel farther and longer than any other human being in the history of our world. Techniques for airway management will need to undergo and be better defined in the coming years. As it stands, an expanding body of research that is trying to provide a better understanding of many aspects of human health in space is already underway. It is imperative for medical science to rapidly expand its body of knowledge when it comes to space travel, if it is to support human quest for space exploration.

Conflict of interest

The author declares no conflict of interest.

Notes/Thanks/Other declarations

Looking up into the night sky is looking into infinity – distance is incomprehensible and therefore meaningless.

–Douglas Adams, A Hitch-hikers Guide to the Galaxy.

Of all milestones and achievements in medicine, conquering pain must be one of the very few that has potentially affected every human being in the world.

–DH Robinson.

Special thanks to Preetam Satish.

Author details

Preethi Reddy
Independent Scientist, Bangalore, India

*Address all correspondence to: preethireddy3108@gmail.com

References

[1] Warnecke T, Tochtermann F, Kerkhoff S, Komorowski M, Neuhaus C, Hinkelbein J. Airway management in microgravity : a systematic review. Acta Anaesthesiol Scand. 2019;63:2-7. DOI: 10.1111/aas.13251

[2] Williams D, Kuipers A, Mukai C, Thirsk R. Acclimation during space flight: effects on human physiology. CMAJ. 2009 Jun 23; 180(13): 1317-1323. DOI: 10.1503/cmaj.090628

[3] Abadie LJ, Lloyd CW, Shelhamer MJ. The human body in space [Internet]. Houston: Johnson Space Center (US), NASA Human Research Program; [cited 2020 June 20]. Available from: https://www.nasa.gov/hrp/bodyinspace

[4] Keller C, Brimacombe J, Giampalmo M, Kleinsasser A, Loeckinger A, Giampalmo G, Pühringer F. Airway management during spaceflight: A comparison of four airway devices in simulated microgravity. Anesthesiology. 2000 May;92(5):1237-1241. DOI: 10.1097/00000542-200005000-00010

[5] LeJeune FE Jr. Laryngeal Problems in Space Travel. Aviat Space Environ Med. 1978 Nov;49(11):1347-1349.

[6] Rabitsch W, Moser D, Inzunza MR, Niedermayr M, Kostler WJ, Staudinger T, Locker GJ, Schellongowski P, Wulkersdorfer B, Rich JM, Meyer B, Benumof JL, Frass M. Airway management with endotracheal tube versus combitube during parabolic flights. Anesthesiology 2006; 105(4): 696 –702. DOI: 10.1097/00000542-200610000-00014

[7] Komorowski M, Fleming S, Mawkin M, Hinkelbein J. Anaesthesia in austere environments: literature review and considerations for future space exploration missions. NPJ Microgravity. 2018 Feb 23; 4:5. DOI: 10.1038/s41526-018-0039-y

[8] Hagberg CA, Artime CA. Airway management in the adult. In: Miller RD, Cohen NH, Eriksson LI, Fleisher LA, Wiener-Kronish JP, Young WL, editors. Miller's Anaesthesia. 8th ed. Philadelphia, PA: Elsevier/Saunders; 2015. p. 1647-1683.

[9] Practice guidelines for preoperative fasting and the use of pharmacologic agents to reduce the risk of pulmonary aspiration: application to healthy patients undergoing elective procedures: an updated report by the American Society of Anesthesiologists task force on preoperative fasting and the use of pharmacologic agents to reduce the risk of pulmonary aspiration. 2017 Mar;126(3):376-93. DOI: 10.1097/ALN.0000000000001452

[10] Combes X, Andriamifidy L, Dufresne E, Suen P, Sauvat S, Scherrer E, Feiss P, Marty J, Duvaldestin P. Comparison of two induction regimens using or not using muscle relaxant: impact on postoperative upper airway discomfort. Br J Anaesth 2007;99(2):276-281. DOI: 10.1093/bja/aem147

[11] Gore MS, Harnagale KD. Evaluation of Intubating Conditions with Varying Doses of Propofol without Muscle Relaxants. J Anaesthesiol Clin Pharmacol 2011; 27(1):27-30.

[12] Erhan E, Ugur G, Gunusen I, Alper I, Ozya B. Propofol - not thiopental or etomidate - with remifentanil provides adequate intubating conditions in the absence of neuromuscular blockade. Can J Anaesth 2003 Feb;50(2):108-115. DOI: 10.1007/BF03017840

[13] Apfelbaum JL, Hagberg CA, Caplan RA, Blitt CD, Connis RT,

Nickinovich DG, et al. Practice guidelines for management of the difficult airway: an updated report by the American Society of Anesthesiologists Task Force on Management of the Difficult Airway. Anesthesiology. 2013 Feb;118(2):251-270. DOI: 10.1097/ALN.0b013e31827773b2

[14] The respiratory pathway. In: Ellis H, Feldman S, Griffiths WH. Anatomy for anaesthetists. 8th ed. Massachusetts: Blackwell Publishing; 2004. p.1-69.

[15] Demontis GC, Germani MM, Caiani EG, Barravecchia I, Passino C, Angeloni D. Human pathophysiological adaptations to the space environment. Front. Physiol. 2017 Aug 2;8:547. DOI: 10.3389/fphys.2017.00547

[16] Komorowski M, Fleming S, Kirkpatrick AW. Fundamentals of Anesthesiology for Spaceflight. J Cardiothorac Vasc Anesth. 2016 Jun;30(3):781-790. DOI: 10.1053/j.jvca.2016.01.007

[17] Norfleet WT. Anesthetic Concerns of Spaceflight. Anesthesiology. 2000 May;92(5):1219-1222. DOI: 10.1097/00000542-200005000-00006

[18] Alfrey CP, Udden MM, Leach-Huntoon C, Driscoll T, Pickett MH. Control of red blood cell mass in spaceflight. J Appl Physiol (1985). 1996 Jul;81(1):98-104. DOI: 10.1152/jappl.1996.81.1.98

[19] Norsk P, Asmar A, Damgaard M, Christensen NJ. Fluid shifts, vasodilatation and ambulatory blood pressure reduction during long duration spaceflight. J Physiol. 2015 Feb;593(3):573-584. DOI: 10.1113/jphysiol.2014.284869

[20] Ade CJ, Bemben DA. Differential MicroRNA expression following head-down tilt bed rest: implications for cardiovascular responses to microgravity. Physiol Rep. 2019 May;7(9):e14061. DOI: 10.14814/phy2.14061

[21] Martin DS, South DA, Wood ML, Bungo MW, Meck JV. Comparison of echocardiographic changes after short- and long-duration spaceflight. Aviat Space Environ Med. 2002 Jun;73(6):532-536.

[22] Perhonen MA, Franco F, Lane LD, Buckey JC, Blomqvist CG, Zerwekh JE, Peshock RM, Weatherall PT, Levine BD. Cardiac atrophy after bed rest and spaceflight. J Appl Physiol (1985). 2001 Aug;91(2):645-653. DOI: 10.1152/jappl.2001.91.2.645

[23] Simanonok KE, Charles JB. Space sickness and fluid shifts: a hypothesis. J Clin Pharmacol. 1994 Jun; 34(6):652-663. DOI: 10.1002/j.1552-4604.1994.tb02020.x

[24] LeBlanc AD, Spector ER, Evans HJ, Sibonga JD. Skeletal responses to space flight and the bed rest analog: a review. J Musculoskelet Neuronal Interact. 2007 Jan-Mar;7(1):33-47.

[25] Smith SM, Wastney ME, Morukov BV, Larina IM, Nyquist LE, Abrams SA, et al. Calcium metabolism before, during, and after a 3-mo spaceflight: kinetic and biochemical changes. Am J Physiol. 1999 Jul;277(1 Pt 2):R1-10. DOI: 10.1152/ajpregu.1999.277.1.r1

[26] Smith SM, Heer M, Shackelford LC, Sibonga JD, Spatz J, Pietrzyk RA, Hudson EK, Zwart SR. Bone metabolism and renal stone risk during International Space Station missions. Bone. 2015 Dec;81:712-720. DOI: 10.1016/j.bone.2015.10.002

[27] Whitson PA, Pietrzyk RA, Morukov BV, Sams CF. The risk of renal stone formation during and after long duration space flight. Nephron. 2001

Nov;89(3):264-270. DOI: 10.1159/000046083

[28] Wantier M, Estenne M, Verbanck S, Prisk GK, Paiva M. Chest wall mechanics in sustained microgravity. Journal of Applied Physiology (Bethesda, Md. : 1985). 1998 Jun;84(6):2060-2065. DOI: 10.1152/jappl.1998.84.6.2060

[29] Prisk GM. Microgravity and the respiratory system. Eur Respir J. 2014 May;43(5):1459-1471. DOI: 10.1183/09031936.00001414

[30] Elliott AR, Prisk GK, Guy HJ, West JB. Lung volumes during sustained microgravity on Spacelab SLS-1. J Appl Physiol (1985). 1994 Oct;77(4):2005-2014. DOI: 10.1152/jappl.1994.77.4.2005

[31] Pierson DL, Stowe RP, Phillips TM, Lugg DJ, Mehta SK. Epstein-Barr virus shedding by astronauts during space flight. Brain Behav Immun. 2005 May;19(3):235-242. DOI: 10.1016/j.bbi.2004.08.001

[32] Wilson JW, Ott CM, Höner zu Bentrup K, Ramamurthy R, Quick L, Porwollik S, et al. Space flight alters bacterial gene expression and virulence and reveals a role for global regulator Hfq. Proc Natl Acad Sci U S A. 2007 Oct 9;104(41):16299-16304. DOI: 10.1073/pnas.0707155104

[33] Heer M, De Santo NG, Cirillo M, Drummer C. Body mass changes, energy, and protein metabolism in space. Am J Kidney Dis. 2001 Sep;38(3):691-695. DOI: 10.1053/ajkd.2001.27767

[34] Smith SM, Zwart SR, Block G, Rice BL, Davis-Street JE. The nutritional status of astronauts is altered after long-term space flight aboard the International Space Station. J Nutr. 2005 Mar;135(3):437-443. DOI: 10.1093/jn/135.3.437

[35] Komorowski M, Fleming S. Intubation after rapid sequence induction performed by non-medical personnel during space exploration missions: a simulation pilot study in a Mars analogue environment. Extrem Physiol Med. 2015 Nov;4:19. DOI: 10.1186/s13728-015-0038-5

[36] Convertino VA, Cooke WH. Evaluation of cardiovascular risks of spaceflight does not support the NASA bioastronautics critical path roadmap. Aviat Space Environ Med. 2005 Sep;76(9):869-876

[37] Komorowski M, Watkins SD, Lebuffe G, Clark JB. Potential anesthesia protocols for space exploration missions. Aviat Space Environ Med. 2013 Mar;84(3):226-233. DOI: 10.3357/asem.3427.2013

[38] Drudi L, Ball CG, Kirkpatrick AW, Saary J, Grenon SM. Surgery in Space: Where are we at now? Acta Astronaut. 2012;79:61-66. DOI: 10.1016/j.actaastro.2012.04.014

[39] Pavy-Le Traon A, Saivin S, Soulez-LaRivière C, Pujos M, Güell A, Houin G. Pharmacology in space: pharmacotherapy. Adv Space Biol Med. 1997;6:93-105. DOI: 10.1016/s1569-2574(08)60079-9

[40] Graebe A, Schuck EL, Lensing P, Putcha L, Derendorf H. Physiological, pharmacokinetic, and pharmaco dynamic changes in space. J Clin Pharmacol. 2004 Aug;44(8):837-853. DOI: 10.1177/0091270004267193

[41] Sørensen MK, Bretlau C, Gätke MR, Sørensen AM, Rasmussen LS. Rapid sequence induction and intubation with rocuronium-sugammadex compared with succinylcholine: a randomized trial. Br J Anaesth. 2012 Apr;108(4):682-689. DOI: 10.1093/bja/aer503

[42] Niazi AU, Haldipur N, Prasad AG, Chan VW. Ultrasound-guided regional

anesthesia performance in the early learning period: effect of simulation training. Reg Anesth Pain Med. 2012 Jan-Feb;37(1):51-54. DOI: 10.1097/AAP.0b013e31823dc340

[43] Salinas FV, Hanson NA. Evidence-based medicine for ultrasound-guided regional anesthesia. Anesthesiol Clin. 2014 Dec;32(4):771-787. DOI: 10.1016/j.anclin.2014.08.001

[44] Ambrosio A, Pfannenstiel T, Bach K, Cornelissen C, Gaconnet C, Brigger MT. Difficult airway management for novice physicians: a randomized trial comparing direct and video-assisted laryngoscopy. Otolaryngol Head Neck Surg. 2014 May;150(5):775-778. DOI: 10.1177/0194599814521380

[45] Maharaj CH, Ni Chonghaile M, Higgins BD, Harte BH, Laffey JG. Tracheal intubation by inexperienced medical residents using the Airtraq and Macintosh laryngoscopes--a manikin study. Am J Emerg Med. 2006 Nov;24(7):769-774. DOI: 10.1016/j.ajem.2006.03.014

[46] McQuillen JB, McKay TL, Griffin DW, Brown DF, Zoldak JT. Final Report for Intravenous Fluid Generation (IVGEN) Spaceflight Experiment. [Internet] Cleveland, Ohio: NASA STI Program; July 2011 [cited 2020 June 25]. 86 p. Report No.: NASA/TM—2011-217033. Available from: https://ntrs.nasa.gov/citations/20110014585

[47] C9 and other microgravity simulations summary report. Houston, Texas: Space Life Sciences Directorate, Human Adaptation and Countermeasures Division, NASA Johnson Space Center; Sep 2009 [cited 2021 Feb 10]. 150 p. Report No.: NASA/TM-2009-214794 Available from: https://www.nasa.gov/centers/johnson/pdf/505838main_FY09_TM-2009-214794.pdf

[48] Campbell MR, Williams DR, Buckey JC Jr, Kirkpatrick AW. Animal surgery during spaceflight on the Neurolab Shuttle mission. Aviat Space Environ Med. 2005 Jun;76(6):589-593.

[49] Campbell MR, Dawson DL, Melton S, Hooker D, Cantu H. Surgical instrument restraint in weightlessness. Aviat Space Environ Med. 2001 Oct;72(10):871-876.

[50] Kirkpatrick AW, LaPorta A, Brien S, Leslie T, Glassberg E, McKee J, et al. Technical innovations that may facilitate real-time telementoring of damage control surgery in austere environments: a proof of concept comparative evaluation of the importance of surgical experience, telepresence, gravity and mentoring in the conduct of damage control laparotomies. Can J Surg. 2015 Jun;58(3):S88-S90. DOI: 10.1503/cjs.014214

[51] Smith HM, Jacob AK, Segura LG, Dilger JA, Torsher LC. Simulation education in anesthesia training: a case report of successful resuscitation of bupivacaine-induced cardiac arrest linked to recent simulation training. Anesth Analg. 2008 May;106(5):1581-1584. DOI: 10.1213/ane.0b013e31816b9478

[52] Galvez JA, Rehman MA. Telemedicine in anesthesia: an update. Curr Opin Anaesthesiol. 2011 Aug;24(4):459-462. DOI: 10.1097/ACO.0b013e328348717b

[53] Murray AW, Beaman ST, Kampik CW, Quinlan JJ. Simulation in the operating room. Best Pract Res Clin Anaesthesiol. 2015 Mar;29(1):41-50. DOI: 10.1016/j.bpa.2015.02.005

[54] Schwid HA, Rooke GA, Carline J, Steadman RH, Murray WB, Olympio M, et al. Anesthesia Simulator Research Consortium. Evaluation of anesthesia residents using mannequin-based simulation: a multi institutional study.

Anesthesiology. 2002 Dec;97(6):1434-1444. DOI: 10.1097/00000542-200212000-00015

[55] Weller JM, Nestel D, Marshall SD, Brooks PM, Conn JJ. Simulation in clinical teaching and learning. Med J Aust 2012;196(9):594. DOI: 10.5694/mja10.11474

[56] Bösenberg AT. Pediatric anesthesia in developing countries. Curr Opin Anaesthesiol. 2007 Jun;20(3):204-210. DOI: 10.1097/ACO.0b013e3280c60c78

[57] Martin J, Tau G, Cherian MN, Vergel de Dios J, Mills D, Fitzpatrick J, et al. Survey of the capacity for essential surgery and anaesthesia services in Papua New Guinea. BMJ Open. 2015 Dec 16;5(12):e009841. DOI: 10.1136/bmjopen-2015-009841.

[58] McQueen K, Coonan T, Ottaway A, Hendel S, Bagutifils PR, Froese A, et al. The Bare Minimum: The Reality of Global Anaesthesia and Patient Safety. World J Surg. 2015 Sep;39(9):2153-2160. DOI: 10.1007/s00268-015-3101-x

[59] Jochberger S, Ismailova F, Lederer W, Mayr VD, Luckner G, Wenzel V, et al. Anesthesia and its allied disciplines in the developing world: a nationwide survey of the Republic of Zambia. Anesth Analg. 2008 Mar;106(3):942-948. DOI: 10.1213/ane.0b013e318166ecb8

[60] Epiu I, Tindimwebwa JV, Mijumbi C, Chokwe TM, Lugazia E, Ndarugirire F, et al. Challenges of Anesthesia in Low- and Middle-Income Countries: A Cross-Sectional Survey of Access to Safe Obstetric Anesthesia in East Africa. Anesth Analg. 2017 Jan;124(1):290-299. DOI: 10.1213/ANE.0000000000001690

[61] Saluja IS, Williams DR, Woodard D, Kaczorowski J, Douglas B, Scarpa PJ, et al. Survey of astronaut opinions on medical crewmembers for a mission to Mars. Acta Astronautica. 2008 Sep;63(5-6): 586-593. DOI: 10.1016/j.actaastro.2008.05.002.

[62] Kuypers MI. Emergency and wilderness medicine training for physician astronauts on exploration class missions. Wilderness Environ Med. 2013 Dec;24(4):445-449. DOI: 10.1016/j.wem.2013.03.024

[63] Stewart LH, Trunkey D, Rebagliati GS. Emergency medicine in space. J Emerg Med. 2007 Jan;32(1):45-54. DOI: 10.1016/j.jemermed.2006.05.031

[64] Keller C, Brimacombe J, A FR, Giampalmo M, Kleinsasser A, Loeckinger A, et al. Airway management during spaceflight: A comparison of four airway devices in simulated microgravity. Anesthesiology. 2000 May;92(5):1237-1241. DOI: 10.1097/00000542-200005000-00010

[65] Deakin CD, Peters R, Tomlinson P, Cassidy M. Securing the prehospital airway: a comparison of laryngeal mask insertion and endotracheal intubation by UK paramedics. Emerg Med J. 2005 Jan;22(1):64-67. DOI: 10.1136/emj.2004.017178

[66] Brimacombe J. The advantages of the LMA over the tracheal tube or facemask: a meta-analysis. Can J Anaesth. 1995 Nov;42(11):1017-1023. DOI: 10.1007/BF03011075

[67] Davies PR, Tighe SQ, Greenslade GL, Evans GH. Laryngeal mask airway and tracheal tube insertion by unskilled personnel. Lancet. 1990 Oct 20;336(8721):977-979. DOI: 10.1016/0140-6736(90)92429-l

[68] Arulkumaran N, Lowe J, Ions R, Mendoza M, Bennett V, Dunser MW. Videolaryngoscopy versus direct laryngoscopy for emergency orotracheal intubation outside the operating room: a systematic review and meta-analysis. Br

J Anaesth. 2018 Apr;120(4):712-724. DOI: 10.1016/j.bja.2017.12.041

[69] Risse J, Volberg C, Kratz T, Plöger B, Jerrentrup A, Pabst D, et al. Comparison of videolaryngoscopy and direct laryngoscopy by German paramedics during out-of-hospital cardiopulmonary resuscitation; an observational prospective study. BMC Emerg Med. 2020 Mar 23;20(1):22. DOI: 10.1186/s12873-020-00316-z

[70] Liu DX, Ye Y, Zhu YH, Li J, He HY, Dong L, et al. Intubation of non-difficult airways using video laryngoscope versus direct laryngoscope: a randomized, parallel-group study. BMC Anesthesiol. 2019 May 15;19(1):75. DOI: 10.1186/s12871-019-0737-3

[71] Groemer GE, Brimacombe J, Haas T, de Negueruela C, Soucek A, Thomsen M, et al. The feasibility of laryngoscope-guided tracheal intubation in microgravity during parabolic flight: a comparison of two techniques. Anesth Analg. 2005 Nov;101(5):1533-1535. DOI: 10.1213/01.ANE.0000181001.25777.53

[72] Rabitsch W, Moser D, Inzunza MR, Niedermayr M, Köstler WJ, Staudinger T, et al. Airway management with endotracheal tube versus Combitube during parabolic flights. Anesthesiology. 2006 Oct;105(4):696-702. DOI: 10.1097/00000542-200610000-00014

Chapter 12

Airway Management in Aviation, Space, and Microgravity

Mohamed Abdelwahab Elarref,
Mogahed Ismail Hassan Hussein, Muhammad Jaffar Khan
and Noran Mohamed Elarif

Abstract

Although medical services in aviation have evolved over years based on our understanding of physiology, advancement in monitoring technology but airway management was only recently studied with a focus on space environment. The barometric pressure of ambient air declines as altitude increases, while the volume of air in a confined space will increase according to Boyle law, and therefore oxygen concentration remains at a constant 21%. Altitude sensitive equipment includes endotracheal and tracheostomy cuffs, pneumatic anti shock garments, air splints, colostomy bags, Foley catheters, orogastric and nasogastric tubes, ventilators, invasive monitors, and intra-aortic balloon pumps. The microgravity reduces the body compensation capacity for hemorrhage, while the redistribution of the blood can affect intubation by causing facial edema. Another change is the decreased gastric emptying during aviation. Acute respiratory failure, hypoxemia or inadequate ventilation and protection of the airway in a patient with impaired consciousness are common indications for advanced airway management in aviation. Airway management requires adequate training to maintain excellent medical care during aviation. Tracheal intubation using laryngoscopy would be difficult in microgravity, since the force exerted by the laryngoscope causes the head and neck move out of the field of vision by lever effect exerted on the head and generated through the laryngoscope blade by hand generating a lack of stability, resulting in the difficulty to insert the tracheal tube. While on the ground with the help of gravity, an adequate positioning of the patient is facilitated to achieve alignment of the laryngeal, pharyngeal and oral axes, which is known as sniffing position that allows visualization of the vocal cords and supraglottic structures allowing the introduction of an endotracheal tube.

Keywords: medical aviation, microgravity, weightless environment, stratosphere, high altitude, near space, space medicine

1. Introduction

Space exploration is rapidly advancing and requiring a parallel advancement of medical services that can be provided in aviation for any kind of medical issues that may arise during the space flight. The physiology of human body is definitely affected by the change in gravity during space flights, this why the extent of physiological changes, the required monitoring and intervention should be carefully tailored based on the physiological response to the space environment and the underlying medical conditions. Although medical services in aviation has evolved over years based on our understanding of physiology, advancement in monitoring technology but airway management was only recently studied with a focus on space environment. Airway management and other hemodynamic goals parameters, especially during medical air transport and aviation put the patient and medical team under unfamiliar and extreme physiological conditions, with detrimental clinical sequalae. In this chapter will cover the airway management in aviation with high emphasis on physiological changes and he preferred airway management techniques during air transport and aviation conditions.

2. Physiological changes in microgravity

The changes occur to human body during aviation can affect the anesthesia delivery if surgery is needed. Almost all the body organs will be affected, but what is more relevant to anesthesia administration is: cardiac systolic and diastolic changes, gastric motility, reduction in blood volume as well as neuromuscular junction changes.

2.1 Pressure related effects

At sea level, barometric pressure is 760 mmHg with a partial pressure of oxygen of 160 mmHg. The barometric pressure of ambient air declines as altitude increases, while the volume of air in a confined space will increase according to Boyle law, and this is why oxygen concentration remains at a constant 21% [1]. The intracranial air volume could be increased by 30% at the usual maximum cabin altitude of 8000 feet. These volume and pressure effects are sometimes associated with hemodynamic compromise (tension pneumothorax), barotrauma (sinuses), equipment malfunction (blood pressure cuffs), and possible injury or compromised monitoring as inflated gas bubble in the arterial line. Certain conditions such as pneumopericardium, subcutaneous emphysema, gas gangrene, systemic air emboli, decompression sickness, and gastric distension may be worsened at altitude [2]. Altitude sensitive equipment includes endotracheal and tracheostomy cuffs, pneumatic antishock garments (eg, medical antishock trousers), air splints, colostomy bags, foley catheters, orogastric and nasogastric tubes, ventilators, invasive monitors, and intra-aortic balloon pumps. Most aircraft cabins are usually pressurized to a pressure equivalent to 5000 to 8000 feet, giving an atmospheric partial pressure of oxygen of 118 mm Hg [3]. Thus, the oxygen requirement (Fio_2) of a patient on mechanical ventilation may increase at altitude. ARDS in animal models were more responsive to increased PEEP, yet resistant to increases of (Fio_2) [4].

Hypoxemia, even at low altitudes (3281–9843 feet), which is the usual flight range for the medical helicopter transport, could lead to global hypoxic pulmonary vasoconstriction and pulmonary edema. Hypoxemia is detrimental to patients with coronary ischemia, pulmonary compromise acute respiratory distress syndrome [ARDS], or neurologic injury. Besides, the hypoxia associated-tachycardia and hypertension increases the cardiac mechanical load and myocardial oxygen consumption.

Flying at low altitude is commonly known as "Altitude restrictions" which mainly for pressure sensitive conditions as in eye trauma, pneumothorax, intracerebral air, and sinusitis [5]. Those low altitude flying restrictions come with the cost of more turbulence and longer transport times, another risk factor for more vibration injury, anxiety and prolonged access to healthcare.

2.2 Cardiovascular changes

The loss of gravity effect of the distribution of blood volume in different body compartments is notable in a microgravity environment. In normal environment at the earth surface there is a pressure gradient created by the gravity and the loss of this gradient during aviation result in more diuresis and by so reduction in blood volume [6–8]. The blood volume is one of the determinants of cardiac output, the reduction in the blood volume in microgravity will result in a 20% reduction in COP [6]. The reduction in these parameters will definitely reduce the body compensation capacity for hemorrhage, while the redistribution of the blood can affect intubation by causing facial edema [6, 9–11].

2.3 Musculoskeletal changes

Two main issues regarding musculoskeletal system changes in microgravity are the reduced bone mass [12] and the muscle atrophy which may lead to increase expression of extra junctional acetylcholine receptors [13, 14]. The abnormally expressed receptors can explain the risk of severe hyperkalemia after succinylcholine in space men [6, 10, 11].

Along with muscle atrophy changes in fat distribution affect the pharmacokinetics of anesthetic medications.

2.4 Gastrointestinal changes

Some studies suggest that there is a decrease gastric emptying during aviation in the first three days [6, 15, 16]. Some studies used paracetamol absorption as an indicator of gastric emptying [17, 18]. In anesthesia, gastric emptying time is very important factor in the assessment of aspiration risk following anesthesia induction.

3. Special consideration in anesthesia and airway management in space and microgravity conditions

The first vehicles carrier used to carry humans to the stratosphere atmosphere, was the Balloons in 1783, the first round across the Earth had been achieved by the hybrid balloon. The increasing advancement of advanced life support programs and control systems progress had allowed to transport humans higher for more plans and the preparation to colonize the Moon and the trip to Mars [19].

Now recently aerospace companies are aiming to give scientists the chance to develop their clinical experience by arranging near space trips [20]. A great progress in Human spaceflight has expanded over the last 40 years leading to a larger, more sophisticated, and more distant journeys. As a result of this continuous advancement, space flight crews might require medical procedures, that mandates anesthesia, so the medical personnel on board should be well experienced to perform surgery and anesthesia during flights in deep space. So anesthesia strategies and techniques have to be adjusted to deal with specific problems and dangers that may rise while patients are under the effects of microgravity [10].

Airway management requires adequate training to maintain excellent medical care during aviation, our knowledge about airway management in microgravity is progressing and numbers of trials that examine the difference between different airway management methods is increasing. This justifies the importance of reviewing this topic to so that a better understanding of all the challenges in microgravity environment is achieved.

The most common indications for advanced airway management in aviation are acute respiratory failure, hypoxemia or inadequate ventilation and protection of the airway in a patient with impaired alertness.

4. Challenges in airway management during space exploration missions

Challenges during space mission are very numerous, it can be classified into: patient related, environmental, and caregivers related. Medical emergency during aviation will more likely to have high risk of morbidity or mortality.

The patient factors are discussed in the physiological changes in microgravity.

The environment during aviation is characterized by the loss of gravity which may make very important simple adjuncts as fluids unavailable, it also affects the actual force that the body control, this render the caregiver with a totally new circumstances while doing intubation. Any practicing Anesthesiologist will be able to appreciate the importance of the ability to create the same effect while holding the laryngoscope with the usual power that the operator tends to use in normal conditions. The weightlessness also creates a big difference in patient positioning, the patient will be in free floating position and precision will be difficult without adequate training as tracheal intubation will be a single-handed technique.

Multiple factors in space are expected to create a challenging environment for airway management and by so affecting patient safety. Stress and cognitive factors, environmental hazards, deficiency in equipment, lack of intubation skills and suboptimal working conditions are not all but most of the challenging factors.

Loss of gravity alter the coordinated effort between the eye and the brain, which will impair eye - hand coordination [10].

Caregivers related factors are mainly related to the lack of expertise in this field, the crew will not likely be accompanied by a trained Anesthetist, and this is why most of the fine anesthesia techniques will be done by non-anesthesiologist during these missions. Facing these challenges, some scientists conducted clinical trials in a simulated environment, they compared the use of video-laryngoscopy in microgravity between the naïve and expertise in airway management. Results suggested that video- laryngoscopy help health care-givers to overcome these factors and it also decreases the difference in intubation efficacy between naive and expertise [21].

4.1 Anesthesia and airway management in microgravity

The approach to provide anesthesia on space flights missions would be necessary to the success of the mission. Physiological accommodation to microgravity may hinder any planning of anesthesia. A previously published assumption for anesthesia airway management reported monitoring, preoxygenation, induction then bag – mask ventilation then they used Rocuronium as a muscle relaxant, followed by endotracheal tube insertion using video laryngoscopy, the tube size was smaller than the proper size to avoid edema [21].

The adaptations of the muscle performance in microgravity particularly the functional changes in acetylcholine receptor variations can have an effect on the administration of depolarizing and non-depolarizing neuromuscular blockers in patients exposed to microgravity promoting their cautiously use [10].

Advance airway management requires adequate skills, knowledge and training to perform in the microgravity setting that add a new difficulty to the existing ones which necessities a proper training and knowledge [22]. Microgravity environments is a significant challenge for the person who is performing airway procedure since it is difficult to position the patient as the body is unsubstantiated, without the gravity of Earth's [23].

Caregiver loaded on the International Space Station (ISS). May be affected with situations that necessitate management of Airway to establish a patent airway for a patient suffering respiratory distress.

4.2 The NASA flight surgeon and NASA space person companions

Airway management procedures had been investigated in a previous study which described using them in inadequate conditions pertaining to space flight. Actually, the optimal way for patient care aboard on space station require that caregiver and patient to be restrained. The Medical Operation Support Team (MOST), 2007 and others previously assessed how to secure airways in microgravity experiments using different techniques for establishing airways in substandard positions by caregiving non-physician – they had accomplished direct laryngoscopy and inserted a cuffed endotracheal tube [24]. As researches are advancing in this field, NASA doctors and companions would be able to provide proper airway management during space trips.

There have been several important studies on airway management in microgravity, with the assumption that a laryngeal airway mask (LMA) had been used. Intubating Laryngeal Mask Airway effectively used which is a supraglottic airway device. Either approach is adequate to perform in substandard situations within a microgravity situation. [23, 25] The challenge to the advanced airway management during space journey is the presence of expertise to be one of the medical onboard team, occasionally the crew physician may had been diseased or incapacitated.

4.3 NASA studies on airway management in microgravity

In studies investigating the efficacy of airway management during air transport. Air medical transport teams are periodically confronted with the responsibility of conducting airways in unexpected and difficult circumstances, meanwhile they should be essentially trained to do the task in a limited field with less resources during their duty in the aircraft.

Unexpected abrupt patient deterioration prominently considered as the prevailing reason for Airway management during aviation. Intubation process achievement was not related to the category of aircraft. The total intubation successfulness rate for advanced airway handling procedures, was 96%. The successful Airway management procedures during flights was conducted with a high achievement percentage in a variety of venues and for a variety of patient status and conditions. Air medical transport teams achievement rates were proportionate to other emergency medical staff [26]. Anatomically the epiglottis lies at the base of tongue and provides an essential reference point for direct laryngoscopy. The epiglottis fulfills the function of gate that covers the glottis, the vallecula is the concavity between the base of the tongue and the epiglottis, shown as reference point where a curved laryngoscope blade is placed. The pressure exerted by the blade tip against the vallecula elevates the epiglottis and this elevation is affected by gravity. In 1978, LeJeune hypothesized that tracheal intubation using laryngoscopy would be difficult in microgravity, since the force exerted by the laryngoscope causes the head and neck move out of the field of vision by lever effect exerted on the head and generated through the laryngoscope blade by hand generating a lack of stability, resulting in the difficulty to insert the tracheal tube [27].

In 2000, a group tried using a deep pool to simulate microgravity and found that the success rate for anesthesiologists in the free-floating condition was 15%, increasing to 92% if the mannequin was tied to a surface [22].

On the ground with the help of gravity, an adequate positioning of the patient is facilitated to achieve alignment of the laryngeal, pharyngeal and oral axes, which is known as sniffing position. This sniffing position allows visualization of the vocal cords and supraglottic structures that allows the introduction of a endotracheal tube (as shown in **Figure 1**).

The need to intubate personnel in the space can arise from traumatic injuries or some other medical condition leading to deterioration of consciousness or respiratory failure and this possibility increases with longer stays in the space that arises with further incursions, and for this it is necessary to evaluate and try to determine probable complications which involves Airway management in non-terrestrial conditions with microgravity or zero gravity, with the complication extra conferred by not having a doctor trained in advanced Airway management and unavailability of an ideal area with the enough space to maneuver comfortably [23].

Intubation and suction techniques used for Airway management in terrestrial conditions are inefficient and of little use in the environment of a space station; so, it is necessary to have special equipment that facilitates endotracheal intubation. In an environment of minimal gravity or zero gravity the main problem will be the proper positioning of the patient to achieve proper alignment and approach of the airway, since without the help of terrestrial gravity the patient's body and personnel attempting Airway management lack adequate support, hence the need for creating a fixation device is paramount. The need to make these attachments has made are tested in simulators that create environments with minimal gravity or zero gravity [24].

Assessment of respiratory failure or the need for airway management can be evaluated by assessment that includes observation of the ventilatory pattern, pulse oximetry and vital signs; after which and if required, the patient must being moved

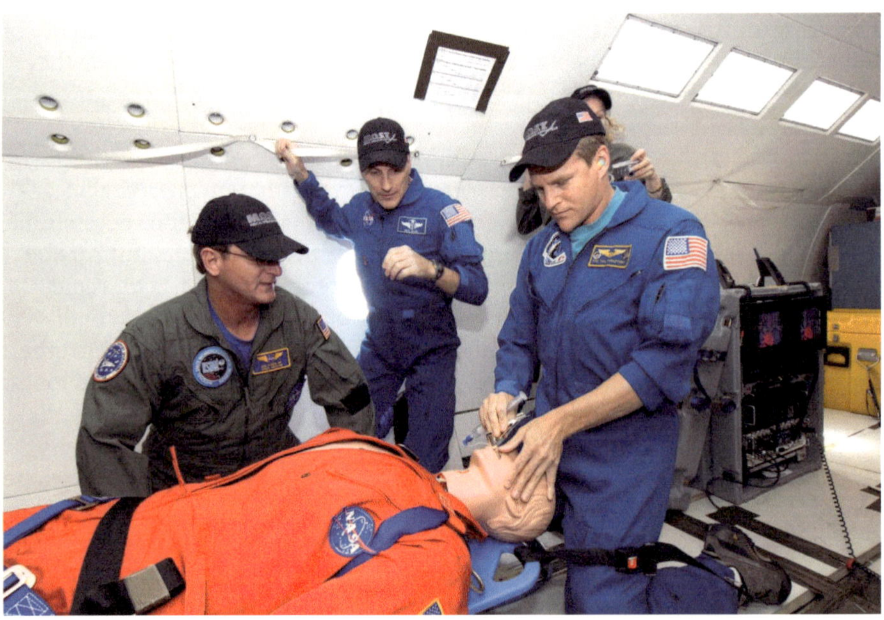

Figure 1.
Simulation of microgravity environment and intubation in restrained mannequin with a demonstration of sniffing position.

to a special area for medical or surgical procedure that indicate airway management, which could be affected in microgravity environments [28]. So it is necessary to provide a mean of fixation of the patient and the person who will secure the airway so that positioning would be easier also decreasing the possibility of complications that might happens during laryngoscopy using a restraint system [24].

A study published in 2005, which simulated a least gravity environment within a deep pool, in which the ability to manage the airway by expert staff and non-expert staff with and without devices holding and optimizing the alignment position; it was found that the success rate for the airway approach was equally rare for inexperienced staff and expert personnel in the free floating condition with the head of the mannequin caught between the knees, and in the fixation condition using a stability device while the dummy tied to a surface, this opens the discussion about using devices to restrain the patient either mandatory or using simple techniques is quite sufficient [25].

So the use of other alternative methods is required to overcome this difficulty like the practice for tracheal intubation as a single hand in free floating attitude or using a device that facilitate intubation indirectly, such as laryngeal masks would be alternatively possibly useful [22].

Studying all the difficulties which is possible to happen in space flights is challenging due to the difficulty of creating a simulated environment, and the research in this field have great limitations. This research field needs an interest to develop the necessary devices, and train flight personnel under these circumstances and manufacture airway approach instruments that makes their approach easier [23].

Moreover, the accessibility of telecare, use of telecommunication and information technologies in order to provide clinical health care assistance at a distance will be unavailable. Managing critical conditions may necessitate some measures, that needs the help of anesthesia provider, but the flight staff might be deficient or unskilled. So, proper training and skills of airway management are essential to perform this procedure during microgravity or aviation circumstances whilst they are in outer space journey.

5. Future consideration

5.1 End of life guidelines

A very important point to raise regarding medical care during aviation is the supportive care and medical resuscitation. A structured protocol needs to be in place to guide medical practice during management of emergency situation in space missions, the development of such protocols must take into account the limited availability restorative care, pain control and psychological adjuncts.

5.2 Health care providers

It is expected that, the increasing demand for a trained personal in space missions will affect the training structure of medical schools and hospitals, and space companies will support this kind of training. In aviation at least one crew member needs to be trained to deal with medical emergencies and the physicians should be skilled and competent in all basic lifesaving procedures. A focus on psychomotor skills and telemedicine is expected as telemedicine in the shape of the future and psychomotor skills is affected by microgravity. The special skills actually required for performance of surgery can be acquired, augmented, or practiced by using simulators and a hybrid technology that has been termed "cybersurgery" Training and retraining in clinical decision-making skills, clinical problem solving, and decision making for multiple casualties or illnesses are also necessary.

5.2.1 Equipment

Coming days and young minds might be able to provide us with a special tool that can be used in the setting of microgravity to safely manage airway. Human mind always get more creative when faced by struggles, so new laryngoscopy with a physical principle that may cancel the effect of microgravity and increase the efficacy of doing the intubation might emerge.

6. Conclusion

The recommended procedure and monitoring during Aviation are aiming to maintain the maximum safety with regards to the requirement of medical services during space flights. However, specific standards for monitoring and airway management are not yet developed.

As planning for future missions targeting distant planets is continuous, all space programs are aiming to include airway management protocols within their plans. Positioning of the patient in microgravity environments is the main problem for proper alignment and Airway management that focus on restraints use in microgravity environment being important for successful endotracheal intubation.

In summary the continuity of the research and Knowledge about accommodation to the space environment would help the crew and other non-anesthesiologist to do some anesthetic procedures that would be lifesaving.

The airway management in the space environment, by non-anesthetist can be improved by using video- laryngoscopes that had been gaining more popularity. A tight balance between: the patient condition, the nature of the medical condition and the safety of the environment, including the monitoring, equipment and back up interventions for unexpected deleterious effects during the trip is needed for a better outcome.

Author details

Mohamed Abdelwahab Elarref[1,2,3]*, Mogahed Ismail Hassan Hussein[4], Muhammad Jaffar Khan[4] and Noran Mohamed Elarif[5]

1 Department of Anesthesiology, ICU and Periop. Medicine, HMC, Qatar

2 Faculty of Medicine, T.U., Egypt

3 Clinical Anesthesiology Weill Cornell Medical College, Qatar

4 HMC, Qatar

5 Heart Institute, Egypt

*Address all correspondence to: melarref@gmail.com

References

[1] G. Chandan and M. Cascella, *Gas Laws and Clinical Application*. StatPearls Publishing, 2019.

[2] G. W. Kaczala and P. W. Skippen, "Air medical evacuation in patients with airleak syndromes," *Air Med. J.*, vol. 27, no. 2, 2008, doi: 10.1016/j.amj.2007.07.004.

[3] M. P. Samuels, "The effects of flight and altitude," *Archives of Disease in Childhood*, vol. 89, no. 5. BMJ Publishing Group, pp. 448-455, May 2004, doi: 10.1136/adc.2003.031708.

[4] N. Lawless, *S. Tobias*, and M. A. Mayorga, "F102 and positive end-expiratory pressure as compensation for altitude-induced hypoxemia in an acute respiratory distress syndrome model: Implications for air transportation of critically ill patients," *Crit. Care Med.*, vol. 29, no. 11, pp. 2149-2155, 2001, doi: 10.1097/00003246-200111000-00017.

[5] B. L. Rish, "Safe practice of our aeromedical evacuation.," *Military Medicine*, vol. 153, no. 1. Mil Med, pp. 51-52, Jan. 1988, Accessed: Feb. 05, 2021. [Online]. Available: https://pubmed.ncbi.nlm.nih.gov/3126428/.

[6] M. Komorowski, S. Fleming, and A. W. Kirkpatrick, "Fundamentals of Anesthesiology for Spaceflight," *Journal of Cardiothoracic and Vascular Anesthesia*, vol. 30, no. 3. W.B. Saunders, pp. 781-790, Jun. 01, 2016, doi: 10.1053/j.jvca.2016.01.007.

[7] R. E. Purdy, M. K. Wilkerson, R. L. Hughson, P. Norsk, and D. E. Watenpaugh, "The Cardiovascular System in Microgravity: Symposium Summary," in *Proceedings of the Western Pharmacology Society*, 2003, vol. 46, pp. 16-27, Accessed: Feb. 05, 2021. [Online]. Available: https://pubmed.ncbi.nlm.nih.gov/14699877/.

[8] Watenpaugh, "Fluid volume control during short-term space flight and implications for human performance - PubMed." https://pubmed.ncbi.nlm.nih.gov/11581336/ (accessed Feb. 05, 2021).

[9] M. Komorowski, S. Fleming, and J. Hinkelbein, "Anaesthesia in outer space: The ultimate ambulatory setting?," *Current Opinion in Anaesthesiology*, vol. 29, no. 6. Lippincott Williams and Wilkins, pp. 649-654, Nov. 28, 2016, doi: 10.1097/ACO.0000000000000390.

[10] J. W. Agnew, E. E. Fibuch, and J. D. Hubbard, "Anesthesia during and after exposure to microgravity," *Aviation Space and Environmental Medicine*, vol. 75, no. 7 SEC. 2. pp. 571-580, Jul. 2004.

[11] M. Komorowski, S. D. Watkins, G. Lebuffe, and J. B. Clark, "Potential anesthesia protocols for space exploration missions," *Aviation Space and Environmental Medicine*, vol. 84, no. 3. Aviat Space Environ Med, pp. 226-233, 2013, doi: 10.3357/ASEM.3427.2013.

[12] S. M. Smith *et al.*, "Bone metabolism and renal stone risk during International Space Station missions," *Bone*, vol. 81, pp. 712-720, Dec. 2015, doi: 10.1016/j.bone.2015.10.002.

[13] C. Ibebunjo and J. A. J. Martyn, "Fiber atrophy, but not changes in acetylcholine receptor expression, contributes to the muscle dysfunction after immobilization," *Crit. Care Med.*, vol. 27, no. 2, pp. 275-285, 1999, doi: 10.1097/00003246-199902000-00031.

[14] I. A. Suliman, J. U. Lindgren, P. G. Gillberg, K. M. Diab, and A. Adem, "Effect of immobilization on skeletal muscle nicotinic cholinergic receptors in the rat," *Neuroreport*, vol. 8, no. 13, pp. 2821-2824, 1997, doi: 10.1097/00001756-199709080-00003.

[15] R. L. Summers, S. L. Johnston, T. H. Marshburn, and D. R. Williams,

"Emergencies in Space," *Ann. Emerg. Med.*, vol. 46, no. 2, pp. 177-184, Aug. 2005, doi: 10.1016/j.annemergmed.2005.02.010.

[16] G. L. Amidon, G. A. DeBrincat, and N. Najib, "Effects of Gravity on Gastric Emptying, Intestinal Transit, and Drug Absorption," *J. Clin. Pharmacol.*, vol. 31, no. 10, pp. 968-973, 1991, doi: 10.1002/j.1552-4604.1991.tb03658.x.

[17] J. Kast, Y. Yu, C. N. Seubert, V. E. Wotring, and H. Derendorf, "Drugs in space: Pharmacokinetics and pharmacodynamics in astronauts," *European Journal of Pharmaceutical Sciences*, vol. 109. Elsevier B.V., pp. S2–S8, Nov. 15, 2017, doi: 10.1016/j.ejps.2017.05.025.

[18] I. V. Kovachevich, S. N. Kondratenko, A. K. Starodubtsev, and L. G. Repenkova, "Pharmacokinetics of acetaminophen administered in tablets and capsules under long-term space flight conditions," *Pharm. Chem. J.*, vol. 43, no. 3, pp. 130-133, Mar. 2009, doi: 10.1007/s11094-009-0255-6.

[19] M. R. Campbell, "A review of surgical care in space," *Journal of the American College of Surgeons*, vol. 194, no. 6. J Am Coll Surg, pp. 802-812, 2002, doi: 10.1016/S1072-7515(02)01145-6.

[20] R. S. Blue *et al.*, "Overview of medical operations for a manned stratospheric balloon flight," *Aviat. Sp. Environ. Med.*, vol. 84, no. 3, pp. 237-241, 2013, doi: 10.3357/ASEM.3537.2013.

[21] S. Benson, G. Cable, and L. Workman, "CHALLENGES IN ANAESTHESIA DURING SPACE EXPLORATION MISSIONS," *J. Australas. Soc. Aerosp. Med.*, vol. 11, pp. 1-10, 2019, doi: 10.21307/asam-2019-002.

[22] C. Keller *et al.*, "Airway management during spaceflight: A comparison of four airway devices in simulated microgravity," *Anesthesiology*, vol. 92, no. 5, pp. 1237-1241, May 2000, doi: 10.1097/00000542-200005000-00010.

[23] "Preliminary Report Regarding NASA's Space Launch System and Multi-Purpose Crew Vehicle Pursuant to Section 309 of the NASA Authorization Act of 2010 (P.L. 111-267)," 2011.

[24] V. I. Hurst, H. K. Doerr, J. D. Polk, S. Parazynksi, and S. Kelly, "Development of Sub-optimal Airway Protocols for the International Space Station (ISS) by the Medical Operation Support Team (MOST)."

[25] G. E. Groemer *et al.*, "The feasibility of laryngoscope-guided tracheal intubation in microgravity during parabolic flight: A comparison of two techniques," *Anesth. Analg.*, vol. 101, no. 5, pp. 1533-1535, 2005, doi: 10.1213/01.ANE.0000181001.25777.53.

[26] S. E. McIntosh, E. R. Swanson, A. McKeone, and E. D. Barton, "Location of airway management in air medical transport," *Prehospital Emerg. Care*, vol. 12, no. 4, pp. 438-442, Sep. 2008, doi: 10.1080/10903120802301518.

[27] F. E. Lejeune, "Laryngoscopy in space travel," *Ann. Otol. Rhinol. Laryngol.*, vol. 88, no. 6, pp. 813-817, 1979, doi: 10.1177/000348947908800613.

[28] M. R. Campbell, "A review of surgical care in space," *Journal of the American College of Surgeons*, vol. 194, no. 6. pp. 802-812, 2002, doi: 10.1016/S1072-7515(02)01145-6.

Chapter 13

Videolaryngoscopy, the Current Role in Airway Management

Tatjana Goranović

Abstract

Videolaryngoscopy has emerged not only as an alternative to direct laryngoscopy for airway intubation in adults and children but also as a new diagnostic and therapeutic tool in head and neck surgery. Videolaryngoscopy has a great advantage over direct laryngoscopy because it has been proven to reduce difficult views of the laryngeal opening (glottis). The success of intubation with a videolaryngoscope depends on both the type of device used and the experience of the operator. Technical details, such as the device's size and blade choice, properly reshaping the endotracheal tube, and customized hand-eye coordination, are all particularly important for targeting the endotracheal tube toward the glottis. Besides its clinical role in airway management, videolaryngoscopy is an excellent tool for education and medicolegal recording.

Keywords: airway management, videolaryngoscopy, direct laryngoscopy, anesthesia, intensive care medicine, emergency, history, education

1. Introduction

Videolaryngoscopy represents a significant improvement in endotracheal intubation and thus an improvement in airway safety. Namely, it is well known that to increase airway safety, it is necessary to apply the appropriate concept of airway visualization on which airway strategies and airway algorithms are based [1]. It is generally believed that improving the visualization of the laryngeal opening (glottis) as the most important airway structure for intubation significantly increases the success of intubation.

The classic concept of endotracheal intubation by direct laryngoscopy is based on the alignment of three axes (oral, pharyngeal, and laryngeal) to expose the laryngeal opening (glottis) to the external observer's eye, who places the tube through the glottis under the full control of eyesight [2]. This requires an appropriate head and neck position, a laryngoscope, and a precise laryngoscope application technique [3]. Often, the position adjustment should be instituted in case of poor visualization of the glottis [4]. Videolaryngoscopy uses optical technology to improve glottis visualization without the need to align the three axes of the airway, which might be especially useful in neck mobility limitations when it is not possible to extend the neck [5, 6]. In addition to better visualization of the glottis, videolaryngoscopy has proven to be a very successful intubation technique in operators with little or no experience [7–9], involves all airway team members [10–12], and is an important tool for perioperative airway assessment, airway care education, and medicolegal intubation recording [12, 13].

 IntechOpen

2. History of videolaryngoscopy

Although videolaryngoscopy as a technique of airway management has been an extremely popular topic for the last decade, the fact is that the principle of indirect airway visualization, on which it is based, is older than direct laryngoscopy. In 1829, Benjamin Guy Babington (1794–1866) described the first "glottoscope" or "glottiscope," which consisted of a speculum to displace the tongue (a tongue depressor) and a system of mirrors to visualize the larynx, with sunlight for illumination [14–16]. Yet since 1895, when Alfred Kirstein (1863–1922) developed the "autoscope" that had an external electrical light source, the developmental pathway of laryngoscopy has focused on direct laryngoscopy [15, 16]. Consequently, since the 1940s, when the Macintosch and Miller blade were introduced [17], direct laryngoscopy has been the gold standard of endotracheal intubation.

In 1998, Markus Weiss incorporated fiberoptic fibers into a direct laryngoscope with a Macintosh blade [18]. In 2001, John Pacey introduced the first videolaryngoscope called the Glidescope®, and since then the number of different devices using videolaryngoscopy has grown [17]. In 2013, the American Society of Anesthesiologists (ASA) suggested the use of videolaryngoscopy as the first choice in airway management in its algorithm of airway management [19]. The Difficult Airway Society (DAS), in the 2015 algorithm, recognized the use of videolaryngoscopy as part of the airway management and suggested to all anesthesiologists the adoption of the videolaringoscopy skills [20]. It is recommended that videolaryngoscope should be immediately available for all obstetric general anesthetics [21]. In 2017, DAS presented videolaryngoscopy as an equivalent technique to direct laryngoscopy in the first attempts of intubation in the airway management algorithm in intensive care units (ICUs) [22].

3. Technique of videolaryngoscopy

The technique of videolaryngoscopy depends on the type of device used. **Table 1** lists some of the videolaryngoscopes. The division of videolaryngoscopes into the channeled and non-channeled devices has practical implications as the technique of videolaryngoscopy also differs significantly whether it is channeled or non-channeled one (**Figures 1–3**).

Non-channeled devices are further divided depending on the type of blade, which can be of the Macintosh, Miller, or hyperangular type, which also further influences the choice of technique (**Figure 4**). Blades can be manufactured from plastic for a single use or from metal for a multiple use. The screen can be on the device itself (**Figure 5**) or on a separate external monitor (**Figure 6**), which can be placed on the side or above the patient's chest. The position of the monitor does not significantly affect the technique, but it requires good eye-hand coordination like all endoscopic techniques.

It is important to note that videolaryngoscopy, in broader meaning, includes all devices that assist laryngoscopy by video technology. Besides the above described videolaryngoscopes, it includes different video intubating stylets and videoendoscopes, too. These devices are equipped with an inbuilt camera and light source [23, 24]. Compared to the older versions of videostylets which were designed as rigid linear rods, the newer intubating stylets are often S-shaped and semiflexible with deflectable tips [25, 26]. The devices can have an eyepiece at their end or can be attached to monitor to allow watching at the screen. **Table 2** lists some video intubating stylets.

Type	Blade type	Name	Manufacturer
Channeled	N/A	Airtraq®	Prodol, Vizcaya, Spain
		Pentax AWS®	Pentax-AWS, Ambu Glen Burnie MD, USA
		King Vision®	King System, Nobesville, IN, USA
		Airway Scope®	Pentax, Tokyo, Japan
		Res-Q-Scope II	N/A
Non-channeled	Angulated blade	Storz V-MAC®/C-MAC®	Karl Storz, Tuttlingen, Germany
		McGrath MAC®	Aircraft Medical, Edinburgh, Scotland
		Glidescope® Core™, Titanium™ Spectrum™	Glidescope, Verathon, WA, USA
		APA™ MAC	Venner Medical, Singapore, Singapore
		Infinium ClearVue®	QuadMed, Inc. Jacksonville, FL, USA
		AP Venerscope®	Intravent Direct, Maidenhead, UK
		Truview PCD™-R	Truphatek International Limited, Netanya, Israel
	Hyperangulated blade	C-MAC D-blade®	Karl Storz, Tuttlingen, Germany
		McGrath Series 5®	Aircraft Medical, Edinburgh, Scotland
		Glidescope® Core™, Titanium™ Spectrum™	Glidescope, Verathon, WA, USA
		APA™ DAB & U-DAB	Venner Medical, Singapore, Singapore
		Infinium Clear Vue®	Quamed, Inc. Jackonsville, FL, USA

N/A, not applicable.

Table 1.
Channeled and non-channeled videolaryngoscopes [10, 15, 23, 24].

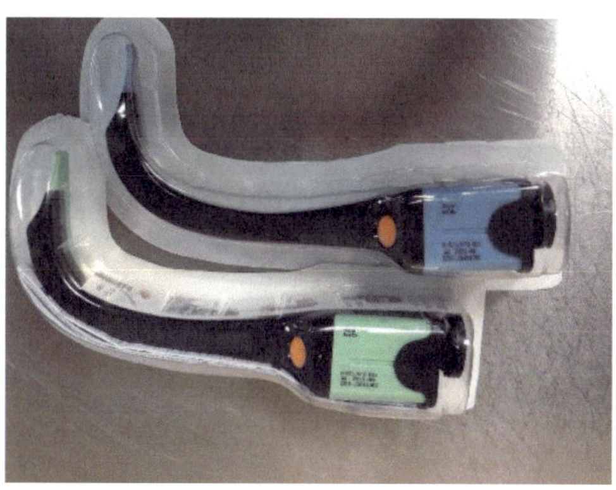

Figure 1.
Airtraq® as an example of the channeled videolaryngoscope (own photography).

3.1 Technique of videolaryngoscopy with a channeled videolaryngoscope

The tube is placed in the dedicated groove of the device (**Figure 7**). The tube or the channel on the device can be lightly lubricated to reduce friction. During this preparation, make sure that the lubricant does not obscure the light source and the outer glass of the screen. The size of the tube should be adjusted to the size of

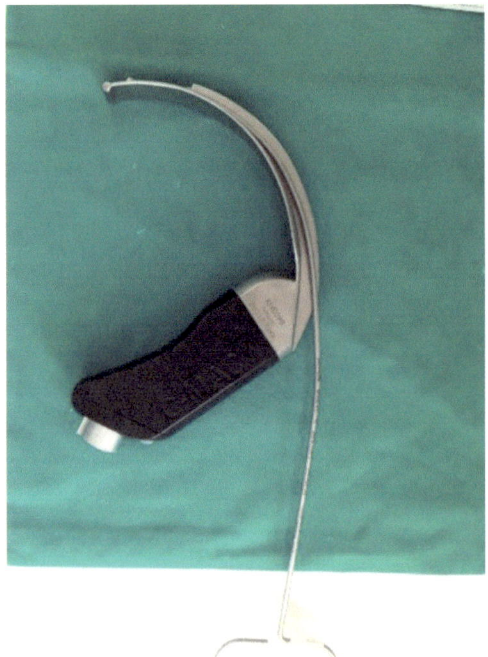

Figure 2.
Storz C-MAC D blade® as an example of the non-channeled videolaryngoscope with a metal reusable blade (own photography).

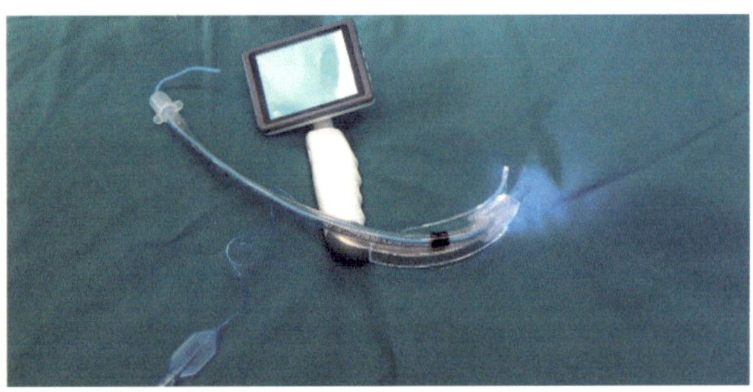

Figure 3.
Infinium ClearVue® as an example of the channeled videolaryngoscope with a plastic single use blade (own photography).

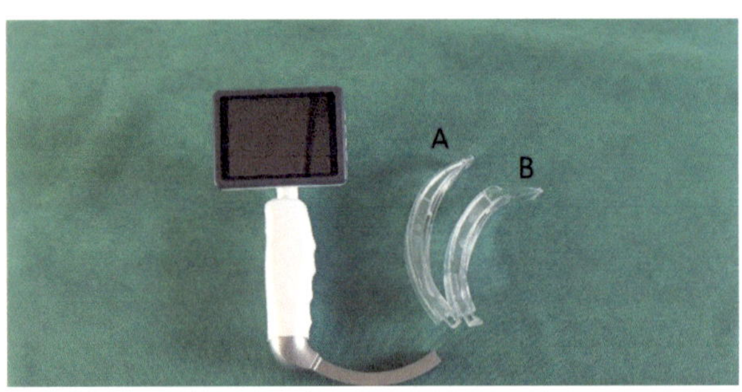

Figure 4.
Different single use plastic blades of the videolaryngoscope (A) Macintosh and (B) hyperangular (own photography).

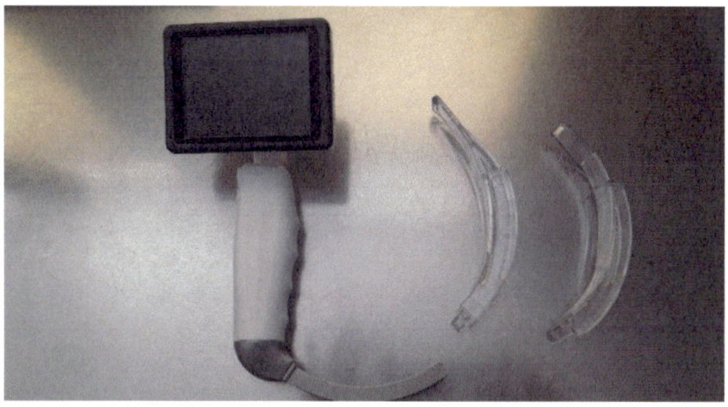

Figure 5.
An incorporated screen of the videolaryngoscope on a device itself (own photography).

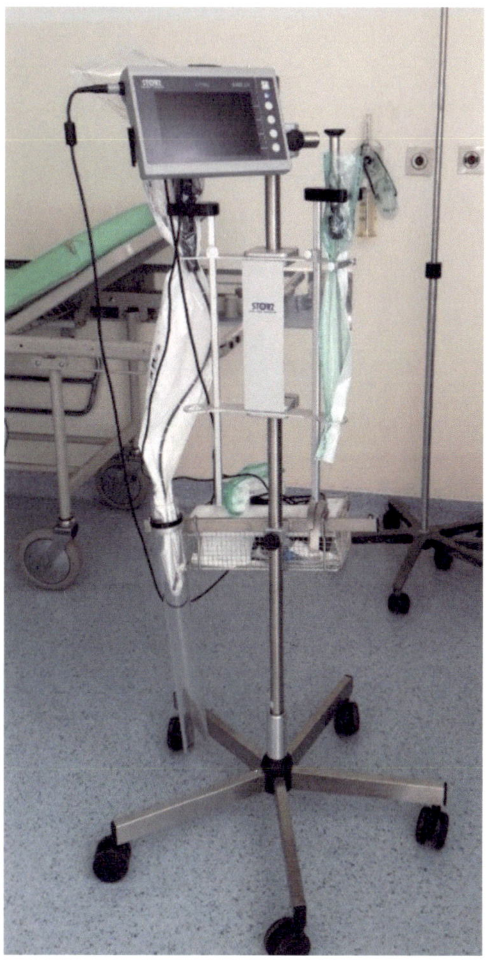

Figure 6.
The screen of the videolaryngoscope on an external monitor (own photography).

the channel. Namely, these devices differ in size, and the size of the channel is also different. When placing the tube, the top of the tube is displayed on the visible screen as a crescent. The entire device with the tube placed in this way is carefully embedded through the open mouth deep into the pharynx with the dominant hand, paying attention to the structures in the mouth (lips, teeth, and palate). If external resistance

Videostylets	Name	Manufacturer
With fixed tip	Bonfils®	Karl Storz, Tuttlingen, Germany
With flexible tip	Rigid and flexible laryngoscope (RIFL)	AI Medical Devices Inc., Williamston, MI, USA
	SensaScope®	Acutronic Medical Systems AG, Hirzel, Switzerland
	C-MAC® VS Video Stylet	Karl Storz, Tuttlingen, Germany

Table 2.
Videostylets [23–26].

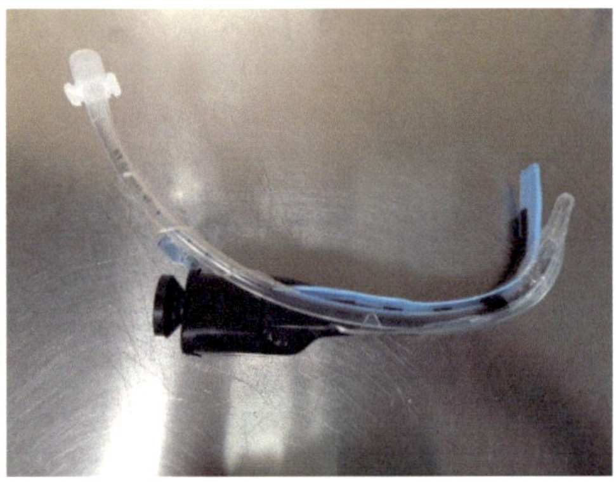

Figure 7.
Tube placed in a dedicated groove in a channeled videolaryngoscope (own photography).

is encountered due to large breasts, etc., the device can be turned with the concave side toward the palate firstly, then it can be placed in the mouth and when it reaches the level of the soft palate, it can be rotated to cover the base of the tongue (similar to positioning a Guedel tube). The device is then grasped with the left hand, the eye of the operator is brought closer to the eyepiece or the gaze is directed to the external screen and the whole device is pulled out vertically to the axis of the pharynx so that the glottis is displayed in the middle of the eyepiece or external screen. A slight rotation of the device to the left or to the right by 90 degrees can also help. When the glottis is displayed in the middle of the screen, the tube is carefully pushed through the channel with the free right hand, targeting the glottis. When the tube passes the vocal cords, the tube is displaced from the channel laterally and separated from the whole device carefully. The whole device is carefully removed from the pharynx and the mouth, taking care not to accidentally pull the tube from the trachea.

3.2 Technique of videolaryngoscopy with a non-channeled videolaryngoscope

The technique of videolaryngoscopy with a non-channeled device largely differs depending on the type of the blade.

If a Macintosh blade (slightly curved) is used (**Figure 8**), the video laryngoscopy technique is similar to direct laryngoscopy with a Macintosh blade, except for watching the progression of the blade and later a tube indirectly on the screen and not directly through the mouth. The mouth is opened, the laryngoscope is taken by the left hand (**Figure 9**), and the tip of the blade is inserted into the right corner of the patient's lip. This step should be watched directly to avoid injuries of the lips and teeth. When the blade is placed in the right corner of the patient's lip, the operator moves his/her gaze toward the screen and from then on keeps watching the screen.

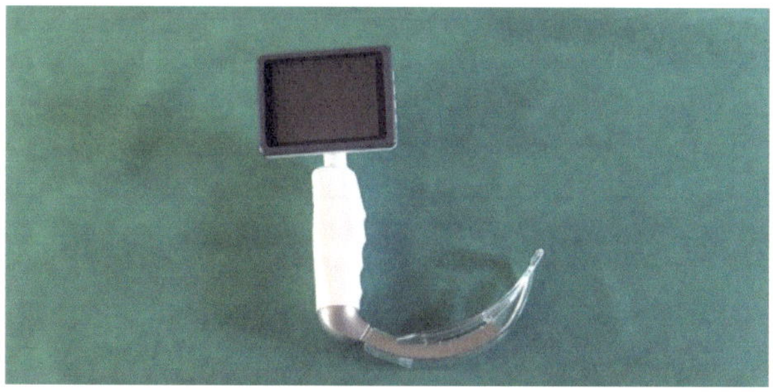

Figure 8.
A videolaryngoscope with a Macintoch blade (own photography).

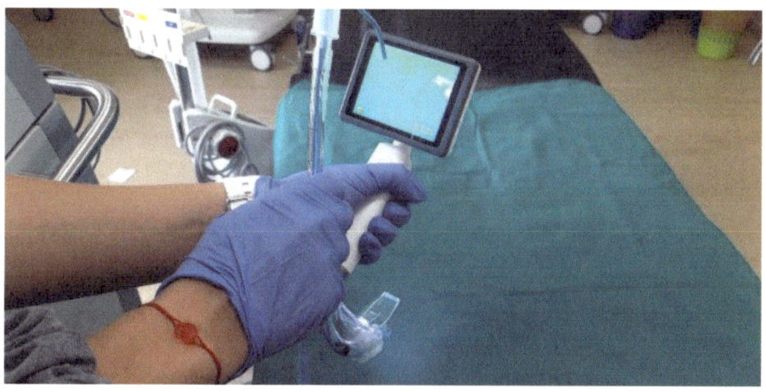

Figure 9.
Grasping a videolaryngoscope with the left hand; a tube is handled with the right hand (own photography).

The lateral left side of the blade encloses the patient's tongue, moving it medially from the buccal mucosa. The moment the tip of the blade reaches the base of the tongue, the blade is straightened in the medial line and the operator should try to display the uvula to be positioned in the middle of the lower edge of the screen. The entire laryngoscope is then gently moved up and forwarded at a 45-degree angle to display the epiglottis and glottis, and the tip of the blade is directed into the vallecula. It is important to position the glottis in the middle of the screen, and if possible, to visualize the space around the glottis including the surrounding lateral wall of the pharynx, without getting too close to the glottis. The tube should be performed with a stylet in such a way that the curve of the tube follows the curve of the blade. The preformed tube with the stylet is lowered with the right hand down the groove of the spatula targeting the opening of the glottis. If it is not possible to reach the opening in this way, then the tube is grasped more freely with the right hand and, regardless of the groove of the blade, is directed at any angle to the laryngeal opening. In order to be able to control the direction of the tube beyond the groove and rotate it in different directions if necessary, it is important to have a wider field of view on the screen; that is, in addition to seeing the glottis, it is advisable to see the cavity of the pharynx and the tip of the tube itself. Instead of a tube, a bougie can be used in the described manner, and when it passes the vocal cords, the tube is pulled over the bougie according to the principle of the Seldinger technique.

If a Miller (straight) blade is used, the video laryngoscopy technique is similar to direct laryngoscopy with a Miller blade. The mouth is opened, the laryngoscope is taken in the left hand, and the tip of the blade is entered into the right corner of the patient's lip. The lateral left side of the blade encloses the tongue, moving it medially from the buccal mucosa. The moment the tip of the blade reaches the base of the tongue, the spatula straightens in the medial line and tries to display the uvula to be positioned in the middle of the lower edge of the screen. The entire laryngoscope is then gently moved up and forward at a 45-degree angle in an effort to display the epiglottis and glottis, and the tip of the blade is directed below the epiglottis to lift it and better display the glottis. The further procedure is as described above.

If a hyperangular blade is used (**Figure 10**), then, unlike the procedures described above, the blade is immediately placed medially in the mouth and progressively directed toward the base of the tongue along the medial line of the tongue. At this point, lifting the base of the tongue attempts to visualize the uvula and place it similar to the one described above by displaying the uvula to the middle of the lower edge of the screen. The further procedure is as described above. To avoid the possible situation of obviously seeing the glottis but not being able to pass the tube through it, it is important to carefully preform the tube according to the hyperangular blade (**Figure 11**). If necessary, a metal stylet can

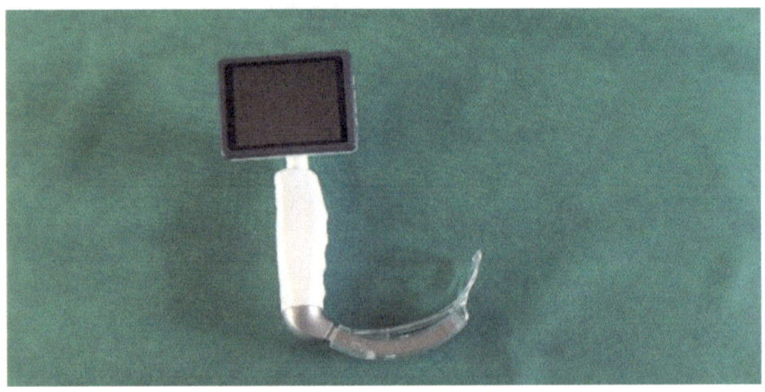

Figure 10.
A videolaryngoscope with a hyperangular blade (own photography).

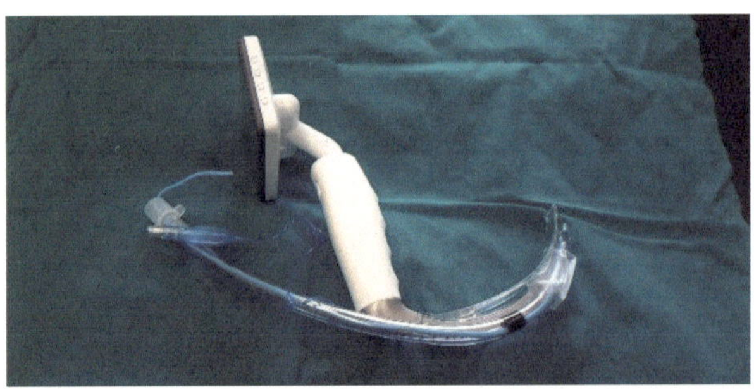

Figure 11.
Preforming a tube by a stylet to adjust the curve of the tube to the hyperangular blade (own photography).

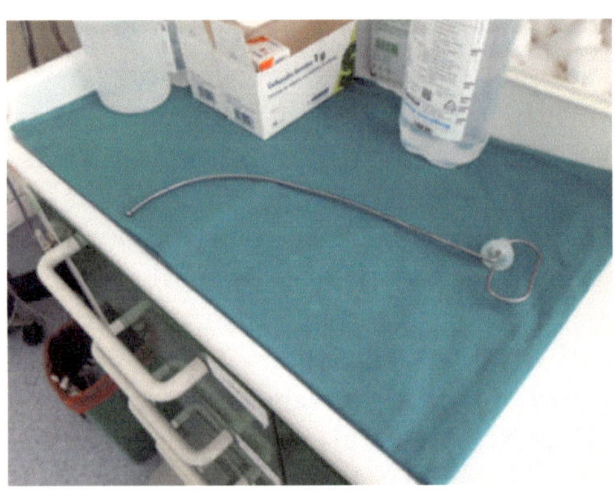

Figure 12.
A metal stylet (own photography).

be used too (**Figure 12**). And again, instead of a tube, a bougie, which is more plastic, can be used in the described manner, and when it passes the vocal cords, the tube is pulled over the bougie according to the principle of the Seldinger technique.

4. Usage of videolaryngoscopy

4.1 Clinical usage of videolaryngoscopy

4.1.1 Single lumen tube orotracheal intubation

The primary use of videolaryngoscopy is the intubation guiding after the induction of general anesthesia in operation theaters, intensive care units, and emergency departments. Various specific pathologies that complicate intubation and represent possible situations of difficult airway management have been successfully overcome by using videolaryngoscopy.

Meta-analyses have shown that videolaryngoscopy compared with direct laryngoscopy reduces impossible intubations in expected difficult intubation in adults [27]. Among individual videolaryngoscopes, regardless of the subjective impressions of clinicians, there is no evidence that a single videolaryngoscope is better than others except specifically only the C-MAC Macintosh blade [27]. Evidence further suggests that videolaryngoscope versus direct laryngoscopy facilitates intubation, improves glottis visualization, and reduces the number of impossible glottis visualizations and reduces laryngeal airway trauma [27]. Cochran's 2016 systematic analysis did not prove that videolaryngoscopy reduces the number of intubation attempts. There were insufficient data to establish a temporal comparison of videolaryngoscopy and direct laryngoscopy of the impact of videolaryngoscopy on hypoxia and respiratory complications, the impact of obesity, and the impact of the site and circumstances of intubation (intensive care unit, emergency medicine) [27]. In children, in contrast to adults, the evidence shows that the number of intubation attempts using videolaryngoscopy is increased compared to direct laryngoscopy, the success of first attempt intubation is not increased, and moreover, the intubation time is extended [28, 29].

Although videolaryngoscopy improves visualization, evidence suggests that traditional direct laryngoscopy is a sufficiently successful method of airway management in intensive care units. Moreover, some evidence suggests that the number of complications when using videolaryngoscopy in intensive care units is higher, especially if used by inexperienced operators [30]. Therefore, for routine airway management in intensive care units, direct laryngoscopy is still recommended as first choice, but videolaryngoscopy is also recommended in a situation of unsuccessful direct laryngoscopy or in the case of expected difficult intubation in the hands of experts [31, 32]. There is a positive trend of using videolaryngoscopy in pediatric ICUs, particularly in older children and those with the positive history of difficult airway. However, there is still no demonstration that this trend has decreased the rate of severe tracheal intubation adverse events or lowered multiple attempts at endotracheal intubation [33].

4.1.2 Double lumen tube orotracheal intubation

Videolaryngoscopy can be used successfully for guiding a double lumen tube. Admittedly, according to some, it prolongs intubation time but improves visualization [34, 35].

4.1.3 Nasotracheal intubation

Although videolaryngoscopy does not improve the overall success of intubation in nasotracheal intubation, it has been shown to improve the success of the first attempt and shorten the intubation time [36].

4.1.4 Intubation of cervical spine pathology

In a clinical scenario of immobilized cervical spine, specifically McGrath®, C-MAC® D- blade, and Airtraq® [37] increase intubation success [38].

4.1.5 Awake intubation

Videolaryngoscopy is proving to be a successful alternative to fiberoptic bronchoscopy in awake intubation because it shortens intubation time, although intubation success and safety profile are indistinguishable [39, 40]. This benefit is recognized for bariatric patients [41, 42] and patients with cervical trauma [43].

4.1.6 Intubation of the patients with suspected or proven COVID-19

Due to less direct contact of the operator with the generated aerosol during the intubation, videolaryngoscopy has been recommended in recent airway management algorithms for the patients with suspected or proven COVID-19 [44]. When this is feasible, it is preferred to use disposable blades and protective shields over the devices to avoid their contaminations and possible cross-transmission of the virus SARS-CoV-2 [45].

4.1.7 Conduit for flexible fiberoptic bronchoscope [video-assisted flexible intubation (VAFI) techniques]

The combined use of flexible bronchoscopy with rigid videolaryngoscopy benefits from the strengths of both techniques in normal and difficult airways. Although first associations were reported for specific videolaryngoscopes [46, 47], this concept seems to be independent of the specific brand or type of videolaryngoscope and flexible bronchoscope [48].

4.1.8 Insertion of different devices into oropharynx

Videolaryngoscopy can be particularly useful for guiding and correcting malposition of different devices through oropharynx such as nasogastric or orogastric tube [49], esophagoscopes, gastroscopes, or transesophageal echocardiography probe [50]. In addition, it can be useful when placing throat packs in oral and maxillofacial surgery. In thyroid surgery, it is useful for the visualization the proper placement of electromyographyic tube since the sensor mark on the tube should be placed exactly at the level of vocal cords [51, 52].

4.1.9 Diagnosis and recording of upper airway pathology

In addition to intubation, videolaryngoscopy has been shown to be successful for diagnostic and therapeutic surgical interventions in head and neck surgery. It has shown even superiority compared to videolaryngostroboscopy in diagnostic of different vocal pathologies [53]. Videolaryngoscopy can assist or replace traditional direct laryngoscopes for diagnostic of vocal pathology and small therapeutic procedures such as vocal polypectomies [54]. In addition, it can be used as an assistance device for small procedures involving the tongue base, such as biopsies, foreign body removal like coins, fish bones, etc., and radiofrequency treatment of obstructive sleep [55–57]. Using the C-MAC and a pair of Magill forceps, some authors reported to be able to successfully remove the duodenal stent dislodged in proximal esophagus [58]. Videolaryngoscopy, in combination with apnoic technique with spontaneous ventilation, was shown to be effective in pediatric cases for a safe, speedy, and successful removal of the foreign body with respect to an unprotected airway, wherein tracheal intubation was not a viable option [59].

4.2 Educational and research usage of videolaryngoscopy

Videolaryngoscopy is an excellent tool for teaching because it allows unhindered supervision of the intubation procedure [60]. In practice, it proves to be a particularly useful tool for introducing beginners to intubation procedures. Moreover, depending on the choice of blade and type of device, it allows the education of different advanced intubation techniques comparable to direct laryngoscopy, including a combination of different techniques [61]. The supervisor follows the procedure performed by the student in a real time with possibility to guide the student verbally or manually with prompt feedback of what has been done. To gain an expertise in situations of unexpected difficult airway, it is necessary to learn how to manage expected difficult airway during routine intubations. Evidence suggests that using videolaryngoscopy during intubation significantly helps in mastering the intubation technique by the trainees even in the most sensitive populations for intubation such as newborns [62, 63].

As a relatively new technique with plenty of new innovative devices, videolaryngoscopy is currently a fruitful subject for the researchers interested in airway management. However, as the indications for its use spread, videolaryngoscopy may be used as an auxiliary tool for the other static and dynamic researches that include visualization of oropharynx and the upper airway.

4.3 Medicolegal usage of videolaryngoscopy

The possibility of recording the videolaryngoscopy procedure and subsequent reviewing of the recorded material offers the possibility of a thorough analysis of the procedure, which itself lasts a limited short time. The first such application was described in 1987 with the purpose of recording the vocal cords during vocal therapies [64]. Recorded material during videolaryngoscopy can be reproduced multiple times, which can be useful in subsequent analyzes that can be done for various medicolegal purposes (Video 1, Video 2, Video 3, and Video 4). It is especially useful to use archived images and videos as the part of preoperative preparation in patients for whom difficult intubation is expected. Another practical indication could be the examination of vocal cords after thyroid surgery and recording for medicolegal issues.

5. Limitations and complications of videolaryngoscopy

Despite the advantages and widespread use of videolaryngoscopy, there are some limitations that may be viewed as absolute or relative contraindications [13]. The only real absolute contraindication for videolaryngoscopy is the significant limitation of opening a mouth which does not allow to insert the blade. In this situation, retromolar intubation with videostylets or fiberoptic intubation, that are comparably smaller devices, may be a good alternative.

Fogging and secretions may obscure view, but they can be solved. Newer devices have additional antifogging adds and one should be aware about it during airway intubation. Adding oxygen may help in antifogging too, while successive early aspiration of secretion may be effective.

The most frustrating situation is when the passage of tube may be difficult despite great view ("laryngoscopic paradox") [13, 24]. However, one must be aware of his/her understanding of the basic videolaryngoscopy concepts. Indeed, as the acute angle is often very sharp, an acutely angled stylet is necessary. In addition, depth perception is lost with a two-dimensional video image, and sometimes, operators may become fixated on the video screen and may not directly observe where the laryngoscope blade or endotracheal tube is being placed [24]. The consequences of this unawareness of the situation are injuries of soft tissues such as soft palate, tonsillar, or pharyngeal wall perforation [65–68]. According to one study female gender, right tonsillar pillars and soft palate were the most frequently injured [69]. The most common repair of these soft tissues' injuries was simple surgical closure with no long-term harm [69].

Additional limitations of videolaryngoscopy are as follows: the need of experience and the time demand for the operator to learn how to use them properly, the rapid deterioration of their display in the presence of a swelling or a secretion, and the fact that they are rather complicated and expensive devices [70].

There are few useful tips that can be practiced to avoid complications. It is particularly important to prepare the tube with the stylet to follow the angle of the blade. As a mnemonic aid, one can remember the abbreviation "CCLL": (1) Choose the right tube, (2) Check the endotracheal tube cuff, (3) Lubricate the stylet and the endotracheal tube (but spare the camera and the light source), and (4) Load the stylet (i.e., band it according to the angle of videolaryngoscopy blade).

To gain great maneuverability with the tube, it is advisable to hold the tube closer to its connector, not to be to too close with the view to the glottis (back it up), and in the case of difficulty, passing through the glottis to use the bougie [71]. In addition, some propose to view videolaryngoscopy as a four-step procedure: First step is to look in the mouth and insert the videolaryngoscopy blade under direct vision. The next step is to look at the screen while gently advancing with the blade toward epiglottis to get the best glottic view. The third step is to move the look again to the mouth while inserting the tube under the direct vision to avoid trauma of soft tissues. And finally, the fourth step, is again to look at the screen to complete intubation. This step will probably need extra rotations and angulations of the tube. It is important that the stylet removal and the tube adjustments are done under direct visualizations [72].

6. Conclusion

Videolaryngoscopy can be used effectively in situations of expected and unexpected difficult airway management. There are several devices for videolaryngoscopy, which differ technically, but with a thorough knowledge of the technical specific details, the success of the use of different videolaryngoscopes in intubation is similar. The choice of a specific videolaryngoscope depends on the individual patient, local resources, and the expertise of the operator. The simplicity and benefits of using videolaryngoscopy lead enthusiasts to entitle videolaryngoscopy as the miracle solution for all possible situations where airway visualization and airway management is required. But, in clinical reality, videolaryngoscopy, like any airway management technique, has its advantages and disadvantages. Its great advantage is that even its shortcomings can be learned faster and more efficiently, because the procedure is widely visible to a larger number of participants gathered in the airway care team in a real time. Therefore, videolaryngoscopy is not only an excellent teaching tool for mastering the airway management with its use but also with other airway devices which can be used as single or in various combinations. In addition, videolaryngoscopy has proven to be a useful technique in other clinical situations besides intubation, such as diagnostics of upper airway and small laryngeal surgeries. Finally, videolaryngoscopy is also an important medicolegal tool for all topics related to airway care as it allows immediate and delayed post-procedure analysis by reproducing its recordings.

Nowadays, many societies' guidelines recommend to use videolaryngoscopy early in intubation attempts in order to aim first-pass intubation success. It is possible that even in close future, it will replace direct intubation as the gold standard. However, for such an evolution, it is necessary for the clinicians to master the videolaryngoscopy technique by daily practicing.

Good preparation makes half of the technique. It is important to be aware of the device characteristics, especially technical details such as the resolution and fogging of the screen, the size and the angle of the blade, and the need to use preformed tube by stylet. During the process of videolaryngoscopy, it is advisable to think about it as a four-step procedure with alternately looking in the mouth and at the screen. Direct and indirect visualization of the upper airway should be complemented with customized hand-eye coordination. If accepted, these routine tips can minimize majority of traumatic complications. Primum nil nocere.

Conflict of interest

The author declares no conflict of interest.

Author details

Tatjana Goranović[1,2]

1 University Department of Anaesthesiology, Resuscitation and Intensive Care Medicine, Sveti Duh University Hospital, Zagreb, Croatia

2 Faculty of Medicine, Josip Juraj Strossmayer University, Osijek, Croatia

*Address all correspondence to: tanjagoranovic@hotmail.com

References

[1] Yang GZ, Xue FS, Sun C, Liu GP. Difficult airway management: Correct concepts and algorithm are important for patient safety. Chinese Medical Journal. 2016;**129**:1886-1887. DOI: 10.4103/0366-6999.186647

[2] Greenland KB, Eley V, Edwards MJ, Allen P, Irwin MG. The origins of the sniffing position and the Three Axes Alignment Theory for direct laryngoscopy. Anaesthesia and Intensive Care. 2008;**36**(Suppl 1):23-27. DOI: 10.1177/0310057X0803601s05

[3] Greenland KB. A proposed model for direct laryngoscopy and tracheal intubation. Anaesthesia. 2008;**63**:156-161. DOI: 10.1111/j.1365-2044.2007.05326.x

[4] El-Orbany M, Woehlck H, Salem MR. Head and neck position for direct laryngoscopy. Anesthesia and Analgesia. 2011;**113**:103-109. DOI: 10.1213/ANE.0b013e31821c7e9c

[5] Farag E. Airway management for cervical spine surgery. Review. Best Practice & Research. Clinical Anaesthesiology. 2016;**30**:13-25. DOI: 10.1016/j.bpa.2016.01.001

[6] Holmes MG, Dagal A, Feinstein BA, Joffe AM. Airway management practice in adults with an unstable cervical spine: The harborview medical center experience. Anesthesia and Analgesia. 2018;**127**:450-454. DOI: 10.1213/ANE.0000000000003374

[7] Howard-Quijano KJ, Huang YM, Matevosian R, Kaplan MB, Steadman RH. Video-assisted instruction improves the success rate for tracheal intubation by novices. British Journal of Anaesthesia. 2008;**101**: 568-572. DOI: 10.1093/bja/aen211

[8] Aghamohammadi H, Massoudi N, Fathi M, Jaffari A, Gharaei B, Moshki A. Intubation learning curve: comparison between video and direct laryngoscopy by inexperienced students. Journal of Medicine and Life. 2015;**8**(Spec Iss 4):150-153

[9] Eismann H, Sieg L, Etti N, Friedrich L, Schröter C, Mommsen P, et al. Improved success rates using videolaryngoscopy in unexperienced users: A randomized crossover study in airway manikins. European Journal of Medical Research. 2017;**22**:27. DOI: 10.1186/s40001-017-0268-7

[10] Paolini JB, Donati F, Drolet P. Review article: Video-laryngoscopy: Another tool for difficult intubation or a new paradigm in airway management? Canadian Journal of Anaesthesia. 2013;**60**:184-191. DOI: 10.1007/s12630-012-9859-5

[11] Jones L, Mulcahy K, Fox J, Cook TM, Kelly FE. C-MAC© videolaryngoscopy: The anaesthetic assistant's view. Journal of Perioperative Practice. 2018;**28**:83-89. DOI: 10.1177/1750458918762314

[12] Cook TM, Boniface NJ, Seller C, Hughes J, Damen C, MacDonald L, et al. Universal videolaryngoscopy: A structured approach to conversion to videolaryngoscopy for all intubations in an anaesthetic and intensive care department. British Journal of Anaesthesia. 2018;**120**:173-180. DOI: 10.1016/j.bja.2017.11.014

[13] Maldini B, Hodžović I, Goranović T, Mesarić J. Challenges in the use of video laryngoscopes. Acta Clinica Croatica. 2016;**55**(Suppl 1):41-50

[14] Lapeña JF. Mirrors and reflections: the evolution of indirect laryngoscopy. Annals of Saudi Medicine. 2013;**33**:177-181. DOI: 10.5144/0256-4947.2013.177

[15] Pieters BM, Eindhoven GB, Acott C, van Zundert AA. Pioneers of

laryngoscopy: Indirect, direct and video laryngoscopy. Anaesthesia and Intensive Care. 2015;**43**(Suppl):4-11. DOI: 10.1177/0310057X150430S103

[16] Toker K. Visualization of airway. Acta Clinica Croatica. 2016;**55**(Suppl 1): 73-75

[17] Treki AA, Straker T. Limitations of the videolaryngoscope: An anesthetic management reality. International Anesthesiology Clinics. 2017;**55**:97-104. DOI: 10.1097/AIA.0000000000000130

[18] Weiss M. Video-intuboscopy: A new aid to routine and difficult tracheal intubation. British Journal of Anaesthesia. 1998;**80**:525-527. DOI: 10.1093/bja/80.4.525

[19] Apfelbaum JL, Hagberg CA, Caplan RA, Blitt CD, Connis RT, Nickinovich DG, et al. Practice guidelines for management of the difficult airway: An updated report by the American Society of Anesthesiologists Task Force on Management of the Difficult Airway. Anesthesiology. 2013;**118**:251-270. DOI: 10.1097/ALN.0b013e31827773b2

[20] Frerk C, Mitchell VS, McNarry AF, Mendonca C, Bhagrath R, Patel A, et al. Difficult Airway Society 2015 guidelines for management of unanticipated difficult intubation in adults. British Journal of Anaesthesia. 2015;**115**: 827-848. DOI: 10.1093/bja/aev371

[21] Mushambi MC, Kinsella SM, Popat M, Swales H, Ramaswamy KK, Winton AL, et al. Obstetric Anaesthetists' Association and Difficult Airway Society guidelines for the management of difficult and failed tracheal intubation in obstetrics. Anaesthesia. 2015;**70**:1286-1306. DOI: 10.1111/anae.13260

[22] Higgs A, McGrath BA, Goddard C, Rangasami J, Suntharalingam G, Gale R, et al. Guidelines for the management of tracheal intubation in critically ill adults. British Journal of Anaesthesia. 2018;**120**:323-352. DOI: 10.1016/j.bja.2017.10.021

[23] Maldini B, Hodžović I, Goranović T. Alternative devices in airway visualization. Acta Clinica Croatica. 2016;**55**(Suppl 1):76-84

[24] Hurford WE. The video revolution: A new view of laryngoscopy. Respiratory Care. 2010;**55**:1036-1045

[25] Setty H, Rawlings JL, Dubin S. Video RIFL: A rigid flexible laryngoscope to facilitate airway management. Journal of Clinical Anesthesia. 2010;**22**:642-647. DOI: 10.1016/j.jclinane.2009.10.019

[26] Biro P. The SensaScope®–A new hybrid video intubation stylet. Saudi Journal of Anaesthesia. 2011;**5**:411-413. DOI: 10.4103/1658-354X.87271

[27] Lewis SR, Butler AR, Parker J, Cook TM, Smith AF. Videolaryngoscopy versus direct laryngoscopy for adult patients requiring tracheal intubation. Cochrane Database of Systematic Reviews. 2016;**11**:CD011136. DOI: 10.1002/14651858.CD011136.pub2

[28] Park R, Peyton JM, Fiadjoe JE, Hunyady AI, Kimball T, Zurakowski D, et al. The efficacy of GlideScope® videolaryngoscopy compared with direct laryngoscopy in children who are difficult to intubate: An analysis from the paediatric difficult intubation registry. British Journal of Anaesthesia. 2017;**119**:984-992. DOI: 10.1093/bja/aex344

[29] Abdelgadir IS, Phillips RS, Singh D, Moncreiff MP, Lumsden JL. Videolaryngoscopy versus direct laryngoscopy for tracheal intubation in children (excluding neonates). Cochrane Database of Systematic Reviews. 2017;**5**:CD011413. DOI: 10.1002/14651858.CD011413.pub2

[30] Cabrini L, Landoni G, Baiardo Redaelli M, Saleh O, Votta CD, Fominskiy E, et al. Tracheal intubation in critically ill patients: a comprehensive systematic review of randomized trials. Critical Care. 2018;**22**:6. DOI: 10.1186/s13054-017-1927-3

[31] Umobong EU, Mayo PH. Critical care airway management. Critical Care Clinics. 2018;**34**:313-324. DOI: 10.1016/j.ccc.2018.03.006

[32] Jaber S, De Jong A, Pelosi P, Cabrini L, Reignier J, Lascarrou JB. Videolaryngoscopy in critically ill patients. Critical Care. 2019;**23**:221. DOI: 10.1186/s13054-019-2487-5

[33] Grunwell JR, Kamat PP, Miksa M, Krishna A, Walson K, Simon D, et al. Trend and outcomes of video laryngoscope use across PICUs. Pediatric Critical Care Medicine. 2017;**18**:741-749. DOI: 10.1097/PCC.0000000000001175

[34] Belze O, Lepage E, Bazin Y, Kerourin P, Fusciardi J, Remérand F, et al. Glidescope versus Airtraq DL for double-lumen tracheal tube insertion in patients with a predicted or known difficult airway: A randomised study. European Journal of Anaesthesiology. 2017;**34**:456-463. DOI: 10.1097/EJA.0000000000000655

[35] Risse J, Schubert AK, Wiesmann T, Huelshoff A, Stay D, Zentgraf M, et al. Videolaryngoscopy versus direct laryngoscopy for double-lumen endotracheal tube intubation in thoracic surgery–A randomised controlled clinical trial. BMC Anesthesiology. 2020;**20**:150. DOI: 10.1186/s12871-020-01067-x

[36] Jiang J, Ma DX, Li B, Wu AS, Xue FS. Videolaryngoscopy versus direct laryngoscopy for nasotracheal intubation: A systematic review and meta-analysis of randomised controlled trials. Journal of Clinical Anesthesia. 2019;**52**:6-16. DOI: 10.1016/j.jclinane.2018.08.029

[37] Suppan L, Tramèr MR, Niquille M, Grosgurin O, Marti C. Alternative intubation techniques vs Macintosh laryngoscopy in patients with cervical spine immobilization: Systematic review and meta-analysis of randomized controlled trials. British Journal of Anaesthesia. 2016;**116**:27-36. DOI: 10.1093/bja/aev205

[38] Kleine-Brueggeney M, Greif R, Schoettker P, Savoldelli GL, Nabecker S, Theiler LG. Evaluation of six videolaryngoscopes in 720 patients with a simulated difficult airway: A multicentre randomized controlled trial. British Journal of Anaesthesia. 2016;**116**:670-679. DOI: 10.1093/bja/aew058

[39] Jiang J, Ma DX, Li B, Wu AS, Xue FS. Videolaryngoscopy versus fiberoptic bronchoscope for awake intubation–A systematic review and meta-analysis of randomized controlled trials. Therapeutics and Clinical Risk Management. 2018;**14**:1955-1963. DOI: 10.2147/TCRM.S172783

[40] Alhomary M, Ramadan E, Curran E, Walsh SR. Videolaryngoscopy vs. fibreoptic bronchoscopy for awake tracheal intubation: A systematic review and meta-analysis. Anaesthesia. 2018;**73**:1151-1161. DOI: 10.1111/anae.14299

[41] Moore AR, Schricker T, Court O. Awake videolaryngoscopy-assisted tracheal intubation of the morbidly obese. Anaesthesia. 2012;**67**:232-235. DOI: 10.1111/j.1365-2044.2011.06979.x

[42] Moore A, El-Bahrawy A, El-Mouallem E, Lattermann R, Hatzakorzian R, LiPishan W, et al. Videolaryngoscopy or fibreoptic bronchoscopy for awake intubation of bariatric patients with predicted difficult airways–A randomised, controlled trial. Anaesthesia. 2017;**72**:538-539. DOI: 10.1111/anae.13850

[43] Dutta K, Sriganesh K, Chakrabarti D, Pruthi N, Reddy M. Cervical spine movement during awake orotracheal intubation with fiberoptic scope and Mcgrath videolaryngoscope in patients undergoing surgery for cervical spine instability: A randomized control trial. Journal of Neurosurgical Anesthesiology. 2020;**32**:249-255. DOI: 10.1097/ANA.0000000000000595

[44] Cook TM, El-Boghdadly K, McGuire B, McNarry AF, Patel A, Higgs A. Consensus guidelines for managing the airway in patients with COVID-19: Guidelines from the Difficult Airway Society, the Association of Anaesthetists the Intensive Care Society, the Faculty of Intensive Care Medicine and the Royal College of Anaesthetists. Anaesthesia. 2020;**75**:785-799. DOI: 10.1111/anae.15054

[45] Brewster DJ, Chrimes N, Do TBT, Frase KR, Groombridge CJ, Higgs A, et al. Consensus statement: Safe Airway Society principles of airway management and tracheal intubation specific to the COVID-19 adult patient group. Medical Journal of Australia. 2020;**212**:472-481. DOI: 10.5694/mja2.50598

[46] Greib N, Stojeba N, Dow WA, Henderson J, Diemunsch PA. A combined rigid videolaryngoscopy-flexible fibrescopy intubation technique under general anesthesia. Canadian Journal of Anaesthesia. 2007;**54**:492-493. DOI: 10.1007/BF03022046

[47] Choi GS, Park SI, Lee EH, Yoon SH. Awake Glidescope(R) intubation in a patient with a huge and fixed supraglottic mass -a case report. Korean Journal of Anesthesiology. 2010;**59**:S26-S29

[48] Boet S, Bould MD, Diemunsch PA. Combined rigid videolaryngoscopy-flexible bronchoscopy for intubation. Korean Journal of Anesthesiology. 2011;**60**:381-382. DOI: 10.4097/kjae.2011.60.5.381

[49] Okabe T, Goto G, Hori Y, Sakamoto A. Gastric tube insertion under direct vision using the king vision™ video laryngoscope: A randomized, prospective, clinical trial. BMC Anesthesiology. 2014;**14**:82. DOI: 10.1186/1471-2253-14-82

[50] Ishida T, Kiuchi C, Sekiguchi T, Tsujimoto T, Kawamata M. McGRATH MAC video laryngoscope for insertion of a transoesophageal echocardiography probe: A randomised controlled trial. Eur J Anaesthesiol. 2016;**33**:263-268. Published online 2015 Nov 15. DOI: 10.1097/EJA.0000000000000367

[51] Berkow L, Dackiw APB, Tufano RP. Use of the GlideScope for placement of a recurrent laryngeal nerve monitoring endotracheal tube. Journal of Clinical Anesthesia. 2011;**23**:81-83. DOI: 10.1016/j.jclinane.2009.12.013

[52] Chang PY, Hu PY, Lin YC, Chen HY, Chiang FY, Wu CW, et al. Trachway video intubating stylet allows for optimization of electromyographic endotracheal tube placement for monitored thyroidectomy. Gland Surgery. 2017;**6**:464-468. DOI: 10.21037/gs.2017.08.08

[53] Kaushik MR, Kole AS, Gupta N, Dhoot S, Dehadaray A. Evaluation of various laryngeal pathologies: Videolaryngoscopy versus videolaryngostroboscopy. Indian Journal of Otolaryngology Head and Neck Surgery. 2018;**70**:244-248. DOI: 10.1007/s12070-017-1115-4

[54] Shenson JA, Marcott S, Dewan K, Lee YJ, Mariano ER, Sirjani DB. Utility of videolaryngoscopy for diagnostic and therapeutic interventions in head and neck surgery. American Journal of Otolaryngology. 2020;**41**:102284. DOI: 10.1016/j.amjoto.2019.102284

[55] Shenoy PK, Aldea M. The use of GlideScope for biopsies of the tongue base. The Journal of Laryngology and Otology. 2013;**127**:215-216

[56] Bruno E, Dauri M, Mauramati S, Viziano A, Micarelli A, Ottaviani F, et al. Utility of Glidescope(®) videolaryngoscopy in surgical procedures involving the larynx. Acta Otorhinolaryngologica Italica. 2015;**35**:45-48

[57] Shamim F, Nafis M, Ikram M. Other clinical applications of videolaryngoscopy besides intubation. Saudi Journal of Anaesthesia. 2018;**12**:491-492. DOI: 10.4103/sja.SJA_697_17

[58] Ho G, Singh N, Andrews J, Westhead P. Novel use of videolaryngoscopy to remove a foreign body. BML Case Reports. 2015;**2015**:bcr2015210011. DOI: 10.1136/bcr-2015-210011

[59] Punnoose SE, Victor J, Hazarika P, SS M. C-MAC® video-laryngoscope assisted removal of pediatric upper airway foreign body via apneic technique: Two case reports. SAGE Open Medical Case Reports. 2019;7:2050313X18823088

[60] Pouppirt NR, Foglia EE, Ades A. A video is worth a thousand words: Innovative uses of videolaryngoscopy. Archives of Disease in Childhood. Fetal and Neonatal Edition. 2018;**103**:F401-F402. DOI: 10.1136/archdischild-2017-314288

[61] Ozgul U, Erdil FA, Erdogan MA, Begec Z, Colak C, Yucel A, et al. Comparison of videolaryngoscope-guided versus standard digital insertion techniques of the ProSeal™ laryngeal mask airway: A prospective randomized study. BMC Anesthesiology. 2019;**19**:244. DOI: 10.1186/s12871-019-0915-3

[62] Lingappan K, Arnold JL, Fernandes CJ, Pammi M. Videolaryngoscopy versus direct laryngoscopy for tracheal intubation in neonates. Cochrane Database of Systematic Reviews. 2018;**6**:CD009975. DOI: 10.1002/14651858.CD009975.pub3

[63] Myatra SN, Doctor JR. Use of videolaryngoscopy as a teaching tool for novices performing tracheal intubation results in greater first pass success in neonates and infants. Indian Journal of Anaesthesia. 2019;**63**:781-783. DOI: 10.4103/ija.IJA_738_19

[64] D'Antonio L, Lotz W, Chait D, Netsell R. Perceptual-physiologic approach to evaluation and treatment of dysphonia. The Annals of Otology, Rhinology, and Laryngology. 1987;**96**(2 Pt 1):187-190. DOI: 10.1177/000348948709600210

[65] Vincent RD Jr, Wimberly MP, Brockwell RC, Magnuson JS. Soft palate perforation during orotracheal intubation facilitated by the GlideScope videolaryngoscope. Journal of Clinical Anesthesia. 2007;**19**:619-621. DOI: 10.1016/j.jclinane.2007.03.010

[66] Malik AM, Frogel JK. Anterior tonsillar pillar perforation during GlideScope video laryngoscopy. Anesthesia and Analgesia. 2007;**104**:1610-1611. DOI: 10.1213/01.ane.0000264321.04403.06

[67] Cooper RM. Complications associated with the use of the GlideScope videolaryngoscope. Canadian Journal of Anaesthesia. 2007;**54**:54-57. DOI: 10.1007/BF03021900

[68] Leong WL, Lim Y, Sia AT. Palatopharyngeal wall perforation during Glidescope intubation. Anaesthesia and Intensive Care. 2008;**36**:870-874. DOI: 10.1177/0310057X0803600620

[69] Greer D, Marshall KE, Bevans S, Standlee A, McAdams P, Harsha W. Review of videolaryngoscopy pharyngeal wall injuries. Laryngoscope. 2017;**127**:349-353. DOI: 10.1002/lary.26134

[70] Saracoglu KT, Eti Z, Gogus FY. Airtraq optical laryngoscope: Advantages and disadvantages. Middle East Journal of Anaesthesiology. 2013;**22**:135-141

[71] Bacon ER, Phelan MP, Doyle DJ. Tips and troubleshooting for use of the GlideScope video laryngoscope for emergency endotracheal intubation. The American Journal of Emergency Medicine. 2015;**33**:1273-1277. DOI: 10.1016/j.ajem.2015.05.003

[72] GlideScope AVL 4-Step Technique. Available from: https://www.youtube.com/watch?v=7jb2tbqQ6VQ [Accessed: 24 July 2020]

Chapter 14

Second Generation Supraglottic Airway (SGA) Devices

Kriti Singh

Abstract

Supraglottic Airways (SGAs) are an integral part of anaesthetic care. Since their introduction, several modifications, additions, and variations have been developed and are currently in clinical practice since the last 25 years. Not only are they useful for difficult ventilation during both in-hospital and out-of-hospital difficult airway management, they also act as a conduit for tracheal intubation. The newer or second-generation SGAs have been designed to provide a better seal of the airway and are relatively safer since they allow gastric aspiration. Thus, the SGAs may be the most versatile component in the airway management cart. Existing literature on SGAs tends to focus on first generation SGAs and their use in OT only. However, the scope and use of these devices is vast. Knowledge regarding specific devices and supporting data for their use is of utmost importance to patient's safety. This chapter addresses various types of commercially available novel SGAs and their use in and out of hospital settings.

Keywords: airway, supraglottic airway devices, laryngeal mask airway, laryngeal tubes, rescue airway

1. Introduction

In spite of tremendous advances in contemporary anaesthetic practice, advances in airway management continue to be of paramount importance to anaesthesiologists. Till some time ago, the cuffed tracheal tube was considered as the gold standard for providing a safe glottic seal [1]. The disadvantages of tracheal intubation, which involves rigid laryngoscopy, are the concomitant hemodynamic responses and damage to the oropharyngeal structures. Postoperative airway morbidity is also a serious concern. This precluded the global utility of the tracheal tube and there was a perceived need for better alternatives [2].

Dr. Archie Brain, a British anaesthesiologist, introduced the laryngeal mask airway (LMA) in 1983 for the first time, designed to be positioned around the laryngeal inlet. LMA is a supraglottic airway (SGA) device with an inflatable cuff forming a low-pressure seal around the laryngeal inlet and permitting ventilation.

Supraglottic Airways (SGAs) have revolutionised the airway management [3]. Besides serving as a rescue device in the difficult airway, and as a conduit for the endotracheal tube insertion, SGAs provide a less invasive and less traumatic means of securing the airway in surgical patients [4, 5].

Careful observations and clinical experience have led to several modifications of the LMA leading to development of newer supraglottic airway devices with better features for airway maintenance [3]. Over a period of time, new airway devices have been added to the anaesthesiologist‘s armamentarium to address specific needs. A wide variety of airway devices are available today which are employed to protect the airway in both elective as well as emergency situations [6].

In 2001, Dr. Archie Brain came up with a modification of the LMA. This device was called the Proseal-Laryngeal mask airway™ (Teleflex®, USA) [7]. This double lumen, double cuff LMA has some clear advantages over its predecessor. The double tube design separated the respiratory and alimentary tracts, providing a safe escape channel for the regurgitated fluids.

Since then, several devices that are able to accommodate nasogastric tubes have been invented. Newer features like better sealing pressures, reduced risk of pulmonary aspiration by stomach contents, single use devices, integrated bite blocks, and the ability to act as conduits for endotracheal tube (ETT) placement have rendered these devices more reliable for routine use. The last decade has seen a rapid rise in the number of clinical studies evaluating these second-generation SGAs.

2. Clinical indications of LMA

2.1 As a substitute for a facemask

LMAs are especially useful when mask fit is difficult as in edentulous or bearded patients. It also frees the hands of the anaesthesia care giver.

2.2 As an alternative to tracheal intubation for routine anaesthesia

The LMA may be used in the spontaneously breathing patient with adequate sedation and topical anaesthesia, or the paralysed, anaesthetised patient with assisted mechanical ventilation.

2.2.1 Laparoscopic surgery

The indications for use of the supraglottic airway devices are expanding. Their routine use in laparoscopic surgeries has almost replaced the endotracheal tubes. Second generation SGAs have proved to provide adequate sealing pressure required to provide adequate ventilation and maintain airway safety [8]. Also, pharyngolaryngeal morbidity (sore throat, dysphagia, dysphonia) are less as compared to endotracheal tube [9, 10].

2.2.2 Obese patients

In today’s era, the number of obese patients undergoing surgeries is increasing. Intubation is known to be more difficult in obese patients [11, 12]. Closed claims analysis shows that obesity, difficult intubation and intubation by inexperienced personnel are risk factors for severe airway injuries and pharyngo-oesophageal perforation [13].

In such cases, SGAs after successful placement can provide better postoperative pulmonary performance if used in very well selected patients. Hence, SGAs may be a simple alternative to intubation in short-term elective surgery in obese patients, as suggested by some randomised controlled trials (RCTs) [14]. These maybe used as conduits for tracheal intubation in obese patients with failed laryngoscopy and expected/unexpected difficult airways [15].

2.2.3 Pregnancy

Maternal morbidity from failed intubation and aspiration remains the biggest concern with general anaesthesia. SGAs can be lifesaving in caesarean deliveries where scenarios of cannot ventilate and cannot intubate is faced. Second generation SGAs have become the gadget of choice in such scenarios [16–18].

2.2.4 Paediatric age group

Being user-friendly, SGAs are now more commonly used in children. They obviate the use of ETTs and avoid many complications associated with endotracheal intubation [19, 20]. The LMA Classic™ and the LMA Proseal™ have established their safety and efficacy for routine as well as in emergency cases in paediatric patients [21–25]. The presence of a drain tube, which helps to empty the stomach in the Second-generation SGAs, has removed the fear of distension of the stomach with gas during controlled or spontaneous ventilation, leading to impairment of respiration, especially in a smaller child.

2.2.5 Prone position

Surgery performed in the prone position require significant OT time and necessitate additional manpower for proper positioning of the patient. Induction and device placement in the prone position avoids the displacement of OT personnel from other tasks as significantly less number of people is required in shifting the patient. Anaesthetic induction of the patient and SGA insertion can be done in prone position, unlike endotracheal intubation. A large cohort study included 1000 patients undergoing surgery under general anaesthesia in prone position where SGAs were safely used to secure the airway [26].

2.3 Aiding blind and fiberoptic-guided endotracheal intubation

SGAs can be used as a conduit for blind and fiberoptic-guided intubation for rescue of failed direct laryngoscopy or failed intubation [27–29]. After inserting the LMA, a well lubricated ETT with deflated cuff is passed over the fiberscope. The fiberscope is then advanced through the LMA. The ETT is advanced around 1.5 cm past the mask aperture. The tip of the ETT lifts the fiberscope away from the bowl of the mask and exposes the glottis. The fiberoptic scope is then advanced up to the distal end of the tracheal tube. The ETT is advanced until the glottis is brought into view and then further advanced into the trachea.

A specific advantage of using an SGA is the ability to continue ventilating and anaesthetising the patient through the SGA until formal tracheal intubation is achieved. The Aintree catheter, a modification of the Cook's airway exchanger may be used to intubate through the SGA. It is loaded over a fiberoptic bronchoscope (FOB) and the trachea is visualised through the SGA [30, 31]. Leaving the Aintree catheter in place, the SGA is then removed. The ETT is then loaded over the catheter and advanced into the trachea.

2.4 Rescue airway

The difficult airway algorithm made by the American Society of Anesthesiologists (ASA) has a prominent place for the use of SGAs in airway rescue [32]. The Difficult Airway Society (DAS) 2015 guidelines suggests the use of SGAs as first line rescue airway for management of a failed intubation [33]. Several case reports support the use of SGAs for supporting ventilation in difficult airways with failed intubation [34–37]. SGAs also aid successful tracheal intubation in situations in which conventional methods have failed.

2.5 Procedures in the critical care units

2.5.1 Paediatric bronchoscopies

Flexible bronchoscopies comprise the major airway procedures performed including bronchoalveolar lavage, transbronchial biopsies, and foreign body removal [38]. LMA use during paediatric bronchscopies is associated with ease of insertion during general anaesthesia with spontaneous or assisted ventilation, as well as a net decrease in procedure time.

2.5.2 Adult bronchoscopies

Certain patients who cannot tolerate the procedure with conscious sedation (i.e., excessive gag response or discomfort) may require general anaesthesia. An LMA is an ideal device in such a scenario.

2.5.3 Percutaneous tracheostomies

Percutaneous tracheostomies are increasingly performed in the critical care setting. It is indicated in patients who are ventilator dependent due to acute illnesses, or if duration of ETT use is expected to exceed 2 weeks [39]. Cattano et al. conducted a study on patients undergoing percutaneous tracheostomy using dilating forceps approach where ETT was replaced by an SGA [40]. They concluded that intubation through SGAs offered a superior view of the trachea without the risk of the bronchoscope or the ETT getting needle punctured.

2.6 Aide to tracheal extubation

Since SGAs cause less cough and rise in intracranial or intraocular pressures compared to the ETT, they may be used for smooth emergence from anaesthesia. The device may be placed after removal of the ETT. This is helpful in situations in which airway and hemodynamic reflexes are undesirable.

2.7 Pre or outside the hospital airway

In the field, securing an airway is of paramount importance. SGAs are lifesaving in the “can’t ventilate, can’t intubate” situation. An SGA can be used for transport until a definitive airway can be obtained [41]. The placement of an SGA is easily mastered by the inexperienced hands with minimal training.

During cardio pulmonary resuscitation (CPR), the first part of the secondary survey includes securing an airway device as soon as possible [42]. SGA use during CPR has increased since SGA insertion is easier to learn than tracheal intubation and feasible with fewer and shorter interruptions in chest compression [43]. Use of SGAs during CPR is associated with a lower incidence of regurgitation of gastric contents than bag-mask ventilation [44].

3. Contraindications

- Patients with risk of gastric aspiration (non-fasted, Gastro Oesophageal Reflux Disease, hiatus hernia)
- Patients with airway morbidities (Respiratory tract infections, COPD etc.)
- Restricted mouth opening (< 2.5 cm)
- Distorted airway anatomy and airway obstruction
- Prolonged duration of surgery (>2 hrs)
- Surgery involving the upper airway
- Maxillo facial trauma
- Morbidly obese patients

3.1 Complications

- Regurgitation and aspiration
- Misplacement of mask and airway obstruction
- Malposition or dislodgement of LMA
- Upper airway trauma
- Inadequate sealing of airway and leaks
- Cough and laryngospasm
- Gastric insufflation
- Vocal cord palsy and nerve injuries (Lingual nerve, Recurrent Laryngeal Nerve, Hypoglossal Nerve, Glossopharyngeal Nerve)

4. Insertion technique

All LMAs consist of four parts, a hollow tube (shaft) continuous with a hollow mask or cuff, inflation line with pilot balloon and drain (gastric access) tube. The broad elliptical inflatable cuff has a smooth upper surface that prevents pharyngeal secretions from entering the airway and an under surface that sits over the larynx to create a seal.

The patient's neck is flexed and head is extended (sniffing position) (**Figure 1**). The LMA is partially deflated and the backside of the LMA is lubricated. The shaft is grasped with the dominant hand like a pen, as near to the mask as possible. The deflated flattened mask is inserted against the hard palate downward into the mouth along the curvature of the back of the pharynx. The index finger follows the tube into the mouth to keep pressing "back" and "down" until the aperture faces the laryngeal inlet. If at any time during insertion the mask fails to stay flattened or starts to fold back, it should be withdrawn and reinserted. Another technique is to

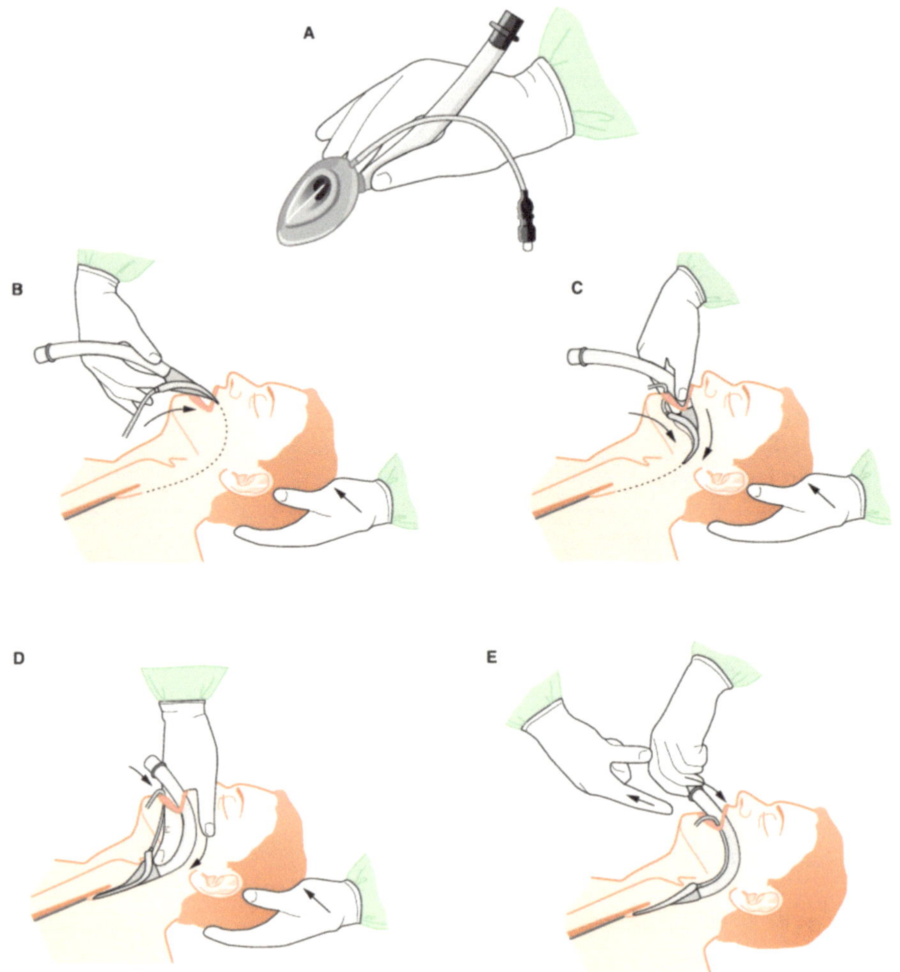

Figure 1.
Technique of LMA insertion. (a) The deflated and lubricated LMA is held by the index finger and thumb of right hand. (b) The left hand stabilizes the occiput. LMA is inserted in the mouth pressed against the hard palate. (c) Using the index finger, it is advanced behind the tongue. (d) It is further pushed into the hypopharynx with the index finger. (e) After removing the index figure, the airway tube of the LMA is pushed further inside with the left hand till a resistance is felt.

allow the dominant hand to guide the shaft and use the nondominant hand to push the tube with or without an introducer [45–47].

Proper placement of the airway is prudent. Cuff should be inflated to achieve adequate tidal volumes with minimal leaks. The cuff inflation pressure should never exceed 60 mm Hg. Higher Cuff pressures may lead to increased pharyngeal mucosal pressures which may lead to mucosal ischemia and airway morbidities [48].

Marjot showed that intracuff pressure increased as cuff volume increases [49]. The pressure exerted on the pharynx by the SGA is usually higher than that of mucosal capillary perfusion pressure when the cuff is inflated with the recommended maximum volume of air.

However, if the cuff is deflated excessively, it may not protect the airway from soiling, due to the regurgitated fluid from the stomach [50]. Therefore. it is desirable to inflate the cuff of the SGA with minimum volume of air which provides a seal around the mask.

In case of malpositioning of the mask, it may have to be replaced or other manoeuvres may have to be tried. A partially or fully inflated SGA cuff may ease insertion [8–10]. Wakeling et al. claim that inserting an SGA with a fully inflated cuff causes less mucosal trauma and leads to fewer airway morbidities. If an assistant is available, he can apply a jaw thrust manoeuvre which moves the tongue forward and prevents compression of the epiglottis [14]. In case of a single operator, a tongue depressor or a laryngoscope may be used to assist insertion of the LMA [15].

5. Size selection

Weight-based selection as per the manufacturer's guideline is done. If unsure, check the package cover for size information. More than one size should always be available, because the correct size cannot always be predicted. Weight-based selection has given way to sex-based selection, especially in adults. The consensus seems to be that the correct size would be a size 4 for most adult women and a size 5 for most adult men [51–57]. Whatever the initial size selected, if malposition or an inadequate seal is present, a larger size LMA should be considered. Alternative formulas based on weight have been proposed [58, 59]. For children, the width of the second to fourth fingers can be matched to the widest part of the mask [60]. If repeated attempts with one type of LMA are unsuccessful, changing to another type may help.

6. Removal technique

Wait for full recovery from anaesthesia. Do not try to pull out the SGA if the patient is biting down on the shaft. Usually, patients emerge smoothly with SGAs.

It is recommended to use a bite block with the LMA in order to prevent damage to the airway tube or pilot balloon during emergence. Manufacturers usually recommend using a wad of gauze swabs rolled into a cylindrical shape and placed along the LMA. Some anaesthesiologists prefer to place the Guedel's airway. The LMA should never be removed if patient is in a light plane of anaesthesia as it may precipitate a laryngospasm.

7. Classification

SGAs have been conventionally classified based on the following characteristics by Miller [61].:

- Whether it is inflatable or anatomically pre-shaped
- Where in the hypopharynx it provides a seal
- Whether or not the sealing effect is directional and
- Whether or not oesophageal sealing occurs

In recent years, devices with oesophageal sealing (Second Generation SGAs) have gained popularity due to presence of a gastric port which allows drainage of stomach contents and reduces the incidence of regurgitation and aspiration pneumonitis.

Modern classification of SGAs is given in **Table 1**.

7.1 Sealing pressure

The airway sealing pressure or the oropharyngeal leak pressure (OLP) is the pressure at which gas leak occurs around the device. It indicates the degree of airway protection. After the successful placement of airway device, OLP can be determined

Oesophageal sealing	Pharyngeal sealer	Perilaryngeal sealers
None (1st generation)	VBM Laryngeal Tube (VBM, Germany)	LMA Classic (Teleflex, USA)
	Cobra PLA (Pulmodyne, USA)	LMA Unique (Teleflex, USA)
		LMA Flexible (Teleflex, USA)
		AuraOnce LMA (Ambu, Denmark)
		Aura-i LMA (Ambu, Denmark)
		Air-Q ILA (Mercury Medical, USA)
Gastric channel (2nd generation)	Combitube (Covidien-Nellcor USA)	LMA ProSeal (Teleflex, USA)
	Rusch Easy Tube (Teleflex, USA)	LMA Supreme (Teleflex, USA)
	VBM LTS II (VBM, Germany)	LMA Guardian (Teleflex, USA)
	King LTS-D (Ambu, Denmark)	LMA Protector (Teleflex, USA)
		AuraGain LMA (Ambu, Denmark)
		i-gel (Intersurgical, UK)
Gastric channel + self-energising mechanism of seal		Baska mask (Baska Versatile Laryngeal Mask Pvt. Ltd., Australia)

LMA: laryngeal mask airway, ILA: intubating laryngeal airway, LTS: Laryngeal Tube Suction, LTS-D: Laryngeal Tube Suction disposable, PLA: perilaryngeal airway.

Table 1.
Classification of supraglottic airways.

by turning off the ventilator and closing the adjustable pressure limiting valve of the circuit. A fixed gas flow of 3 L/min is started and the pressure allowed to rise.

There are various methods of assessment of OLP [62].:

a. Audible noise over the patient's mouth

b. Auscultation just lateral to the thyroid cartilage for an audible noise

c. Manometer stability test- The fresh gas flow is set at 3 l/minute of oxygen and the adjustable pressure limiting valve of the circle system is closed. As the pressure from the breathing system increases, the aneroid manometer dial is observed to note airway pressure at which the dial attains stability and no further rise in pressure is seen. A maximum pressure of 40 cm H2O is allowed.

Correct placement of the LMA can be checked by a simple test. A soap bubble solution is placed over the tip of the drain tube. If the tip of the LMA is in the laryngopharynx, bubbling or bursting of soap solution column will occur during positive pressure ventilation.

7.2 First generation SGA

7.2.1 LMA classic ™ (cLMA)

The original Laryngeal Mask Airway (cLMA, Intavent Direct, Maidenhead, UK) was the first SGAs introduced into clinical practice. It was invented by Dr. Archie Brain in the United Kingdom 1981 and was introduced into clinical practice in 1988.

In 1992 a task force was commissioned by the ASA to establish practice guidelines for management of difficult airway scenarios. In 1993, the ASA published the algorithm for difficult airways. They stressed on an early attempt at LMA insertion in case of inadequate face mask ventilation. cLMA has revolutionised anaesthetic practice ever since [63].

7.2.2 Device description, technical aspects

The cLMA consists of the following parts (**Figure 2**):

- Curved airway tube (shaft)
- Pilot tube
- Elliptical mask

The angle between the mask and shaft is 30°. The machine end of the shaft has a standard 15-mm adapter. Two flexible vertical bars at the junction of the shaft and mask prevent obstruction of the ventilating lumen by the epiglottis (**Figure 3**). Reusable devices are constructed of medical grade silicone designed to provide an oval seal around the laryngeal inlet and act as a sleeve joint at the upper oesophagus. The single use devices have a cuff constructed of polyvinyl-chloride.

The classic laryngeal mask is available in eight sizes, as shown in **Table 2**.

7.2.3 Limitations of the LMA classic™

Although the cLMA is used in a large number of cases requiring airway management, it has some limitations

- It has a moderate pharyngeal seal (~20 cm H_2O)
- It may be associated with pulmonary aspiration of regurgitated fluid

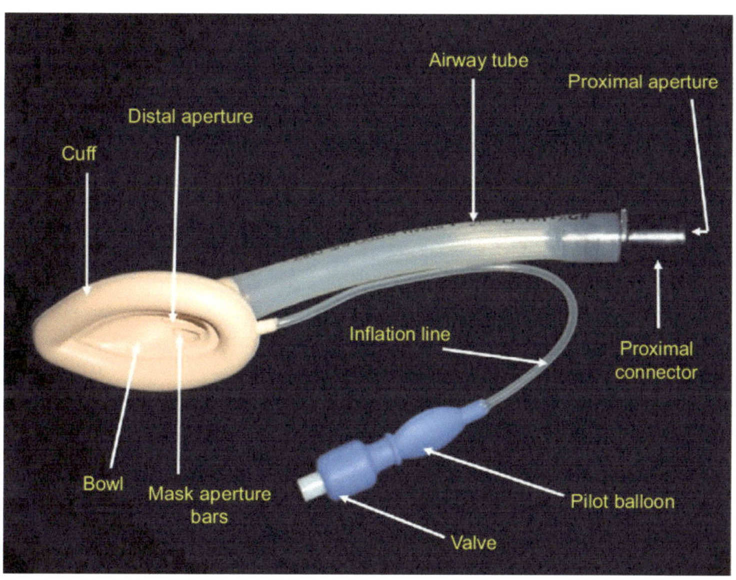

Figure 2.
Classic LMA.

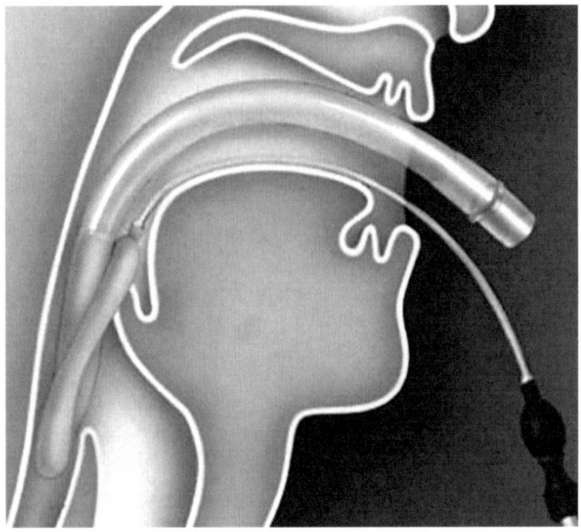

Figure 3.
Classic LMA in-situ.

Mask size	Patient weight	Maximum cuff volume of air (ml)
1	Neonates/infants up to 5 kg	4
1.5	Infants 5–10 kg	7
2	Infants/children 10–20 kg	10
2.5	Children 20–30 kg	14
3	Children 30–50 kg	20
4	Adults 50–70 kg	30
5	Adults 70–100 kg	40
6	Large adults over 100 kg	50

Table 2.
Available classic LMAs.

First generation SGAs have only a single lumen for ventilation. There is risk of regurgitation of gastric contents and aspiration with positive pressure ventilation. To combat this risk, a separate channel was incorporated into this design to allow for gastric drainage and provide better seal. Several modifications of the Classic LMA were done and lead to the invention of second-generation SGAs.

7.3 Second generation SGA

A second-generation SGA is one with design features (higher oropharyngeal seal pressures and oesophageal drain tubes) specifically intended to reduce the risk of aspiration [33].

7.3.1 LMA Proseal™ (pLMA)

7.3.1.1 Introduction

The Proseal LMA™ (Teleflex®, USA) designed by Dr. Archie Brain, is based on the cLMA. It was introduced in the year 2001. In comparison to the cLMA, it has a larger and deeper bowl without aperture bars, second drainage tube placed lateral to the airway tube that ends at the tip of the mask, posterior extension of the mask cuff, integral silicone bite block, and an anterior pocket for seating an introducer or finger during insertion.

7.3.1.2 Device description, technical aspects and practicalities of use

The pLMA has four main components (**Figure 4**):

- Mask
- Inflation line with pilot balloon.
- Airway tube
- Drain tube.

The mask conforms to the contours of the hypopharynx. The mask has a main cuff that seals around the glottic aperture. The rear cuff pushes the mask anteriorly which helps to increase the seal. A pilot balloon with valve is used to inflate or deflate the device.

A drain tube (DT) passes parallel and lateral to the airway tube. It continues to enter the cuff bowl and terminates at the mask tip. Cuff tip lies at the origin of the upper oesophageal sphincter if device is positioned correctly. The wire reinforced airway tube prevents collapse and terminates with a standard 15 mm connector [7]. The pLMA can also be used for FOB guided intubation.

7.3.1.3 Size selection, practical aspect, adjuncts

Sizes 3 to 5 were introduced in 2000 and sizes 1½-2½ in 2004. Sizes 1½-2½ have no dorsal cuff. Device properties and recommendations for use are given in **Table 3**. The pLMA is reusable and recommended product life is 40 sterilisations. Not all protein material can be removed by routine cleaning of laryngeal masks and this raises theoretical concerns over cross-infection risk, hence steam autoclaving is the recommended method of sterilising this device.

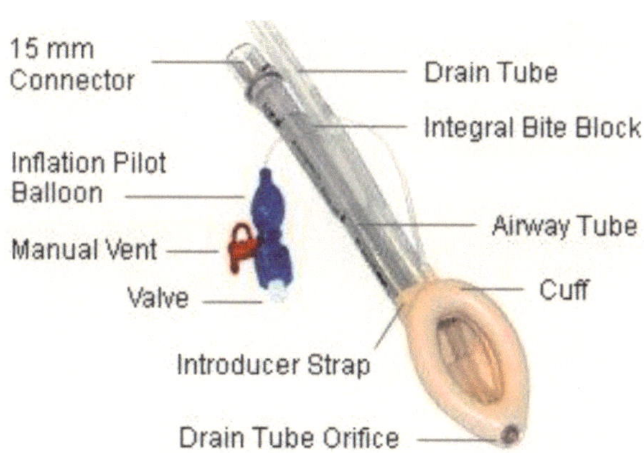

Figure 4.
Parts of Proseal LMA.

Mask size	Patient weight	Maximum cuff volume of air (ml)	Gastric tube size (French)	Largest ETT ID (mm)
1	Neonates/infants up to 5 kg	4	8	3.5
1.5	Infants 5–10 kg	7	10	4
2	Infants/children 10–20 kg	10	10	4.5
2.5	Children 20–30 kg	14	14	5
3	Children 30–50 kg	20	16	6
4	Adults 50–70 kg	30	16	6
5	Adults 70–100 kg	40	18	7

Table 3.
Available Proseal LMAs.

The pLMA is accompanied by a cuff deflator (**Figure 5**) and insertion tool (**Figures 6** and 7). The cuff deflator assists complete deflation and flattening the device tip before insertion to improve insertion success.

7.3.2 The LMA-supreme™ (SLMA)

7.3.2.1 Introduction

LMA Supreme™(Teleflex®, USA) is a second generation, single use, SGA device which facilitate ease of placement and in-situ airway stability. It forms an effective seal first with the oropharynx (oropharyngeal seal) and a second seal with the upper oesophageal sphincter (the oesophageal seal). This devise is designed incorporating features of a cLMA, pLMA, and LMA Fastrach [64–66]. SLMA delivers measured oropharyngeal leak pressures up to 37 cm H2 O [67].

7.3.2.2 Device description, technical aspects and practicalities of use

The SLMA has following components (**Figure 8**):

- Modified cuff
- Elliptical airway tube
- Drain tube

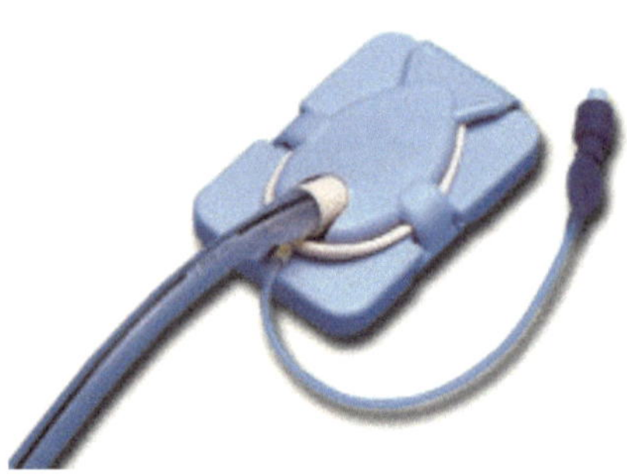

Figure 5.
PLMA cuff deflator.

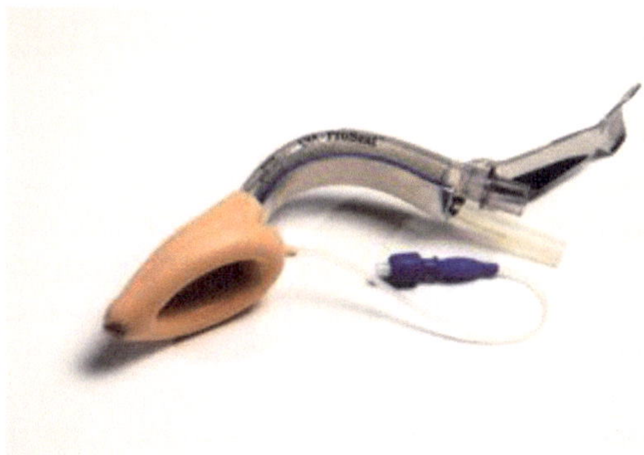

Figure 6.
pLMA with insertion tool.

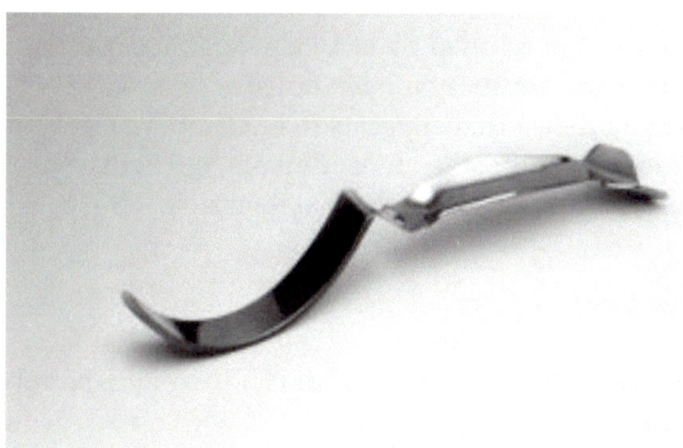

Figure 7.
Insertion tool.

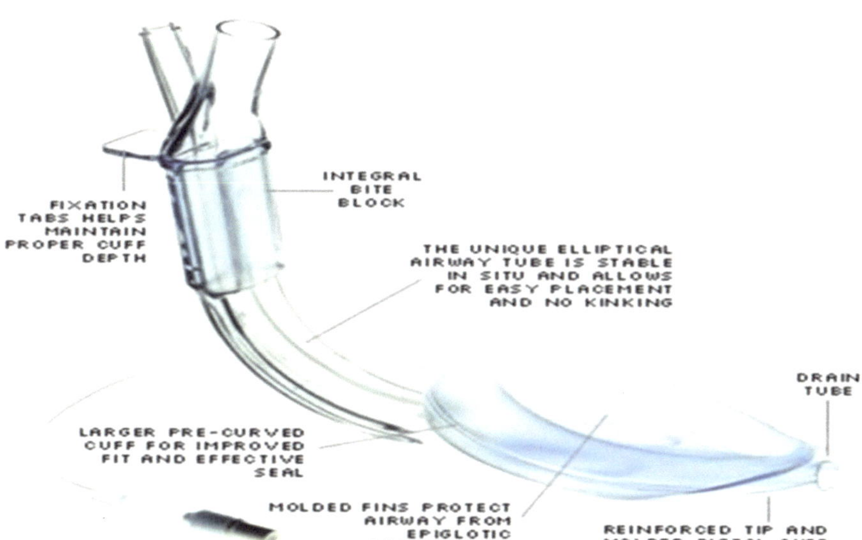

Figure 8.
Parts of LMA supreme.

- Integrated bite block
- Inflation line with pilot balloon
- Fixation tab

The device is preformed and anatomically shaped. The stiffness of SLMA is intended to guide the airway into the correct position during insertion (**Figure 9**). This also eliminates the need for placing the clinician's fingers into the patient's mouth. Also, rotational mal-positioning of the airway becomes unlikely owing to this feature. The integrated bite block reduces the potential for damage to, or obstruction of the airway tube in the event of biting. The airway also has a fixation tab designed to facilitate easy fixation and improve drain tube position. These improvisations render it suited for inexperienced users in an emergency situation.

Primarily, the SLMA has been recommended for securing airway in routine and emergency surgical procedures. It may also be used to secure an immediate airway when tracheal intubation is precluded by lack of available expertise or equipment, or when attempts at tracheal intubation have failed.

There is increasing evidence that suggests that it may be used for airway rescue in emergency situations and in hostile environments, particularly when tracheal intubation may be challenging or may delay oxygenation [68–70].

7.3.2.3 Size selection, practical aspect, adjuncts

Size 1 to 5 are commercially available (**Table 4**). A weight-based size selection is suggested by the manufacturer. The cuff is inflated with air as recommended for that specific size. The intra-cuff pressure should never exceed 60 cm H_2O. The cuff should be inflated with just enough air to achieve a seal sufficient to permit ventilation without leaks, if no manometer is available.

Some studies advocate an anatomical-related size selection method. The patient's thyromental distance is measured by the palm side of patient's hand. If it is four

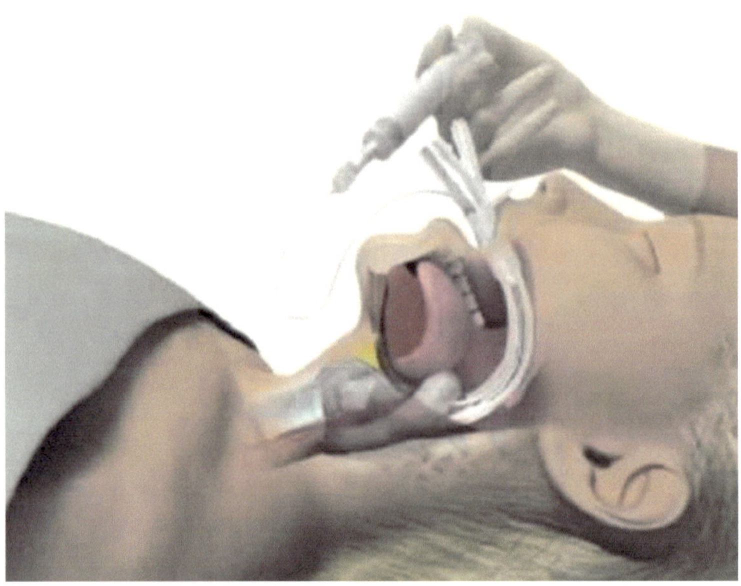

Figure 9.
LMA supreme in-situ.

Mask size	Patient weight	Maximum cuff volume of air (ml)	Gastric tube size (French)
1	Neonates/infants up to 5 kg	5	6
1.5	Infants 5–10 kg	8	6
2	Infants/children 10–20 kg	12	10
2.5	Children 20–30 kg	20	10
3	Children 30–50 kg	30	14
4	Adults 50–70 kg	45	14
5	Adults 70–100 kg	45	14

Table 4.
Available supreme LMAs.

fingers wide (index, middle, ring and little fingers), they suggest size 4 SLMA; If it is three fingers wide (index, middle, ring fingers), they suggest size 3 SLMA [71].

7.3.3 The LMA Guardian™ (GLMA)

The Guardian laryngeal mask airway™ (GLMA) (Teleflex®, USA) is a new disposable silicone SGA device. The cuff forms a seal with the glottis for ventilation, and with the hypopharynx for airway protection. The gastric drainage port helps to suction the stomach contents. Also, it has a port for suctioning material from the hypopharynx. The pilot balloon valve with pressure logo indicates visual intracuff pressure (Yellow <40 cmH2O, Green 40–60 cmH2O and Red >60 cmH2O) (**Figure 10**). A study suggests that it provides sealing pressures as high as 32 cm H2O [72, 73].

7.3.4 LMA protector and LMA protector™ cuff pilot™

7.3.4.1 Introduction

The LMA-Protector™ (Teleflex®, USA) is a novel SGA made of medical-grade silicone (**Figure 11**). In comparison to other devices made of

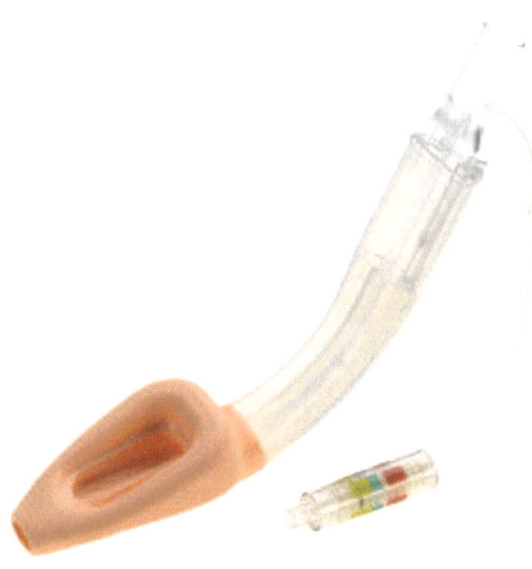

Figure 10.
LMA guardian.

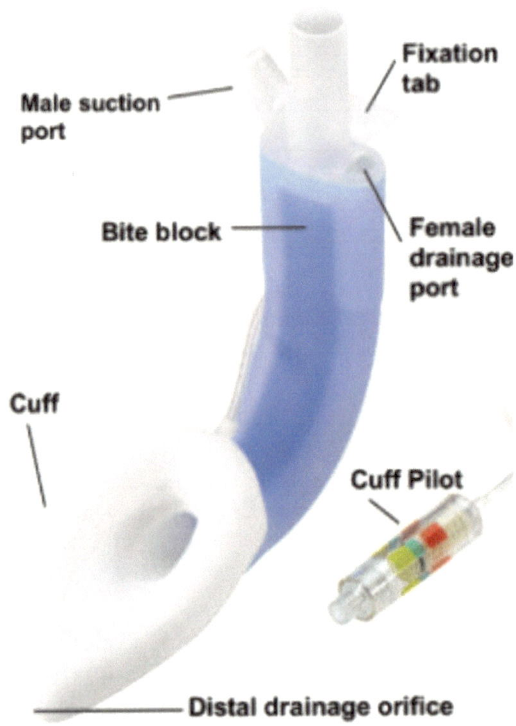

Figure 11.
LMA protector cuff pilot.

polyvinylchloride, it is more flexible and less traumatic. Its fixed, anatomically curved shape is elliptical in cross section and aids easier insertion. It has two separate drain channels. At the machine end, they begin as the male and female suction ports. The channels then enter a chamber behind the cuff bowl. At the patient end, the chamber ends at the tip of the cuff. The device is flexible and stays in place if the patient's head is mobilised. A built-in bite block reduces the potential for damage to, or obstruction of the airway tube in the event of biting. Additionally, the LMA-Protector™ is available with a pilot balloon or the integrated Cuff Pilot™. The Cuff Pilot™ enables constant visualisation of intracuff pressure inside the mask cuff that provides easier adjustment and is colour coded for inflation pressure [74].

7.3.4.2 Size selection, practical aspect, adjuncts

It is commercially available in size 3, 4 and 5. The manufacturer recommends using a size 4 device for normal adults. After insertion, the device is fixed in place and inflated to the recommended pressure. There should be a minimum of a 1 cm gap between the fixation tab and the patient's upper lip. The cuff should be inflated with sufficient air to prevent a leak with positive pressure ventilation, but it must not exceed either a pressure of 60 cm H2O or the specific device cuff volume maxima. If no manometer is available, inflate with just enough air to achieve a seal sufficient to permit ventilation without leaks. It provides high first attempt and overall insertion success rate. It helps rapidly achieve effective ventilation with reliable airway seal. Additionally, it acts as a conduit for FOB guided intubation [75, 76].

7.3.5 Ambu AuraGain

7.3.5.1 Introduction

The AuraGain™ (Ambu®, Denmark) is intended for use as an alternative to a face mask for achieving and maintaining control of the airway during routine and emergency anaesthetic procedures. The gastric channel of AuraGain™ may be used as a conduit for passing a gastric tube into the stomach for removal of air and gastric fluids.

It is intended for use as a conduit for an endotracheal tube in “can’t intubate – can’t ventilate” scenarios. It may also be used to establish a clear airway during resuscitation in profoundly unconscious patients with absent glossopharyngeal and laryngeal reflexes who may need artificial ventilation [77].

7.3.5.2 Device description

The parts of AuraGain are as follows (**Figures 12** and **13**):

- Inflatable Mask
- Inflation line with pilot balloon.
- Airway tube with integrated bite block
- Gastric channel

The mask is designed to conform to the contours of the hypopharynx with its lumen facing the laryngeal opening. When correctly inserted, the distal tip of the cuff rests against the upper oesophageal sphincter. It is anatomically shaped with an integrated bite block.

7.3.5.3 Size selection, practical aspect

The AuraGain™ comes in eight different sizes for use in patients of different weight (**Table 5**). This device is meant to be used only once. Studies suggest that AuraGain™ provides adequate sealing of the airway [78–80].

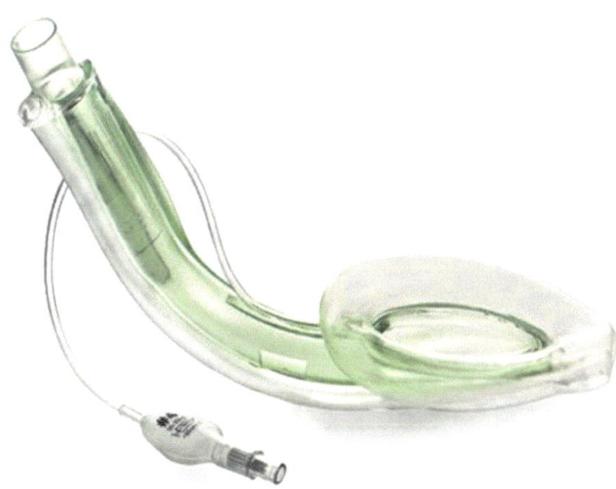

Figure 12.
Ambu AuraGain.

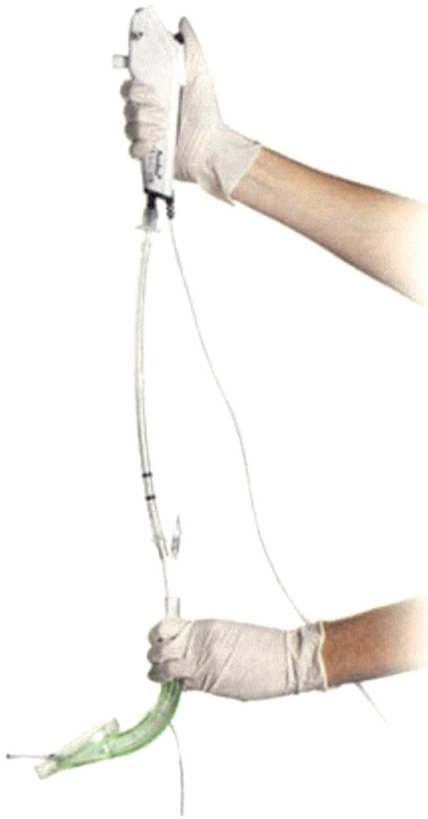

Figure 13.
FOB guided intubation.

Mask size	Patient weight	Maximum cuff volume of air (ml)	Gastric tube size (French)	Largest ETT ID (mm)
1	Neonates/infants up to 5 kg	4	6	3.5
1.5	Infants 5–10 kg	7	8	4
2	Infants/children 10–20 kg	10	10	5
2.5	Children 20–30 kg	14	10	5.5
3	Children 30–50 kg	20	16	6.5
4	Adults 50–70 kg	30	16	7.5
5	Adults 70–100 kg	40	16	8
6	Adults more than 100 kg	50	16	8

Table 5.
Available Auragain LMAs.

7.3.6 i-gel®

7.3.6.1 Introduction

The i-gel® (Intersurgical®, UK) is the innovative second generation supraglottic airway device from Intersurgical launched in 2007. Made from a medical grade thermoplastic elastomer, i-gel has been designed to create a non-inflatable, anatomical seal of the pharyngeal, laryngeal and perilaryngeal structures whilst avoiding compression trauma.

7.3.6.2 Device description

The igel has the following parts (**Figure 14**):

- Soft non-inflatable cuff
- Gastric channel
- Epiglottic rest
- Buccal cavity stabiliser
- Airway tube
- Gastric tube

A horizontal line (Adult sizes 3,4 and 5 only) at the middle of the integral bite-block represents the correct position of the teeth. The soft design of the i-gel is able to retain its shape to facilitate ease of insertion. In a known difficult or unexpectedly difficult intubation, for intubating the patient, by passing an ETT through the device under fibre optic guidance.

7.3.6.3 Size selection, practical aspect, adjuncts

Size selection is done on a weight basis (**Table 6**). However, individual anatomical variations should always be considered. Patients with cylindrical necks or wide thyroid/cricoid cartilages may require a larger size i-gel than would normally be recommended on a weight basis [81, 82].

The i-gel can be used in difficult or unanticipated difficult intubations. Owing to its ease of insertion, it can quickly establish and maintain a clear airway in a pre-hospital setting [83, 84]. In a study it was observed that hemodynamic parameters, ease of insertion and postoperative complications were comparable among the i-gel, pLMA and cLMA but airway sealing pressure was significantly higher with i-gel [85].

A modification of this device is the i-gel O2. It contains a supplementary oxygen port for passive oxygen administration. It may be utilised for cardiopulmonary resuscitation. The i-gel O2 Resus Pack is a resuscitation pack provided by the manufacturer. It contains the i-gel O2 LMA, an airway support strap to fix and secure the device in place, a suction tube (12 Fr) and a pack of lubricant. The Resus Pack is available in three adult sizes (3, 4 and 5). The presence of a colour coded hook ring on the LMA allows easy identification of the size during resuscitation.

7.3.7 Combitube®

7.3.7.1 Introduction

The Combitube® (Covidien-Nellcor®, Pleaseton, USA) is a single use, double-lumen tube that combines the features of a conventional ETT with those of an oesophageal obturator airway.

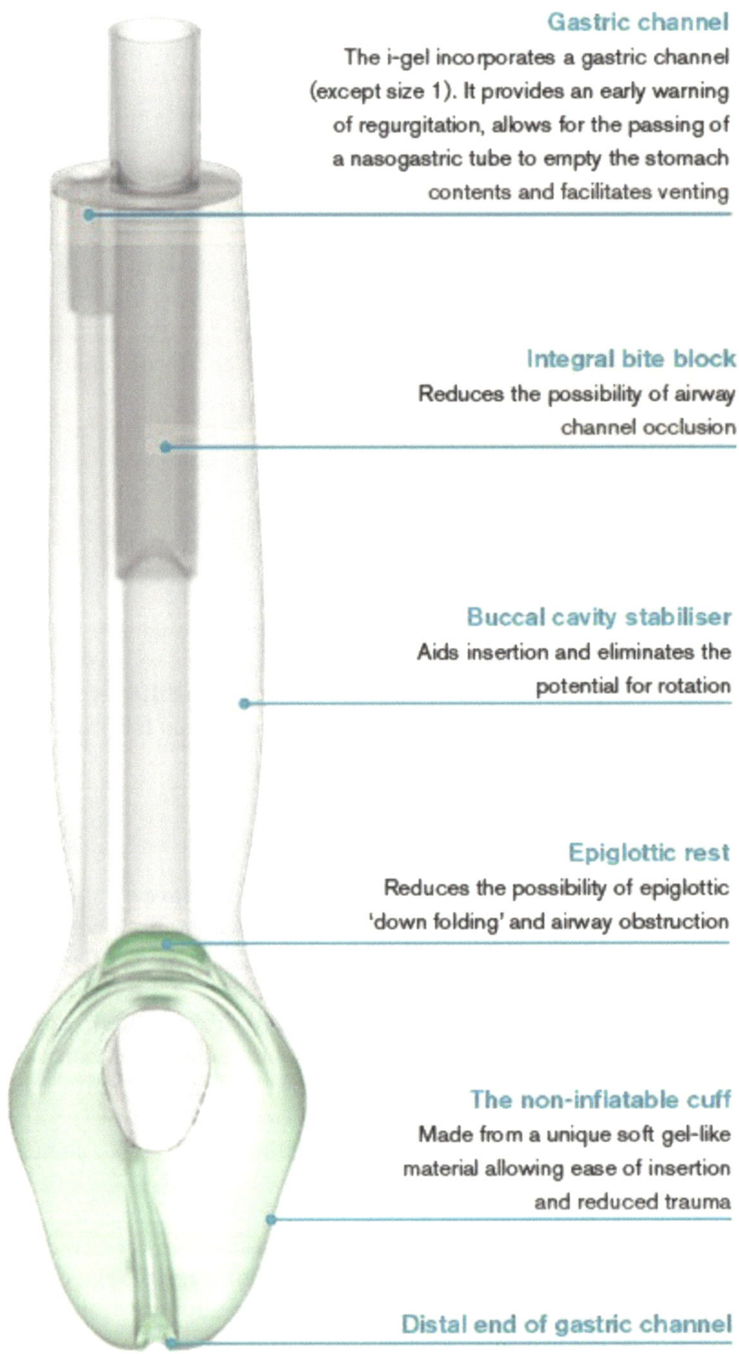

Figure 14.
Parts of i-gel.

7.3.7.2 Device description

The Combitube® has the following parts (**Figure 15**):

- A large proximal balloon cuff seals the hypopharynx
- A ventilating, proximal lumen terminates at side ports overlying the laryngeal inlet

Mask size	Patient weight	Largest ETT ID (mm)	Gastric tube size (French)
1	Neonates 2-5 kg	3	NA
1.5	Infants 5–12 kg	4	10
2	Infants/children 10–25 kg	5	12
2.5	Children 25–35 kg	5	12
3	Children, Small adult 30–60 kg	6	12
4	Adults 50–90 kg	7	12
5	Adults >90 kg	8	14

Table 6.
Available i-gel LMAs.

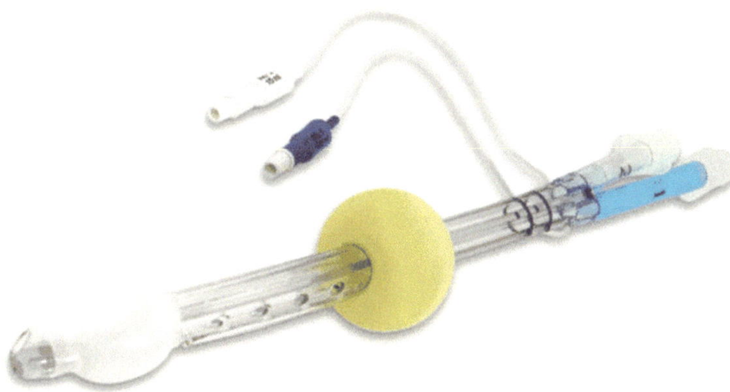

Figure 15.
Combitube.

- A distal lumen and its smaller balloon cuff terminate in and seal the upper oesophagus (in >90% of insertions)

The device commonly enters the oesophagus on insertion. Ventilation is achieved through multiple proximal apertures situated above the distal cuff (**Figure 16**). Both the proximal and distal cuffs have to be inflated to prevent air from escaping through the oesophagus. If the tube enters the trachea, ventilation is achieved through the distal lumen.

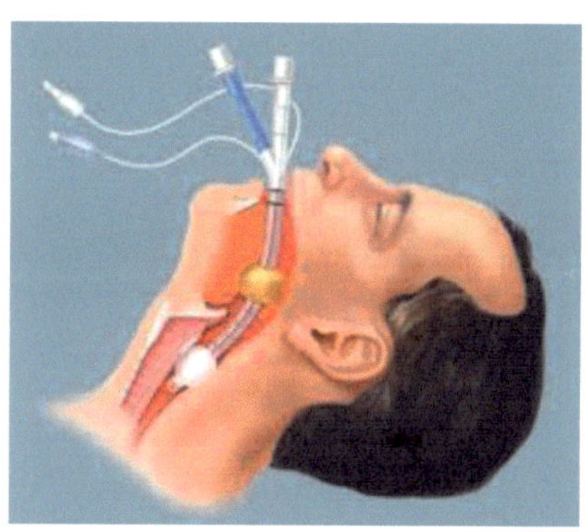

Figure 16.
Combitube in-situ.

7.3.7.3 Size selection, practical aspect, adjuncts

Combitube® is commercially available in two sizes (**Table 7**). It has a major advantage over conventional ETT as it can be inserted without head and neck movement, which may be an important consideration in trauma patients [86]. Situations where ETT placement is not immediately possible, it is used for emergency airway control [87]. The Combitube® has been used effectively in cardiopulmonary resuscitation [88, 89]. It has been used successfully in difficult airway situations owing to severe facial burns, trauma, upper airway bleeding and vomiting where there was an inability to visualise the vocal cords [90–92].

7.3.8 Ambu® king LTS-D™ (disposable laryngeal tube)

7.3.8.1 Introduction

The King Laryngeal Tube Suction-D™ (Ambu®, Denmark) is a disposable, double-lumen, supralaryngeal device for airway management introduced in 2005. A single pilot tube can be used to inflate both oropharyngeal and oesophageal soft silicon cuff. A ventilating outlet opens in front of the vocal cords. It is present between these cuffs. It is available in six sizes to fit patients from neonates to large adults.

7.3.8.2 Device description

Parts of the LTS-D (**Figures 17** and **18**):

- Proximal cuff.
- Distal cuff
- Inflation line with pilot balloon
- Ventilation holes
- Drain tube

The Proximal cuff stabilises the device and seals the oropharynx. Distal cuff blocks entry of the oesophagus, reducing the possibility of gastric insufflation. Multiple distal ventilatory openings and bilateral ventilation eyelets facilitate air flow. The device has a curvature of 60 degrees. Sealing pressures of 30 cm H20 or more are achievable.

7.3.8.3 Size selection, practical aspect

Size selection is done on a weight basis (**Table 8**). The slim profile allows easy insertion; thus, it can be considered for airway management in patients with

Patient's height	Combitube size
4 to 6 feet tall	37 French
5 feet and above	41 French

Table 7.
Available combitube.

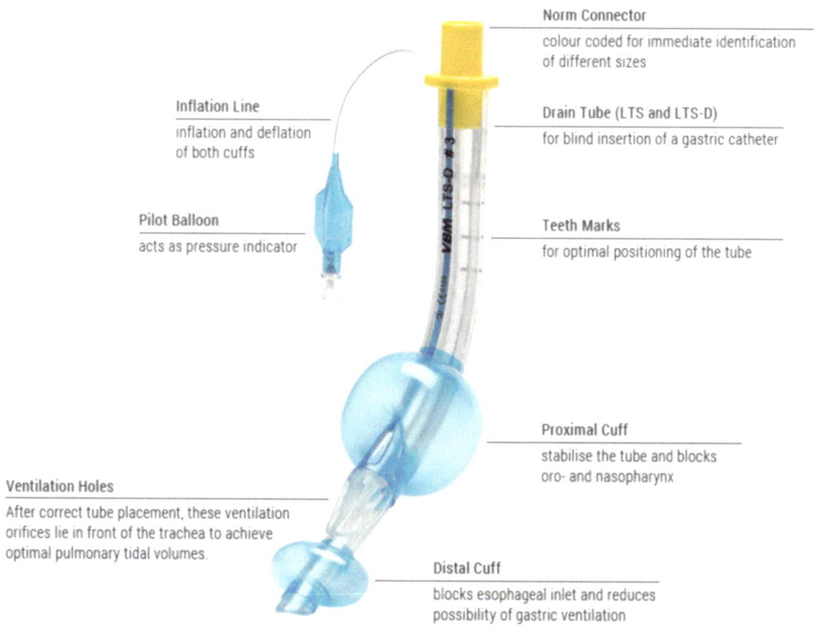

Figure 17.
Parts of LTS-D.

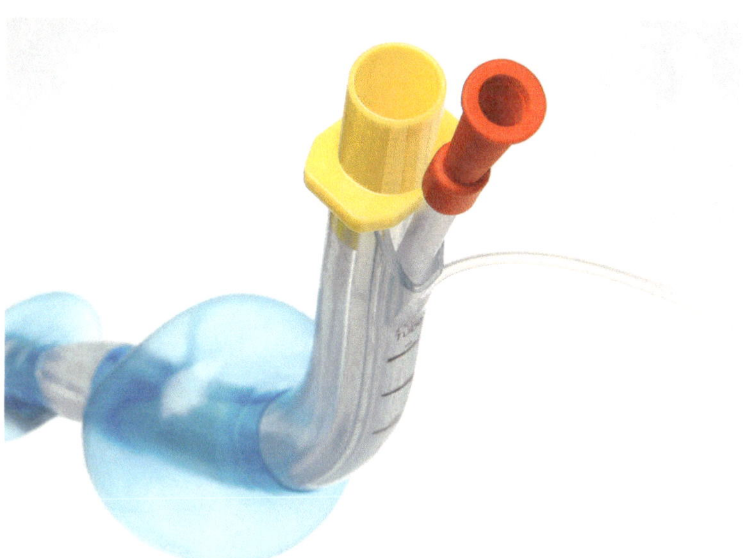

Figure 18.
LTS-D drain tube.

restricted mouth opening. Since insertion is relatively easy and guarantees a clear airway in most patients on the first attempt extensive training is not necessary [93].

It can be used during spontaneous or controlled ventilation. The LTS-D has been recommended as an emergency device to be used in cases of difficult intubation and cannot intubate, cannot ventilate situations while one is preparing to perform a surgical airway [94–96]. A modification of this device, the Intubating Laryngeal Tube Suction-D(iLTS-D™) is a novel device which may also be used as a conduit for intubation.

Size	Patient weight	Maximum cuff volume of air (ml)	Colour of Connector
0	Neonates<6 kg	15	TRANSPARENT
1	Infants 6–15 kg	40	WHITE
2	Children 15–30 kg	60	GREEN
3	Small Adult 30–60 kg	120	YELLOW
4	Medium Adult50–90 kg	130	RED
5	Large Adults >90 kg	150	VIOLET

Table 8.
Available LTS-D tubes.

7.3.9 Baska mask®

7.3.9.1 Introduction

The Baska Mask® (Baska Versatile Laryngeal Mask Pty Ltd., Australia) has been designed by Australian anesthesists, Kanag and Meenakshi Baska. It obviates the need of an orogastric tube and replaces this with a sump and two drains. It brings together features of PLMA, SLMA, SLIPA and i-gel. The biggest advantage of Baska mask lies in the fact that cuff deflation or inflation is not required prior to insertion [97].

7.3.9.2 Device description

Parts of the Baska mask® (**Figures 19** and **20**):

- Self-sealing variable pressure cuff
- Insertion tab
- Integrated bite block
- Airway tube
- Suction attachment
- Sump area

It is made of medical grade silicone. It differs in several ways from the conventional LMA, including; a cuff-less self-sealing membranous bowl which inflates and deflates with each positive pressure inspiration and expiration respectively, an inbuilt "tab" that permits to increase its angulation for easy negotiation of the oropharyngeal curve during placement, a bite block. It has a dual high flow suction drainage system. The distal aperture at oesophageal end is aspirated using two vents running along the entire length of the stem. One tube is connected to high pressure suction whereas the other is left open.

7.3.9.3 Size selection, practical aspect

Size selection is given below (**Table 9**). Zundert *et al*. in their study concluded that Baska mask® improves safety when used in both intermittent positive pressure

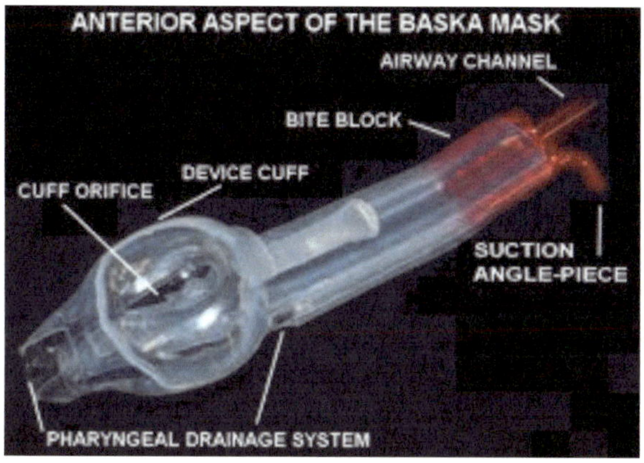

Figure 19.
Baska mask-anterior.

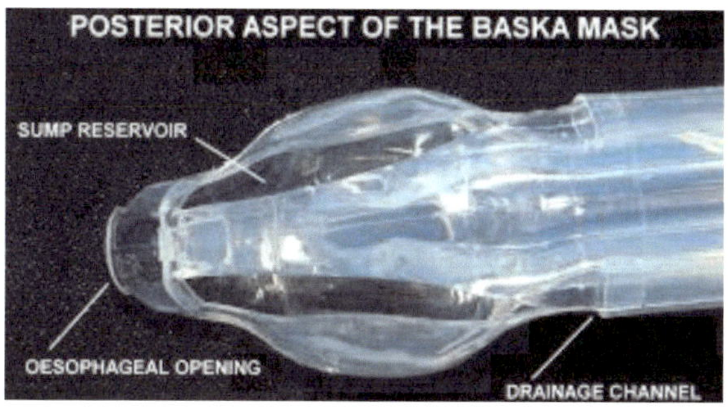

Figure 20.
Baska mask-posterior.

Mask size	Patient	Colour coded connector
1	Neonates	PURPLE
1.5	Infants 1–2 yrs	ORANGE
2	Children 2-5 yrs	DARK BLUE
2.5	Large child or small female	WHITE
3	Large female or small man	GREEN
4	Average adult man	YELLOW
5	Large man	RED

Table 9.
Available Baska LMAs.

ventilation (IPPV) and spontaneous breathing [98]. Another study found its safety profile comparable to i-gel [99].

7.3.10 Air-Q® blocker™ intubating laryngeal airway

7.3.10.1 Introduction

The Air-Q® Blocker™ ILA (Cookgas® LLC, Mercury Medical, USA) was introduced by Daniel Cook in 2005. It is a disposable, anatomically shaped device ideal for use in pre-hospital and critical care settings.

7.3.10.2 Device description

Parts of the Air-Q® Blocker™ ILA (**Figure 21**):

- Inflatable cuff with elevation ramp
- Built up mask heel
- Airway tube
- Integrated bite block
- Blocker Channel
- Thethered Colour Coded connector

The Air-Q® Blocker™ airway outlet is keyhole-shaped. The anatomical shape facilitates ease of insertion. The soft blocker channel accepts naso-gastric tube to suction stomach contents. Alternatively, a blocker tube may be inserted through the blocker channel and helps to suction the pharynx or suction and block the upper oesophagus. The tethered colour coded connector avoids misplacements. In a known difficult or unexpectedly difficult intubation, it may be used as a conduit for intubation. The elevation ramp directs ETT midline and upward toward the laryngeal inlet. The Air-Q Removal Stylet helps easily remove the Air-Q® Blocker™ after intubation without ETT dislodgement.

7.3.10.3 Size selection, practical aspect, adjuncts

Size selection is done on a weight basis (**Table 10**). It is available in three sizes. Device placement is easy and offers less resistance. The major advantage of the device design is

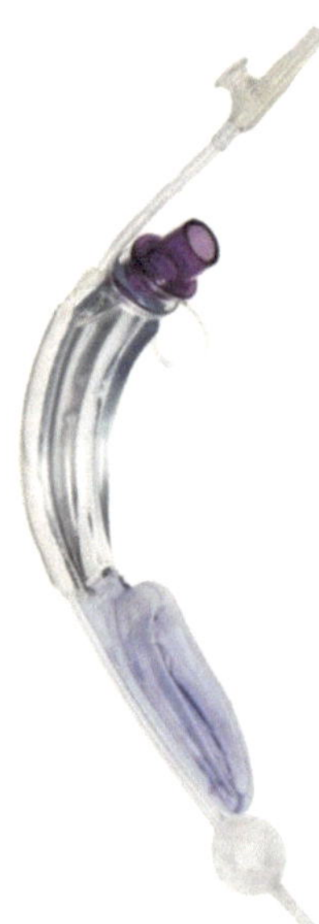

Figure 21.
Air-Q blocker.

that conventional PVC endotracheal tube can be passed through it without the use of conventional laryngoscope. It is useful in delivery of anaesthesia, resuscitation, critical care and difficult airway management in and out of hospital. It has a self-pressurising cuff which inflates to adequate pressure during positive pressure ventilation. This prevents airway trauma and morbidity associated with excessive cuff inflation [100].

7.3.11 LMA gastro™ airway

7.3.11.1 Introduction

The LMA® Gastro™ Airway with Cuff Pilot™ Technology (Teleflex®, USA) is the first SGA designed to enable active management of the airway while facilitating direct endoscopic access via the integrated endoscope channel. It is a soft, disposable, anatomically shaped device made up of silicone.

7.3.11.2 Device description

Parts of the LMA® Gastro™ Airway (**Figure 22**):

- Inflatable cuff
- Gastric drain tube or Endoscope channel
- Silicone airway tube
- Integrated bite block
- Adjustable holder and strap
- Cuff pilot

Being anatomically shaped, it conforms to the patients's airway creating a better seal. Cuff Pilot™ Technology prevents cuff over inflation and reduces airway morbidity. The gastric channel provides as a conduit for passage of gastro-duodenoscope.

7.3.11.3 Size selection, practical aspect

Size selection is done on a weight basis (**Table 11**). It is available in three sizes. Moderate to deep sedation if often required for endoscopic procedures. This can lead to hypoxemia and warrants the need of rescue airway. LMA® Gastro™ can be successfully employed as a primary airway technique for such procedures [101].

Mask size	Patient ideal body weight(kg)	Internal cuff volume (ml)	Cuff inflation volume (ml)	Largest ETT ID (mm)
2.5	30–50	12	2–3	6.5
3.5	50–70	18	3–4	7.5
4.5	70–100	25	4–5	8.5

Table 10.
Available air-Q blocker LMAs.

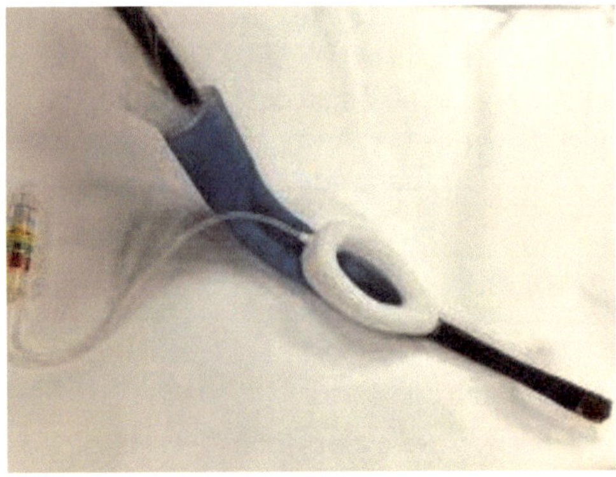

Figure 22.
Gastro LMA.

Mask size	Patient weight (kg)	Maximum intracuff pressure (cm H2O)	Maximum endoscope size (mm)
3	30–50	60	14
4	50–70	60	14
5	70–100	60	14

Table 11.
Available gastro LMAs.

8. Conclusion

The first clinically useful SGA was introduced more than 3 decades ago.

The clinical utility of various SGAs has significantly increased over this period. Different designs have specific advantages in different clinical scenarios. Insertion is easy to learn, and with adequate training nonphysicians are capable of securing an airway.

The use of SGAs for expanded indications has been described in many ways. The expanded spectrum of indications including airway instrumentation, surgeries in prone position, paediatric age group and use in critical care settings. The position of SGAs for rescue airway management is prominent in guidelines issued by various authorities. SGAs continue to be an important mode of rescue ventilation in patients in "can't ventilate can't intubate" scenarios. The ability to aspirate gastric contents renders them a safe alternative to the conventional ETTs. The ability to act as a conduit for intubation in elective and emergency patients is a valuable rescue technique.

Knowledge about the indications and contraindications of using an SGA is prudent for its appropriate use. SGAs with enough documented evidence of safety and efficacy should be used. Increasing recognition of an SGA's applications should expand its role in airway management for the anesthesiologist.

Conflict of interest

The author declares no conflict of interest.

Abbreviations

SGA	Supraglottic Airway
LMA	Laryngeal Mask Airway
ETT	Endotracheal Tube
OT	Operation Theatre
FOB	Fibreoptic Bronchoscopy
CPR	Cardiopulmonary Resuscitation
ID	Internal Diameter
mmHg	millimetres of mercury
L	Litre
Min	Minute
mm	millimetre
cmH2O	centimetre of water
Kg	kilogramme
ml	millilitre

Author details

Kriti Singh
ESIC Hospital and PGIMSR, Basaidarapur, New Delhi, India

*Address all correspondence to: drkritisingh@gmail.com

References

[1] Sharma B, Sahai C, Bhattacharya A, Kumar VP, Sood J. ProSeal laryngeal mask airway: A study of 100 consecutive cases of laparoscopic surgery. Indian J Anaesth. 2003;47:467–72.

[2] Misra MN, Ramamurthy B. The Pro-Seal LMATM and the tracheal tube: A comparison of events at insertion of the airway device. Internet J Anesthesiol. 2008;16.

[3] Pennant JH,White PF. The laryngeal mask airway. Its uses in anesthesiology. Anesthesiology. 1993;79:144–63.

[4] Kovac AL. Controlling the hemodynamic response to laryngoscopy and endotracheal intubation. J Clin Anesth. 1996;8:63–79.

[5] Prys-Roberts C, Greene LT, Meloche R, Foëx P. Studies of anaesthesia in relation to hypertension. II. Haemodynamic consequences of induction and endotracheal intubation. Br J Anaesth. 1971;43:531–47.

[6] Helmy AM, Atef HM, El-Taher EM, Henidak AM. Comparative study between i-gel, a new supraglottic airway device, and classical laryngeal mask airway in anesthetized spontaneously ventilated patients. Saudi J Anaesth. 2010;4(3):131–6.

[7] Brain AIJ, Verghese C, Strube PJ. The LMA 'Proseal' – A laryngeal mask with an oesophageal vent. Br J Anaesth. 2000; 84:650–654.

[8] Wakeling HG, Butler PJ, Baxter PJ. The laryngeal mask airway: a comparison between two insertion techniques. Anesth Analg. 1997; 85:687–690.

[9] Matta BF, Marsh DS, Nevin M. Laryngeal mask airway: a more successful method of insertion. J Clin Anesth. 1995; 7:132–135

[10] Brimacombe J. Laryngeal mask insertion techniques. Anesth Analg. 1998;86:1337–38.

[11] Gonzalez H, Minville V, Delanoue K, Mazerolles M, Concina D, Fourcade O. The importance of increased neck circumference to intubation difficulties in obese patients. Anesth Analg.2008; 106: 1132–6.

[12] Lavi R, Sega l D, Ziser A. Predicting difficult airways using the intubation difficulty scale: a study comparing obese and non-obese patients. Journal of Clinical Anesthesia. 2009; 21: 264–7.

[13] Domino KB, Posner K, Caplan RA, Cheney FW. Airway injury during anesthesia: a closed claims analysis. Anesthesiology. 1999; 91: 1703–11.

[14] Aoyama K, Takenaka I, Sata T, et al. The triple airway manoeuvre for insertion of the laryngeal mask airway in paralyzed patients. Can J Anaesth. 1995; 42:1010–16.

[15] Campbell RL, Biddle C, Assudme N, et al. Fiberoptic assessment of laryngeal mask airway placement: blind insertion versus direct visual epiglottoscopy. J Oral Maxillofac Surg. 2004; 62:1108–13.

[16] Brain AJ. The Intavent Laryngeal Mask Instruction Manual. London: Intavent; 1991.

[17] Awan R, Nolan JP, Cook TM. Use of a ProSeal laryngeal mask airway for airway maintenance during emergency Caesarean section after failed tracheal intubation. Br J Anaesth 2004; 92:144–6.

[18] Cook TM, Brooks TS, Van der Westhuizen J, Clarke M. The Proseal LMA is a useful rescue device during failed rapid sequence intubation: Two additional cases. Can J Anaesth. 2005; 52:630–3.

[19] Brimacombe J, Holyoake L, Keller C, et al. Emergence characteristics and postoperative laryngopharyngeal morbidity with the laryngeal mask airway: a comparison of high versus low initial cuff volume. Anaesthesia. 2000; 55:338–343.

[20] Cook T, Howes B. Supraglottic airway devices: recent advances. Continuing Educ Anaesth Crit Care Pain 11(2): 56–61.

[21] Carron M, Veronese S, Gomiero W, Foletto M, Nitti D, et al. Hemodynamic and hormonal stress responses to endotracheal tube and ProSeal Laryngeal Mask Airway TM for laparoscopic gastric banding. J Am Soc Anesthesiol. 2012; 117(2): 309–20.

[22] Ulrich-Pur H, Hrska F, Krafft P, Friehs H, Wulkersdorfer B, et al. Comparison of mucosal pressures induced by cuffs of different airway devices. J Am Soc Anesthesiol. 2006; 104(5): 933–938.

[23] Nicholson A, Cook TM, Smith AF, Lewis SR, Reed SS. Supraglottic airway devices versus tracheal intubation for airway management during general anaesthesia in obese patients. Cochrane Database Syst Rev. 2013. 9(9): CD010105.

[24] Henderson JJ, Popat MT, Lotto IP, Pearce AC. Difficult Airway Society guidelines for management of the unanticipated difficult intubation. Anaesthesia. 2004. 59(7): 675694.

[25] Verghese C, Brimacombe JR.Survey of laryngeal mask airway usage in 11,910 patients: safety and efficacy for conventional and nonconventional usage. Anesth Analg. 1996. 82(1): 129–133.

[26] Gable A, Whitaker E. E, Tobias J. D. Use of the laryngeal mask airway in the prone position. Pediatric Anesthesia and Critical Care Journal.2015; 3(2):118–123.

[27] Sinha PK, Misra S. Supraglottic airway devices other than laryngeal mask airway and its prototypes. Ind J Anaesth.2005 ;49:281–92.

[28] Luba PP, Brain AI. The laryngeal mask—a new concept in airway management. Br J Anaesth.1983;55: 801–5.

[29] Dorsch JA, Dorsch SE. Supraglottic airway devices. In: Dorsch JA, Dorsch SE editors. Understanding Anesthesia Equipment. 5th ed. Philadelphia: Williams L, Wilkins; 2008. p. 491s

[30] Atherton DP, O'Sullivan E, Lowe D, Charters P. A ventilation exchange bougie for fibreoptic intubations with the laryngeal mask airway. Anaesthesia. 1996;51(12):1123–26.

[31] Higgs A, Clark E, Premraj K. Low-skill fibreoptic intubation: use of the Aintree Catheter with the classic LMA. Anaesthesia. 2005;60(9): 915–920.

[32] Practice Guidelines for Management of the Difficult Airway: An Updated Report by the American Society of Anesthesiologists Task Force on Management of the Difficult Airway. Anesthesiology.2003;98(5):1269–1277.

[33] Frerk C, Mitchell VSS, McNarry AFF, et al. Difficult Airway Society 2015 guidelines for management of unanticipated difficult intubation in adults. British Journal of Anaesthesia.2015; 115: 827–48.

[34] Augoustides JG, Groff BE, Mann DG, Johansson JS. Difficult airway management after carotid endarterectomy: utility and limitations of the Laryngeal Mask Airway. J Clin Anesth. 2007;19(3):218–221.

[35] Fundingsland BW, Benumof JL. Difficulty using a laryngeal mask airway in a patient with lingual tonsil hyperplasia. Anesthesiology.1996;84(5): 1265–6.

[36] Kidani DC, Shah NK. The use of a laryngeal mask airway after a prolonged suspension laryngoscopy to preserve a vocal cord fat graft. Anesth Analg.2007; 105(6):1753–4.

[37] Parmet JL, Colonna-Romano P, Horrow JC, Miller F, Gonzales J, Rosenberg H. The laryngeal mask airway reliably provides rescue ventilation in cases of unanticipated difficult tracheal intubation along with difficult mask ventilation. Anesth Analg.1998;87(3):661–5.

[38] Swanson KL. Airway foreign bodies: what's new? Semin Respir Crit Care Med. 2004;25:405–411.

[39] Heffner JE. Tracheotomy application and timing. Clin Chest Med. 2003;24:389–98.

[40] Cattano D, Abramson S, Buzzigoli S, et al. The use of the laryngeal mask airway during guidewire dilating forceps tracheostomy. Anesth Analg. 2006;103:453–457.

[41] Martin SE, Ochsner MG, Jarman RH, et al. Use of the laryngeal mask airway in air transport when intubation fails. J Trauma-Injury Infection Crit Care. 1999;47:352–7.

[42] The American Heart Association in Collaboration with the International Liaison Committee on Resuscitation. Guidelines for cardiopulmonary resuscitation and emergency cardiovascular care. Circulation. 2000; 102(suppl 1):95–104.

[43] Wang HE, Simeone SJ, Weaver MD, Callaway CW. Interruptions in cardiopulmonary resuscitation from paramedic endotracheal intubation. Ann Emerg Med. 2009;54(5):645–52.

[44] Stone BJ, Chantler PJ, Baskett PJ. The incidence of regurgitation during cardiopulmonary resuscitation: a comparison between the bag valve mask and laryngeal mask airway. Resuscitation. 1998;38(1):3–6.

[45] Brimacombe J, Keller C. Insertion of The Lma-UniqueTM with and without digital intraoral manipulation by inexperienced personnel after manikin only training. J Emerg Med. 2004;26:1–5.

[46] Dingley J, Baynham P, Swart M, et al. Ease of insertion of the laryngeal mask airway by inexperienced personnel when using an introducer. Anaesthesia. 1997;52:756–60.

[47] Omi A, Fukuhara T, Isshiki A, et al. The effectiveness of the Fukuhara laryngeal mask airway holding forceps (F Forceps). Anesth Analg. 1997;85:697–700.

[48] Brimacombe J, Keller C, Puehringer F. Pharyngeal mucosal pressure and perfusion. A fiberoptic evaluation of the posterior pharynx in anesthetized adult patients with a modified cuffed oropharyngeal airway. Anesthesiology. 1999 Dec; 91(6): 661–5.

[49] Marjot R. Pressure exerted by the laryngeal mask airway cuff upon the pharyngeal mucosa. Br J Anaesth. 1993 Jan; 70(1):25–29.

[50] Brimacombe J, Berry A, Brain AIJ. Optimal intracuff pressures with the laryngeal mask. Br J Anaesth. 1996 Aug; 77(2):295–96.

[51] Asai T. Appropriate size of the laryngeal mask airway in adults. Br J Anaesth.1998;81:656–657.

[52] Asai T, Murao K, Yukawa H, et al. Re-evaluation of appropriate size of the laryngeal mask airway. Br J Anaesth.1999;83:478–479.

[53] Berry AM, Brimacombe J, McManus KF, et al. An evaluation of the factors influencing selection of the optimal size of laryngeal mask airway in normal adults. Anaesthesia.1998;53:565–570.

[54] Voyagis GS, Batzioulis PC, Secha-Doussaitou P. Selection of the proper size of laryngeal mask airway in adults. Anesth Analg. 1996;83:663–664.

[55] Voyagis GS. Appropriate size of the laryngeal mask airway in adults. Br J Anaesth.1998;81:656.

[56] Brimacombe, JR, Berry AM, Campbell RC, et al. In response. Anesth Analg.1996;83:664.

[57] Brimacombe J, Keller C. Laryngeal mask airway size selection in males and females: ease of insertion, oropharyngeal leak pressure, pharyngeal mucosal pressures and anatomical position. Br J Anaesth. 1999;82:703–707.

[58] Brimacombe J, Berry AM, Campbell RC, et al. Selection of the proper size of laryngeal mask airway in adults. Anesth Analg. 1996;83:664.

[59] Hirai S, Nakamura R, Mackawa N. Alternative formula for laryngeal mask airway size selection. Anesthesiology. 2004;100:460.

[60] Gallart LM, Mases A, Martinez-Perez JA, et al. An alternative method to determine the size of laryngeal mask airway in children. Br J Anaesth.1998;80: A486.

[61] Miller DM. A proposed classification and scoring system for supraglottic sealing airways: a brief review. Anesth Analg. 2004;99(5).

[62] Keller C, Brimacombe JR, Keller K, et al. Comparison of four methods for assessing airway sealing pressure with the laryngeal mask airway in adult patients. Br J Anaesth.1999; 82: 286–7.

[63] Joseph R. Brimacombe, Laryngeal Mask Airway: Principles and Practice, Second Edition (2005), pp. 23–26.

[64] van Zundert A, Brimacombe J. The LMA Supreme-a pilot study. Anaesthesia.2008;63:209–10.

[65] Hosten T, Gurkan Y, Ozdamar D, Tekin M, Toker K, Solak M. A new supraglottic airway device: LMA-Supreme™, comparison with LMA-Proseal™. Acta Anaesthesiol Scand.2009;53:852–7.

[66] Cook TM, Gatward JJ, Handel J, Hardy R, Thompson C, Srivastava R, et al. Evaluation of the LMA Supreme™ in 100 non-paralysed patients. Anaesthesia.2009;64:555–62.

[67] C. Verghese, B. Ramaswamy, LMA-SupremeTM—a new single-use LMATM with gastric access: a report on its clinical efficacy. BJA.2008; 101(3):405–410.

[68] Andrew JW Fletcher, Ramai Santhirapala, Peter J. Young, Introducing the LMA Supreme into clinical practice: use by experienced and inexperienced LMA users. BJA.2008; 101: eLetters Supplement.

[69] Länkimäki, Sami et al. "Feasibility of LMA Supreme for airway management in unconscious patients by ALS paramedics." Scandinavian journal of trauma, resuscitation and emergency medicine. 2015; 23 24. 26.

[70] Wong DT, Yang JJ, Jagannathan N. Brief review: The LMA Supreme™ supraglottic airway. Can J Anaesth. 2012;59(5):483–493.

[71] Changhong Miao, Meilin Weng, A novel way to choose the size of Laryngeal Mask Airway Supreme in adults, BJA.2015; 115, eLetters Supplement.

[72] Pajiyar AK, Wen Z, Wang H, Ma L, Miao L, Wang G. Comparisons of clinical performance of Guardian laryngeal mask with laryngeal mask airway ProSeal. BMC Anesthesiol. 2015 1;15:69.

[73] Tiefenthaler W, Eschertzhuber S, Brimacombe J, Fricke E, Keller C,

Kaufmann M. A randomised, non-crossover study of the GuardianCPV laryngeal Mask versus the LMA Supreme in paralysed, anaesthetised female patients. Anaesthesia. 2013;68 (6):600–4.

[74] LMA-Protector Instructions for use, Athlone, Ireland, Teleflex Medical, 2015.

[75] Chang, J., Kim, H., Lee, J. et al. A prospective, randomized comparison of the LMA-protector™ and i-gel™ in paralyzed, anesthetized patients. BMC Anesthesiol. 2019; 19: 118.

[76] Sng, B.L., Ithnin, F.B., Mathur, D. et al. A preliminary assessment of the LMA protector™ in non-paralysed patients. BMC Anesthesiol. 2017; 17: 26.

[77] AMBU (DK). AuraGain™ Disposable Laryngeal Mask [Internet]. Baltorpbakken (DK): ABMU A/S; Nov 2015[Cited 2016 Dec 19] Available from: http://www.ambu.com/corp/products/anaesthesia/product/auragain% E2%84%A2_disposable_laryngeal_mask-prod18315.aspx

[78] Lopez AM, Agusti M, Gambus P, Pons M, Anglada T, Valero R. A randomized comparison of the Ambu AuraGain versus the LMA supreme in patients undergoing gynaecologic laparoscopic surgery. J Clin Monit Comput. 2017;31(6):1255–62.

[79] Shariffuddin II, Teoh WH, Tang E, Hashim N, Loh PS. Ambu® AuraGain™ versus LMA Supreme™ Second Seal™: a randomised controlled trial comparing oropharyngeal leak pressures and gastric drain functionality in spontaneously breathing patients. Anaesth Intensive Care. 2017;45(2):244–50.

[80] Singh K, Gurha P. Comparative evaluation of Ambu AuraGain™ with ProSeal™ laryngeal mask airway in patients undergoing laparoscopic cholecystectomy. Indian J Anaesth. 2017;61:469–74.

[81] Richez B, Saltel L, Banchereau F, Torrielli, Cros AM: A new single use supraglottic airway with a noninflatable cuff and an esophageal vent: An observational study of the i-gel: Anesth Analg. 2008 Apr;106(4):1137–9.

[82] I-gel user guide, Berkshire, uk, Intersurgical Ltd, 2020.

[83] Gabbott DA, Beringer R: The i-gel supraglottic airway: A potential role for resuscitation? Resuscitation. 2007 Apr; 73(1):161–2.

[84] Soar J: The i-gel supraglottic airway and resuscitation - some initial thoughts: Resuscitation. 2007 Jul;74(1):197.

[85] Das B, Mitra S, Jamil SN, Varshney RK. Comparison of three supraglottic devices in anesthetised paralyzed children undergoing elective surgery. Saudi J Anaesth 2012;6: 224–8.

[86] Mercer MH, Gabbott DA. Insertion of the Combitube airway with the cervical spine immobilised in a rigid cervical collar. Anaesthesia. 1998;53: 971–4.

[87] Calkins MD, Robinson TD. Combat trauma airway management: Endotracheal intubation versus laryngeal mask airway versus combitube use by Navy SEAL and Reconnaissance combat corpsmen. J Trauma. 1999;46:927–32.

[88] Frass M, Frenzer R, Rauscha F, Schuster E, Glogar D. Ventilation with the esophageal tracheal combitube in cardiopulmonary resuscitation. Promptness and effectiveness. Chest. 1988 Apr;93(4):781–4.

[89] Frass M, Frenzer R, Rauscha F, Weber H, Pacher R, Leithner C. Evaluation of esophageal tracheal combitube in cardiopulmonary resuscitation. Crit Care Med. 1987;15(6): 609–11.

[90] Wagner A, Roeggla M, Roeggla G, Weiss K, Marosi C, Locker GJ, Knapp S, Staudinger T, Metnitz PG, Frass M. Emergency intubation with the combitube in a case of severe facial burn. Am J Emerg Med. 1995;13(6):681–3.

[91] Staudinger T, Tesinsky P, Klappacher G, Brugger S, Rintelen C, Locker G, Weiss K, Frass M. Emergency intubation with the Combitube in two cases of difficult airway management. Eur J Anaesthesiol. 1995;12(2):189–93.

[92] Eichinger S, Schreiber W, Heinz T, Kier P, Dufek V, Goldin M, Leithner C, Frass M. Airway management in a case of neck impalement: use of the oesophageal tracheal combitube airway. Br J Anaesth. 1992;68(5):534–5.

[93] Jokela, Jorma & Nurmi, Jouni & Genzwürker, Harald & Castrén, Maaret. Laryngeal tube and intubating laryngeal mask insertion in a manikin by first-responder trainees after a short video-clip demonstration. Prehospital Disast Med. 2009; 24: 63–6.

[94] Mihai R, Knottenbelt G, Cook TM. Evaluation of the revised laryngeal tube suction: the laryngeal tube suction II in 100 patients. Br J Anaesth.2007;99:734–9.

[95] Genzwuerker HV, Altmayer S, Hinkelbein J, Gernoth C, Viergutz T, Ocker H. Prospective randomized comparison of the new Laryngeal Tube Suction LTS II and the LMA-ProSeal for elective surgical interventions. Acta Anaesthesiol Scand. 2007;51:1373–7.

[96] Gaitini LA, Vaida SJ, Somri M, Yanovski B, Ben-David B, Hagberg CA. A randomized controlled trial comparing the ProSeal Laryngeal Mask Airway with the Laryngeal Tube Suction in mechanically ventilated patients. Anesthesiology. 2004;101:316–20.

[97] Baska K, Baska M. Baska Mask. The new generation supraglottic airway with high volume suction clearance. Available on http://www.baskamask.com.au/main/page_about_the_mask.html [Accessed 30 July 2020].

[98] van Zundert T, Gatt S. The Baska Mask – A new concept in self-sealing membrane cuff extraglottic airway devices using a sump and two gastric drains: A critical evaluation. J Obstet Anaesth Crit Care.2012;2:23–30.

[99] Sachidananda R, Shaikh SI, Mitragotri MV, Joshi V, Ladhad DA, Mallappa M, Bhat VK. Comparison between the Baska Mask® and I-Gel for Minor Surgical Procedures Under General Anaesthesia. Turk J Anaesthesiol Reanim. 2019 Feb;47(1): 24–30.

[100] The Air- Q® Intubating Laryngeal Airway (ILA™, Cookgas® LLC, Mercury Medical, Clearwater, FL, USA): Information for Use [Package insert]

[101] Tran A, Thiruvenkatarajan V, Wahba M et al. LMA® Gastro™ Airway for endoscopic retrograde cholangiopancreatography: a retrospective observational analysis. BMC Anesthesiol. 2020;20: 113.

Chapter 15

Management of New Special Devices for Intubation in Difficult Airway Situations

Demetrio Pérez-Civantos, Alicia Muñoz-Cantero, Francisco Fuentes Morillas, Pablo Nieto Sánchez, María Ángeles Santiago Triviño and Natalia Durán Caballero

Abstract

Difficult airway management in critically ill patients has serious implications, as failing to secure a stable airway can lead to a brain injury or even death. Early recognition of a difficult airway can allow the clinician to minimize the potential morbid-mortality. In this chapter, we describe all about the common scenarios that we may tackle when we need to secure a patent airway. It is important to know common definitions about the airway, pre-visualize potential problems and knowing how to be aware of the different pathways on managing and solving the different problems that clinicians may face. It is highlighted to know all the different medical equipment and medication used when an airway is suspected not to be easy to manage or when problems arrive without warning and the practitioner needs to rapidly change the plan on the go. We discuss the current most relevant guidelines and literature about this subject trying to give a practical approach.

Keywords: difficult airway, airway management, ventilation, intubation, airway devices

1. Introduction

One of the most stressful situations that all anesthetists, intensivists and emergency physicians can face is the management of a difficult airway (DA). That stressful situation can turn into a tragedy if the team is not well trained, not ready, and the plans are not well established or known.

The prediction of a DA is essential to anticipate all the strategy that the team has to deploy to successfully manage that situation.

Different guidelines and much literature have been published on this topic in recent years, all these articles try to establish a structured approach and facilitate in the simplest way the different steps to follow in this problematic scenario.

Airway management was considered inappropriate in a high percentage of complaints, including inadequate evaluation, lack of planning for difficult intubation, failure to use the supraglottic airway for rescue, delay in requesting help, and perseveration in failed techniques.

IntechOpen

A thoroughly well-designed plan needs to be established and summarized in the airway approach algorithm and foresight all possible situations that may be encountered during the clinical practice of a serious and threatening airway crisis, all of them should be discussed in advance. Awake intubation, intubation after induction of anesthesia, and the "can't intubate, can't oxygenate" (CICO) situation should be planned and well known to all team members.

2. Definition of difficult airway

There is no universal definition of difficult airway in the literature. However, We can define the DA such as some clinical factors that make ventilation of the mask difficult or some anatomical factors that make tracheal intubation difficult for a trained specialist [1]. Difficult airway encompasses the interaction of various circumstances: patient factors, clinical settings, and specialized skills.

Difficult ventilation is the inability of an experienced specialist (intensivist or anesthesiologist) to maintain oxygen saturation above 90% with a 100% FiO2 face mask. We know that with some indirect signs such as absence or inadequate respiratory sound, inadequate chest movement, haemodynamic changes such as hypertension or hypotension, arrhythmias associated with hypoxaemia, cyanosis, etc.

Difficult orotracheal intubation (DOTI) is defined as three or more attempts to perform tracheal intubation or more than ten minutes to perform it. It occurs in 1.5–8% of general anesthesia procedures [2, 3]. The cause of these may be due to difficulty in laryngoscopy: we cannot visualize any portion of the vocal cords, failed intubation: the place of the endotracheal tube is incorrect after multiple attempts, presence of tracheal pathology that prevents correct tracheal intubation.

3. Purposes of the guidelines for difficult airway management

DOTI is a common cause of anesthetic morbidity and mortality, so it is important to anticipate these difficulties before the process. Up to 30% of death from anesthesia could be due to a difficult airway. That is why it is very important to have high prognosis tests to identify difficulties in the airways [4, 5] and make a universal definition to classify the DA and teach the management of this. The main adverse outcomes include brain injuries that can be related to dental damage, trauma to the airways, unnecessary surgical airways or some injuries related to cardiopulmonary arrest, hypoxia, brain injury, or even death. The use of one method and another for the management of the DA, the hierarchy of categories made according to the level of scientific evidence collected will be carried out hereunder.

4. Assessment of the airway

The experienced clinician can anticipate when intubation may be difficult by taking a proper history and complete physical examination. In emergencies, a brief but comprehensive airway assessment is essential to treat patients who require advanced airway management.

4.1 History of the respiratory tract

The physician should take a history of the patient's airway, investigating in detail the medical, surgical, and anesthetic factors that may indicate the presence of a

DA. Many disease states have been associated with DA (**Table 1**). Additionally, lung problems such as asthma, chronic obstructive pulmonary disease (COPD), bronchitis, recent upper respiratory infection, or the presence of pneumonia can affect oxygenation and ventilation. Most patients presenting for emergency procedures are at increased risk of aspiration (**Table 2**) [6].

Congenital	Acquired
Pierre Robin syndrome	Morbid obesity
Treacher-Collins syndrome	Acromegaly
Goldenhar syndrome	Infections involving the airway (Ludwig's angina, epiglottitis, croup, etc.)
Mucopolysaccharidoses	Rheumatoid arthritis
Achondroplasia	Ankylosing spondylitis
Micrognathia	Obstructive sleep apnea
Down syndrome	Tumors involving the airway
Cretinism	Trauma or burns of the face, head, or neck
Beckwith syndrome	Radiation of face or neck

Table 1.
Diseases associated with difficult airway management.

Full stomach – nonfasted, emergency surgery or trauma
Pregnancy after 12 to 20 weeks gestation (gestational age for increased risk is controversial) Symptomatic gastroesophageal reflux
Diabetic or another gastroparesis
Hiatal hernia
Gastric outlet obstruction
Oesophagal pathology
Bowel obstruction
Increased intra-abdominal pressure – ascites, abdominal mass

Table 2.
Conditions that increased risk of aspiration.

4.2 Examination of the respiratory tract

The purpose of this evaluation is to detect physical characteristics that may indicate the presence of a DA.

The sight assessment provides very useful information. Obesity, facial hair, thick and short neck, and neck collars are immediately apparent and suggest a possible DA.

Mouth. The jaw opening should be at least 4 centimeters in adults, which is roughly three to four fingers. A mouth opening of fewer than three fingers is considered limited. Patients with temporomandibular joint (TMJ) disease or previous surgery may have a very limited mouth opening or trismus. The movement of the TMJ must allow at least a maximum opening of the mouth of 50 to 60 mm. A small or large jaw can affect vision when intubated. The dentition should be evaluated, paying particular attention to the presence of caps, crowns, implants, veneers, dentures, braces, or loose teeth. The small space between incisors suggests possible DA management [7–9]. The Mallampati classification was first described in 1985 as a test to predict difficult laryngoscopy [10]. The Mallampati classification involves the size of the tongue concerning the oral cavity. The more the tongue obstructs the view of the pharyngeal structure, the more difficult the migration of the device:

Class I: The entire tonsillar pillars, uvula, hard and soft palates are visualized.

Class II: Partial uvula and soft palate are visualized.

Class III: Only the soft palate is visualized.
Class IV: No visualization of any structures beyond the tongue.

Neck range of motion decreases with age, neck arthritis, cervical spine disease, or previous spinal surgery. Patients with restricted neck extension may be more difficult to position optimally for induction of anesthesia and intubation [11]. Airway management must be based on the fact that DA cannot be predicted reliably. This is a particularly important consideration in the intensive care setting [12]. Recognition of patients at particular risk of DA management helps planning and is recommended, even in the most urgent situations. The only validated airway assessment tool in critically ill patients is the MACOCHA score (**Table 3**). A score of ≥3 predicts difficult intubation in critically ill patients. However, to reject difficult intubation with certainty, the main value of the score comes from the negative predictive value of the parameter. It is wise to be prepared for DOTI, even if intubation is ultimately not difficult [13].

Mallampati 3 or 4	5
Obstructive Sleep **A**pnea	2
Cervical-spine movement limited	1
Mouth **O**pening < 3 cm	1
Coma	1
Hypoxemia (<80%)	1
Non-**A**nesthetist intubator	1

Table 3.
MACOCHA score.

5. Basic preparation for difficult airway management

A difficult airway management protocol includes several well-organized strategies to achieve sufficient ventilation and apply various intubation techniques to have the best chance of success and decrease the chance of injury to the patient. Although the airway approach is a challenge for the emergency team, airway management is even more difficult in critically ill patients. Decision-making, interaction within the team, use of resources, and motor skills can all be affected under stress. The goal is to ensure oxygenation in life-threatening and rapidly changing situations that require agile decision making, thereby reducing the number and severity of critical incidents and complications.

5.1 Recommendations for the management of the difficult airway

There should be at least one portable storage unit containing all specialized equipment for managing DA. A variety of standard and alternative airway devices should be readily available, including masks, appropriate sizes and types of laryngoscopes (direct, indirect, flexible), oral and nasal airways, supraglottic airways (SGA), spark plugs and equipment. For the front of the mouth neck access (FONA). Make sure there is at least one additional person who must be immediately available to serve as an assistant in managing DA.

All patients must be pre-oxygenated before induction of general anesthesia. Pre-oxygenation increases oxygen reserve delays the onset of hypoxia and allows more time for laryngoscopy, tracheal intubation, and airway rescue in the event of intubation failure [14]. The duration of apnea without desaturation can also be prolonged by passive oxygenation during the apneic period (apneic oxygenation). This can be achieved by administering up to 15 liters/min of oxygen through nasal cannulas. Nasal administration of oxygen during intubation management has been shown to prolong apnea time in obese patients with a DA [15]. High-flow nasal cannulas (with humidified high-flow oxygen (up to 70 liters/min) have been shown to prolong apnea time, although their ability to improve preoxygenation has not yet been elucidated [16, 17].

5.2 Recommendations for basic DA management

There should be a portable chart unit containing all specialized pieces of equipment for the management DA. The following steps are highly recommended [16]: • Inform the patient (or responsible person, if possible) about the risks and special procedures related to the management of DA. • Make sure there is at least one person available to operate as an assistant. • Pre-oxygenate with a mask before starting DA management. In the uncooperative or pediatric patient may result impossible to achieve. • Actively seek any opportunity to supply supplemental oxygen throughout the DA management. These include the delivery of oxygen via nasal cannulas, mask or LMA, and oxygen supply through any applied device. Airway management is safer when potential problems are identified in advance in case of urgent intubation, allowing planning and reducing the risk of complications [17]. Airway assessment should be performed routinely to identify factors that may cause difficulties with face mask ventilation, SAD insertion, tracheal intubation, or front neck access (FONA). The prediction of DA management is not always completely reliable. Basic management preparation for DA management includes (1) availability of DA management equipment, (2) informing the patient or relatives of a known or suspected DA, (3) assigning a person for help and assistance, (4) mask pre-oxygenation, and (5) supplemental oxygen administration throughout the DA management.

6. Difficult airway intubation strategy

A well pre-planned strategy before induction includes several interventions, designed to facilitate intubation in the event of DA. Non-invasive maneuvers targeted at treating DA include [17]: (1) awake intubation, (2) video-assisted laryngoscopy, (3) intubation stylet or tube changers, (4) SGA for ventilation (eg. LMA, laryngeal tube), (5) PEG for intubation (eg. ILMA), (6) rigid laryngoscopy, (7) fibreoptic-guided intubation, and (8) stylets with light or light wands. Following the Difficult Airway Society, we will proceed with a structured detailed plan that consists of several considerations.

6.1 Plan A. Mask ventilation and tracheal intubation

The very essence of Plan A is to maximize the chance of successful intubation on the first attempt or, failing that, limit the number and duration of laryngoscopy attempts to prevent airway injury and progression to a " cannot intubate, cannot oxygenate "(CICO). Patients must be in an optimal position and well pre-oxygenated before the administration of anesthetic medication. The use of neuromuscular blockade facilitates mask ventilation and tracheal intubation. Any attempt at laryngoscopy and tracheal intubation is potentially harmful. A suboptimal attempt is a vain attempt and carries the possibility that success diminishes with each subsequent attempt [18–20]. Repeated attempts at tracheal intubation reduce the likelihood of effective airway rescue with SAD [21]. Current guidelines recommend a maximum of three intubation attempts; a fourth attempt can be done by a more experienced colleague. If unsuccessful, a failed intubation should be stated and proceed to Plan B.

6.2 Plan B. SAD

Maintaining of oxygenation: supraglottic airway device (SAD) insertion is in the guidelines. The emphasis of Plan B is to maintain oxygenation using a SAD. If we succeed in the placement of a SAD, it brings the opportunity to stop and consider whether to wake the patient, try a new attempt at intubation, continue without a tracheal tube, or, in rare cases, proceed to a cricothyroidotomy. If we cannot achieve oxygenation via SAD after a maximum of three attempts, proceed to Plan C.

6.3 Plan C. Awakening or total paralysis

Final attempt at mask ventilation. If effective ventilation has not been established after three attempts at SAD insertion, Plan C proceeds directly. At this stage, several possible scenarios can be developed. During Plans A and B, it will be determined whether mask ventilation was easy, difficult, or impossible, but the situation may have changed if attempts at intubation and SAD placement have traumatized the airway. If mask ventilation results in inadequate oxygenation, the patient should be awakened in all but exceptional circumstances, and this situation will require total antagonism of the neuromuscular block. If oxygenation cannot be maintained using a face-mask, ensuring complete paralysis before critical hypoxia develops and we will have one last chance to rescue the airway without resorting to Plan D. Sugammadex has been used to antagonize neuromuscular block during the situation of CICO, but does not guarantee a patent and manageable upper airway. Residual neuro-depressant medication, airway laceration, or pre-existing upper airway disease may contribute to airway obstruction [17, 21].

6.4 Plan D. Front neck emergency access (FONA)

A CICO situation arises when attempts to manage the airway by tracheal intubation, mask ventilation, and SAD have failed. Hypoxic brain damage and death can occur if the situation is not resolved quickly. NAP4 report provided feedback on a cohort of emergency surgical airway and cannula cricothyroidotomies performed when other methods of securing the airway had failed [22, 23]. The report highlighted several issues, including decision making (delayed progression to cricothyroidotomy), knowledge gaps (not understanding how the available equipment worked), system failures (specific equipment not available), and technical failures (not placing a cannula in the airway). After NAP4, the discussion focused largely on the choice of technique and equipment used when airway rescue failed, but the report also highlighted the importance of human factors (discussed elsewhere) [16, 17]. Regular training in technical and non-technical elements is needed to reinforce and retain skills. Success depends on decision-making, planning, preparation, and skill acquisition, all of which can be developed and refined with repeated practice [24, 25].

FONA consists of surgical airway access employing an emergency cricothyroidotomy. This technique is presented and discussed elsewhere in this book.

7. Different techniques and devices for approaching intubation in DA

7.1 Intubation stylets or tube exchangers

7.1.1 Stylets

We define the classic stylet as a malleable metal wire designed to be inserted into the endotracheal tube to facilitate tracheal placement at the time of intubation with difficult laryngoscopy. Mild mucosal bleeding and a sore throat are complications associated with stylets (**Figure 1**).

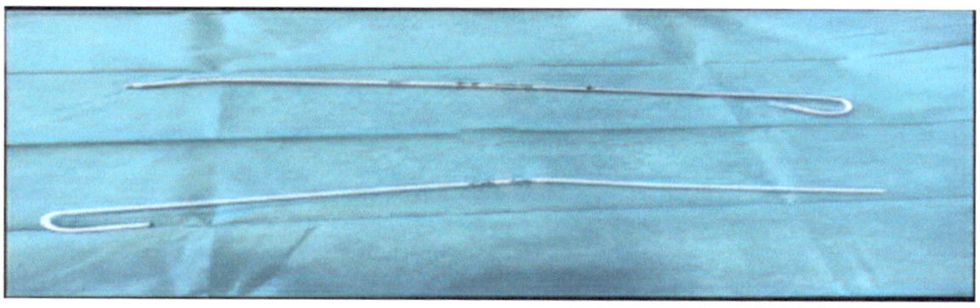

Figure 1.
Classical stylets.

We can find several commercialized types that differ in curvature and size. There are also specialized stylets available known as endotracheal tube introducers or "rubber elastic plug" which consist of a 50 to 60 cm stylet with the distal tip bent at a 30-degree angle. They are indicated in a grade III Cormack-Lehane view because they allow the physician to direct forward under the epiglottis and through the vocal cords and then a tracheal tube can be inserted over it. Some of them are single-use like **Frova,** whose tip is fenestrated to allow oxygenation. However, Eschmann introducer can be sterilized and reused [26].

Today there are also disposable optical lighted stylets or light wands that incorporate a video or fiber-optic display element at the distal end. The viewing element provides the clinician with an adequate view from outside the mouth with direct laryngoscopy to the region near the glottis. Common examples include; the **Clarus video system**, the **Shikani video system**, the **Bonfires retromolar intubation fibrescope**, and the **Leviton FPS telescope** (**Table 4**) [27, 28]. They are not indicated for use in patients with laryngeal trauma, tumors, and foreign bodies. It is also not indicated for patients with thick necks or limited neck extension.

Instructions for use [28]:

Introduce the ET over the stylet having previously lubricated the inner face of the ET. Choose the desired stylet angle. Using the index finger of the left hand or the laryngoscope, move the tongue to the left and insert the tip of the pencil into the right side of the mouth with the right hand. Try to direct the tip of the stylet towards the midline of the neck trying to pass the glottis. Once the tip of the stylet passes the glottis, we will appreciate light in the midline of the neck by transillumination. We then advance the ETT through the stylet to the trachea.

CLASSICAL	SINGLE USED	REUSED	
SPECIALIZED	LIGHTED	BOUGIE	OPTICAL

Table 4.
Stylets.

7.1.2 Tube exchangers

Airway exchange catheters are long, hollow catheters that allow clinicians to remove and replace tracheal tubes without the need for laryngoscopy (**Figure 2**). These catheters often have connectors for manual and jet ventilation or oxygen insufflation. Cook's Airway Exchange Catheter (CAEC) is one example [26].

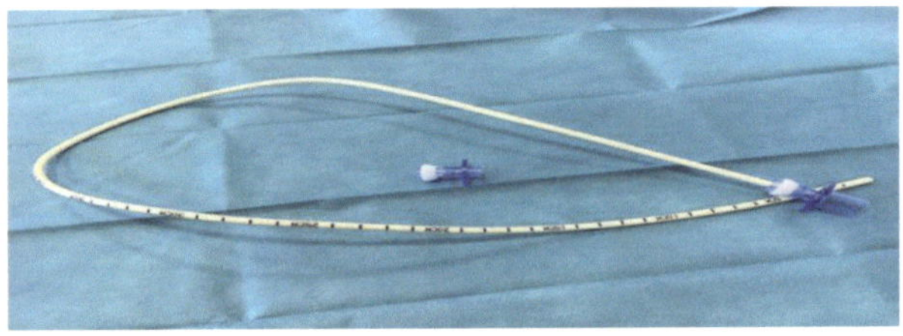

Figure 2.
Cook airway exchange catheter.

7.2 Extraglottic devices for ventilation

Extraglottic airway devices are used to establish an airway for oxygenation and ventilation without entering the trachea. They are important tools that are frequently used in the pre-hospital setting, the emergency department, the operating room, and other settings [26, 29].

These devices are useful in cases of DA management in patients who cannot be intubated or ventilated. Contraindications to the use of extra-glottic airway devices include obstructive airway diseases, traumatized airways, gag reflex, etc.

These types of devices should be used under sedation to reduce pharyngeal spasms/reflexes that can impair ventilation (**Table 5**).

7.2.1 Supraglottic devices

They are laryngeal masks that seal around the glottis and remain superior to the larynx. The laryngeal mask airway (LMA) is a useful supraglottic device added to emergent airway management. Its use is extended by 3 or 4 degrees Cormack-Lehane of laryngoscopic view and Difficult Bag Ventilation Mask (DBVM). This device allows clinicians to provide adequate ventilation in severely hypoxic patients facilitating subsequent treatment. It is very important to correctly fix the LMA as its dislocation is easier compared to endotracheal intubation. However, the LMA does not increase the risk of aspiration if its fixation is ensured.

We can consider LMA as the milestone in the field of supraglottic airway approach. It was first described by Archie Brain in 1983 and has become a commonly accepted device for rescue airway management and is included in the major societal recommendations and DA management algorithms [29].

Supraglottic devices	Retroglottic devices
LMA. (Laryngeal mask airway).	Combitube.
ILMA. (Intubating laryngeal mask airway).	King LT (King laryngeal tube).
Air-Q.	
i-Gel.	

Table 5.
Common extra-glottic devices.

There are multiple types of laryngeal masks, each with specific characteristics. Therefore, the placement of a laryngeal mask (**Figure 3**) is an important tool in adults with a DA, especially in the case of a high anterior larynx, which represents a substantial advance as a rescue device in situations of CICO [29, 30].

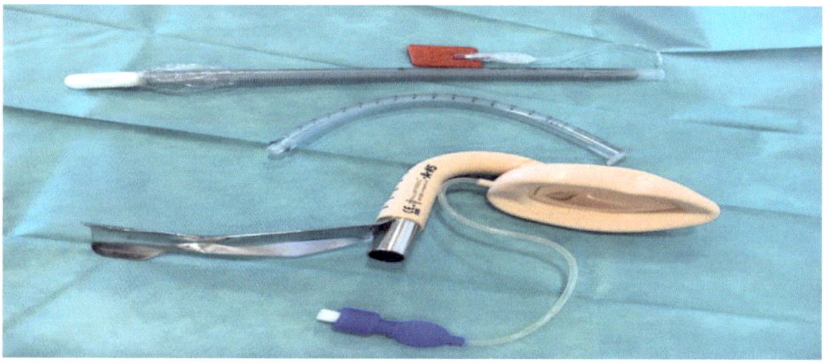

Figure 3.
ILMA (FASTRACH).

7.2.2 Retroglottic devices

They are laryngeal tubes that end in the upper part of the esophagus, posterior to the glottis, and have two balloons, one pharyngeal and the other oesophagal, with ventilation fenestrations in the middle that line up with the glottic opening (**Table 6**).

7.3 Rigid laryngoscopic blades of alternative design and size

The purpose of the laryngoscope is to move the oral anatomical structures out of the laryngoscopist's line of vision to expose the glottic opening. The blade of a laryngoscope consists of a flat element (spatula), a vertical element (flange), and a light source. Straight and curved blades are the most common.

Both the Macintosh (curve) and Miller (straight) blades are available in sizes 0 (neonatal) to 4 (large adult), although we commonly prefer to use the straight blade for infant intubations and curved blades for adults.

7.3.1 Fiber-optic guided intubation (FBO) and awake tracheal intubation (ATI)

Fiber-optic intubation is a technique in which a flexible endoscope with an endotracheal tube loaded along its length is passed through the glottis. The tracheal tube is then pushed out of the endoscope and into the trachea and the endoscope is removed. The nasotracheal route is used frequently and requires the use of nasal vasoconstrictors. A nebulized local anesthetic is delivered to the airways through a mask. Sedation can be given, but ideally, the patient should breathe spontaneously and respond to verbal commands [31].

Curve blade	Straight blade
Macintosh.	Miller.
Adults.	Infants.
Indirectly rising the epiglottis.	Improve lifting of the epiglottis.

Table 6.
Common types of blades.

7.3.1.1 Advantages of FBO-guided intubation

- Avoid the stress of direct laryngoscopy.
- Direct visualization of the vocal cords.
- Short intubation time according to training.
- Less traumatic and less repeated intubation attempts.
- Maximum incidence of success.
- Minimal risk of injury.
- Allows the administration of oxygen through the suction channel.
- Maximum safety in awake patients.
- Definitive control of the ET position.
- Endoscopic study before intubation.
- Possibility of oral or nasal application.
- Possibility of execution in extreme positions [31–33].

Due to all these advantages, intubation with FBO is the cornerstone of DA management as well as its ultimate goal: suspect and identify a DA, perform intubation with the patient awake to avoid unnecessary risks.

Intubation with an awake patient while maintaining spontaneous breathing is the "gold standard" in the treatment of "predicted difficult airway."

Awake fiber-optic intubation is reported to be successful in 88–100% of DA patients. Case reports using other techniques for awake intubation (blind tracheal intubation, intubation through supraglottic devices, optically guided intubation) report not so high odds of success with DA patients [21].

Awake intubation has the following advantages [28, 34]: the patient retains the ability to keep the ventilation and airway patent and the muscle tone that keeps the pharynx clean and preserved; the collaboration of the patient and helps us pass the ET with deep breathing; with good local anesthesia, it facilitates a poor haemodynamic response.

FBOs also have disadvantages [33]: necessary training, skill, patient cooperation, longer execution time, optical fibers are fragile and require rigorous precautions.

The route for tracheal intubation should take into account the patient's anatomy, surgical access, and the tracheal extubation plan. In patients with limited mouth opening, the nasal approach is the only option, while in patients who had nasal surgical interventions, the oral approach should be preferred. No evidence or consensus is found among experts on the superiority of a route if both are feasible. Awake tracheal intubation (ATI) by using video-laryngoscopy has the same success rate and safety as ATI: FBO (98.3% each) [35]. Careful selection of the tracheal tube is critical to the success of any ATI technique. It is advisable to use the tracheal tube with a smaller external diameter, as it can reduce the incidence of injury [36]. A checklist of all the supplies needed should be disposable.

Oxygenation: Desaturation (SpO2 $\leq$ 90%) with low-flow (< 30 l/min-1) oxygen techniques during ATI ranges between 12% and 16% [37, 38]. When using warmed and humidified high-flow nasal oxygen, desaturation plummets to 0–1.5% [39]. Administration of supplemental oxygen during ATI is highly recommended. It should be commenced on patient arrival before the procedure and continued throughout. High-flow nasal oxygen should be the technique of choice for pre-oxygenation.

Airway topical anesthesia: An effective topicalization with local anesthetics the key point for a successful ATI. The use of topical endonasal vasoconstrictors before nasotracheal intubation is highly recommended. Lidocaine has benefits when compared to other local anesthetic agents due to a safety cardiovascular and systemic reduced toxicity risk profile [16, 17, 21]; perhaps this is the most used local anesthetic drug for ATI. The dose of topical lidocaine should not exceed 9 mg/kg^{-1} lean body weight [40]. Nebulised lidocaine can be used but the absorption is variable. The adequacy of topicalisation should be tested before airway instrumentation, for example, with a soft suction catheter. The use of an antisialogogue is not mandatory and may be associated with undesirable clinical consequences [41].

Sedation:

ATI may be safe and effective even performed in the absence of sedation [42, 43]. Its use during ATI can reduce patient anxiety and discomfort and increase procedural tolerance. In certain patient populations, the risk of over-sedation is particularly hazardous, thus an independent practitioner delivering sedation is strongly recommended. Based on our experience, we can recommend the use of minimal sedation. Two drugs, remifentanil and dexmedetomidine have been associated with high levels of patient satisfaction and low risk of over-sedation and airway obstruction. Complications are reduced when using capnography.

7.3.1.2 Indications and contraindications for FBO-guided intubation

- Suspicion of difficult airway management.
- Knowledge of the difficult airway.
- Risk of aspiration.
- Teaching, learning or consolidation of experiences.
- Unstable cervical spine injury or I. vertebrobasilar.
- Patients with recent voice disorders, stridor, goiter, tracheal stenosis, flexed and fixed neck, use of accessory muscles to breathe, need to sit up to breathe.
- High risk of dental damage.
- Morbid obesity.
- Contraindication to anesthesia or muscle relaxants.
- Improve the safety of airway procedures, such as endotracheal tube changes and percutaneous tracheostomy [33, 34, 44].

7.3.1.3 Contraindications to FBO-guided intubation

- Non-collaboration of the patient.
- Children.
- Allergy to local anesthetics.
- Rejection of the technique.
- Lack of experience or insufficient time.

- Blood or discharge.
- Major fractures.
- Fungal tumors in the larynx.
- Coagulation disorders.
- Full stomach with risk of aspiration.
- Emergencies [33, 34, 44].

7.3.1.4 Complications of FBO-guided intubation

- Hypoxemia.
- Laryngospasm and bronchospasm.
- Haemodynamic disorders and arrhythmias.
- Esophageal intubation.
- Sore throat.
- Tissue trauma.
- Regurgitation or vomiting. Aspiration.
- Stridor or oedema of the glottis.
- Esophageal perforation.
- Gastric distension. Rupture of the stomach.
- Bleeding, epistaxis.
- Eye trauma.
- Pulmonary barotrauma.
- Arrhythmias: bradycardia due to nasal stimulation (naso-cardial reflex) or stimulation of the region of the recurrent and superior laryngeal nerve.
- Haemodynamic disorders: hypertension or hypotension is justified by a diminished stimulus.
- Barotrauma: in the narrow upper respiratory tract.
- Esophageal intubation.
- Regurgitation and vomiting.
- Gastric distension: stomach rupture [45].

8. Confirmation of tracheal intubation

Confirmation of the correct position of the endotracheal tube (ET) is mandatory for all patients during initial intubation. There are several methods [27, 31, 32]:

- Direct visualization of ET passing between the vocal cords.

- Auscultation of respiratory sounds in six areas: apex, bases, trachea and epigastrium.
- Measurement of expired CO2 by capnography.
- Use of self-inflating esophageal detectors.

The most reliable methods are direct visualization of ET placement in the trachea (by direct laryngoscopy or fiber-optic bronchoscopy) and measurement of expired CO2 by capnography. Even if the tracheal tube is observed to pass through the vocal cords and its position is verified by chest expansion and auscultation during positive pressure ventilation, staff should obtain additional confirmation of the location of the tracheal tube in three ways: capnography, a CO2 wave at the end of the exhalation, or with an esophageal sensing device [27, 31].

Capnography measures and displays exhaled CO2 throughout the respiratory cycle. A persistent waveform with ventilation should be observed: during expiration, the capnography does not initially read CO2, but as the anatomical dead space is exhaled, there is an increase in exhaled CO2 to a plateau, which falls to 0% with the start of inspiration. The presence of exhaled CO2 confirms the placement of the endotracheal tube. However, capnography can produce false positives and false negatives. If gastric insufflation has occurred by mask ventilation or after ingestion of carbonated fluids, capnography may produce a false positive after esophageal intubation. In cardiac arrest, states of low cardiac output, and extremely low pulmonary blood flow, a false negative can occur [31, 32].

Esophageal sensing devices aid in detecting the location of the ET based on the anatomical difference between the trachea (a firm spine) and the esophagus (a folding spine). A self-inflating bulb is in ET after placement. Air must collapse the esophagus, while the trachea must remain permeable.

Other imprecise methods include visualization of condensed water vapor in ET, chest wall movement, and Cheney test.

Cheney test: A spark plug or catheter-like device is passed distally into the trachea. The purpose of this test is to detect the impact of the tip in the carinal or bronchial lumen. Generally, the advancement of a spark plug to a depth of 30 to 35 cm can allow appreciation of blockage of distal structures compared to unrestricted advancement if the ET is in the esophagus [27, 31].

9. DA extubation strategy: Recommendations for extubation

There is not a sufficient basis to evaluate the benefits of an extubation strategy for DA. For the DA management guidelines, an extubation strategy is considered a logical extension of the intubation strategy.

The extubation strategy will depend on the surgery or situation that led to ICU hospitalization, in addition to the patient's condition and the skill of the physician.

The recommended strategy for extubation of the DA, according to the literature, includes:

- The relative merit of extubation awake versus extubation under the effects of sedation.
- Various situations can harm ventilation after the extubation of the patient.
- An airway management plan should be implemented if the patient cannot maintain adequate ventilation after extubation.
- Short-term use of a device that can serve as a guide for accelerated re- intubation.

This type of device can be a stylet (intubation plug) or a conduit. Intubation stylets or spark plugs are generally inserted through the lumen of the tracheal tube and into the trachea before removing the tracheal tube; they can be used to provide a temporary means of oxygenation and ventilation. The tubes are inserted through the mouth and can be used for supraglottic ventilation and intubation. The intubating laryngeal mask airway and the laryngeal mask airway are examples of conduits.

10. Other considerations in DA management

10.1 Human factors

Human factors (HF) issues have been considered to have contributed to adverse outcomes in 40% of the instances reported to the National Audit Project (NAP4) [22, 23]; however, HF influences in every instance. It has been identified as latent threats (poor communication, poor training and fragile teamwork, deficiencies in equipment, and inadequate systems and protocols) predisposing to loss of situation awareness and subsequent poor decision-making that lead to final errors. Developing guidelines and a professional willingness to follow them are not enough to avoid serious complications of airway management during the procedure. During a crisis, it is common to receive more information than can be processed. An information overload impairs decision-making and can make clinicians 'lose sight of the big picture. It is of huge importance for the team to stop and think to help reduce this risk. For any plan to work well in an emergency, it must be known to all members of the team and should be rehearsed. For rare events, such as CICO, this rehearsal can be achieved with simulation training [17, 21].

10.2 Rapid sequence induction (RSI)

Intubation of the trachea with a cuffed tube offers the greatest protection against aspiration. Suxamethonium is the U.K. and other European countries the neuromuscular blocking agent of choice due to its rapid onset that allows early intubation without the need for bag-mask-ventilation (BMV). Suxamethonium has been compared with rocuronium for RSI, and both are very similar in properties [46]. The ability to antagonize the effect of rocuronium with sugammadex may be a great advantage. Sugammadex can be used as a part of the failed intubation plan, (the correct dose is 16 mg kg – 1.) Cricoid pressure can be applied to protect the airway from gastric content aspiration during the period between the loss of consciousness and placement of the tube (BURP). This is a standard maneuver of an RSI in many countries. Gentle mask ventilation after BURP and before tracheal intubation prolongs the time to desaturation. In case of initial attempts at laryngoscopy are difficult during RSI, cricoid pressure should be released. This should be done only under vision with the laryngoscope and suction available; in the event of gastric regurgitation cricoid pressure should be immediately reapplied [16, 17, 21].

10.3 Position

Adequate patient positioning maximizes the chance of successful laryngoscopy and tracheal intubation. The best position for direct laryngoscopy with a Macintosh-style blade is performed with the neck flexed and the head extended at the atlanto-occipital joint; the classic 'sniffing' position [21]. In the obese patient, the 'ramped' position must be used to ensure horizontal alignment of the external auditory meatus and the suprasternal notch because this improves the view during direct laryngoscopy [47, 48]. This position improves airway patency and respiratory mechanics, facilitating passive oxygenation during apnoea [49]. All patients must be pre-oxygenated before the induction of general anesthesia. De-nitrogenation can be achieved with an appropriate flow of 100% oxygen into the breathing system while maintaining a total face-mask seal [17, 21]. Preoxygenation increases the oxygen reserve delays the onset of hypoxia and allows more time for laryngoscopy, tracheal intubation, and airway rescue in case of a failed intubation. In healthy adults, the duration of apnoea without desaturation (defined as the interval between the onset of apnoea and the time peripheral capillary oxygen saturation reaches a value of ≤90%) is limited to 1–2 min whilst breathing room air but can be extended to up 8 min when using pre-oxygenation. The duration of apnoea without desaturation can also be prolonged by passive oxygenation during the apnoeic period, delivering up to 15 liters min − 1 of oxygen through nasal cannulae. Nasal Oxygenation During Efforts Of Securing A Tube (NODESAT) has been shown to extend the apnoea time in obese patients and patients with DA. Transnasal humidified high-flow oxygen (up to 70 liters min − 1) via nasal cannulae has been shown to extend the apnoea time.

10.4 Choice of induction agent

The induction agent should be selected according to the clinical condition of the patient. Propofol, the most commonly used induction agent in the UK, suppresses laryngeal reflexes and provides better conditions for airway management than other agents. The National Audit Project of the Royal College of Anesthetists highlighted the relationship between DA management and awareness [22, 23]. Several other agents are used depending on the clinical status, these are Midazolam, Ketamine, Etomidate, etc. It is important to ensure that the patient is anesthetized during repeated attempts at intubation. Neuromuscular block (NMB) if intubation is difficult, further attempts should not proceed without full neuromuscular block. NMB abolishes laryngeal reflexes, improves chest compliance, and facilitates face-mask ventilation. A complete NMB should be used if any difficulty is encountered with airway management. Rocuronium has a rapid onset and can be antagonized immediately with sugammadex, but the incidence of anaphylaxis may be higher than with other types of non-depolarizing NMB agents. Mask ventilation with 100% oxygen should begin as soon as possible after the induction of anesthesia. If some difficulty is encountered, the airway position should be optimized and airway maneuvers such as a chin lift or jaw thrust should be ensured.

10.5 Choice of laryngoscope

The choice of laryngoscope greatly influences the reaching a successful tracheal intubation. Video-laryngoscopes (VAL) offer an improved view when compared with traditional direct laryngoscopy and are currently the first choice or default device for many anesthetists, intensivists and emergency practitioners. Meta-analyses of RCTs comparing both types of laringoscopes in patients with predicted DA report better results with VAL but no differences in time to intubation, airway trauma, gum/lip trauma, dental trauma, or sore throat has been reported.

Airtraq is employed regularly daily in our environment even by our colleagues' Anesthesia on many patients with excellent results. We have a very good experience with this device in cases of DA. Airtraq has a lot of endorsing literature showing better results than the traditional Macintosh and Miller laryngoscopy, as well as with other VAL, reporting excellent intubation rates, less cardiac and haemodynamic alterations, better results in obese patients, a better curve of learning for novice personnel, and very good results when combined with fiber-optic bronchoscope intubation [50–52]. Regular practice is required to ensure that the improved view translates reliably into successful tracheal intubation. All intensivists, anesthetists and emergency practitioners should be trained to use VAL, and have immediate access to, a video-laryngoscope [16–21]. There are available several other interesting models of VAL as **GlideScope Video Laryngoscope, C-Mac Video Laryngoscope, Pentax Airway Scope, McGrath Video Laryngoscope, AirTraq Optical Laryngoscope, King Vision Laryngoscope**, etc. (**Figure 4**).

10.6 Tube selection

Endotracheal tubes should be selected according to the nature of the surgical procedure, age and body weight, but their size, composition material, length, etc. can influence the ease of intubation. A smaller tube usually is easier to be inserted because of a better view of the laryngeal inlet during the passage of the tube between the cords. Smaller tubes are less likely to cause trauma [53]. 'Hold-up' at the arytenoids is a feature of the left-facing bevel of most tracheal tubes and can occur whilst railroading larger tubes over a bougie, stylet, or fibrescope [54]. This problem can be solved by rotating the tube anticlockwise to change the orientation of the bevel (**Figure 5**).

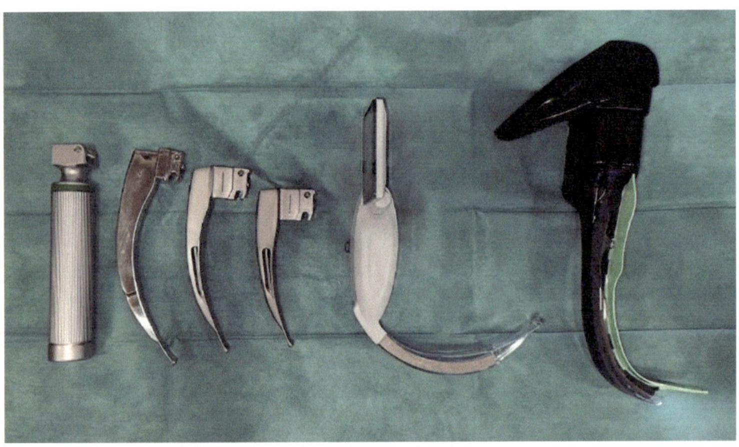

Figure 4.
Different laryngoscopes. From left to right: Traditional Macintosh, McGrath Videolaryngoscope and Airtraq Videolaryngospe.

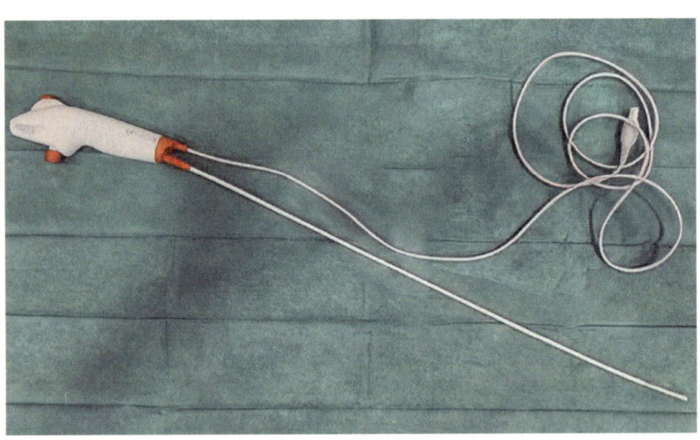

Figure 5.
Single-use fiberoptic bronchoscope.

10.7 Special situations such as Covid-19 pandemia

Managing the airway in Covid-19 pandemia have led intensivists to a point of maximum risk of exposition to the virus due to aerosols and high proximity to the patient's airway. It has been endorsed by many studies and many medical scientific societies the safety use of all personal protective equipment throughout the intubation process. It is also advised to avoid BMV if possible and when the situation allows to pre-oxygenate with a high-flow non-rebreathing mask or high-flow humidified nasal cannulae, then using RSI with a hypnotic drug and rapid depolarizing NBA. Small endotracheal tubes are not recommended due to the predicted long period of mechanical intubation and frequent plugs of mucous that interfere with the patient's adequate ventilation and oxygenation.

11. Conclusions

Intubation, the approach to a DA and the management of the different aspects of the human airway is an intrinsic domain that is supposed to be mastered by the anesthesiologist, the intensivist and the emergency physician, since all of them can face any difficult situation and life-threatening situation involving the airway.

It is also of utmost importance to have an experienced and rehearsed team, as well as a revised and well-equipped mobile chart with all the necessary material to successfully face any potentially threatening situation related to airway management. Knowing and practising under a well-coordinated guide or protocol is the best way to overcome any potential airway life-threatening situation.

We have updated and compiled relevant information on how to manage a DA crisis knowing the best available possibilities to prevail in such problematic situations.

Author details

Demetrio Pérez-Civantos*, Alicia Muñoz-Cantero, Francisco Fuentes Morillas, Pablo Nieto Sánchez, María Ángeles Santiago Triviño and Natalia Durán Caballero
Faculty of Medicine, Intensive Care Department, Badajoz University Hospital, University of Extremadura, Society of Intensive and Critical Care Medicine of Extremadura (SEXMICYUC), Badajoz, Spain

*Address all correspondence to: dpcivantos@gmail.com

References

[1] Orozco-Diaz E, Alvarez-Rios JJ, Arceo-Diaz JL, OrnelasAguirre JM. Predictive factors of difficult airway with known assessment scales. Cir Cir 2010; 78: 393-399.

[2] Domino, KB, Posner, KL, Caplan, RA, Cheney, FW Airway injury during anesthesia: A closed claims analysis.. *Anesthesiology*. (1999). *91* 1703-11 [Article] [PubMed]

[3] Paix AD, Williamson JA, Runciman WB. Crisis management during anaesthesia: Difficult intubation. Qual Saf Health Care 2005;14:e5.

[4] Salimi A, Farzanegan B, Rastegarpour A, Kolahi AA. Comparison of the upper lip bite test with measurement of thyromental distance for prediction of difficult intubations. Acta Anaesthesiol Taiwan 2008;46:61-65.

[5] Shiga T, Wajima Z, Inoue T, Sakamoto A. Predicting difficult intubation in apparently normal patients: a meta-analysis of bedside screening test performance. Anesthesiology 2005;103:429-437[a]

[6] Rosenblatt WH, Sukhupragarn W. Airway management. In: Clinical Anesthesia, 6th ed, Barash PG, Cullen BF, Stoelting RK, et al (Eds), Lippincott, Williams and Wilkins, Philadelphia 2009. p.751.

[7] Butler PJ, Dhara SS. Prediction of difficult laryngoscopy: An assessment of the thyromental distance and Mallampati predictive tests. Anaesth Intensive Care 1992; 20:139.

[8] Janssens M, Hartstein G. Management of difficult intubation. Eur J Anaesthesiol 2001; 18:3.

[9] Qudaisat IY, Al-Ghanem SM. Short thyromental distance is a surrogate for inadequate head extension, rather than small submandibular space, when indicating possible difficult direct laryngoscopy. Eur J Anaesthesiol 2011; 28:600.

[10] Mallampati SR, Gatt SP, Gugino LD, et al. A clinical sign to predict difficult tracheal intubation: A prospective study. Can Anaesth Soc J 1985; 32:429.

[11] Updated by the Committee on Standards and Practice Parameters, Jeffrey L. Apfelbaum, Carin A. Hagberg, et al, Practice Guidelines for Management of the Difficult Airway: An Updated Report by the American Society of Anesthesiologists Task Force on management of the Difficult Airway. *Anesthesiology* 2013;118(2):251-270.doi: https://doi.org/10.1097/ALN.0b013e31827773b2.

[12] Naguib M, Scamman FL, O'Sullivan C, Aker J, Ross AF, Kosmach S, Ensor JE. Predictive performance of three multivariate difficult tracheal intubation models: A double-blind, case-controlled study. Anesth Analg 2006;102:818-824.

[13] De Jong A, Molinari N, Terzi N, et al. Early identification of patients at risk for difficult intubation in the intensive care unit: Development and validation of the MACOCHA score in a multicenter cohort study. Am J Respir Crit Care Med. 2013;187(8):832-839. doi:10.1164/rccm.201210-1851OC

[14] Bell MDD. Routine pre-oxygenation – A new 'minimum standard' of care? Anaesthesia 2004; 59: 943-945

[15] Tanoubi I, Drolet P, Donati F. Optimizing preoxygenation in adults. Can J Anaesth 2009; 56: 449-466

[16] American Society of Anesthesiologists Task Force on Management of the Difficult Airway.

Practice guidelines for Management of the Difficult airway. An Updated Report. Anesthesiology 2013; 118: 251-270.

[17] Difficult Airway Society 2015 Guidelines for management of unanticipated difficult intubation in adults. Frerk C, Mitchell VS, McNarry AF, Mendonca C, R Bhagrath, Patel a, O'Sullivan E P, Woodall NM, Ahmad I and difficult airway Society intubation guidelines working group. Bri J Anaesth 2015, 115 (6): 827-848.

[18] Haynes SR, Allsop JR, Gillies GW: Arterial oxygen saturation during induction of anaesthesia and laryngeal mask insertion: Prospective evaluation of four techniques. Br J Anaesth 1992; 68:519-522.

[19] Connelly NR, Ghandour K, Robbins L, Dunn S, Gibson C. Management of unexpected difficult airway at a teaching institution over a 7-year period. J Clin Anesth 2006; 18: 198-204 56.

[20] SaklesJC,ChiuS,MosierJ,WalkerC,StolzU.Theimportance of first pass success when performing orotracheal intubation in the emergency department. Acad Emerg Med 2013; 20: 71 –8.

[21] Ahmad I, El-Boghdadly K, Bhagrath R, Hodzovic I, McNarry AF, Mir F, O'Sullivan EP, Patel A, Stacey M,Vaughan D. Difficult airway Society guidelines for awake tracheal intubation (ATI) in adults. Anaesthesia 2020; 75:509-552.

[22] Cook TM, Woodall N, Frerk C on behalf of the Royal College of Anaesthetists fourth National Audit Project. Major complications of airway management in the UK: Results of the fourth National Audit Project of the Royal College of Anaesthetists and the difficult airway Society. Part 1: Anaesthesia. Bri J Anaesth 2011; 106: 617-631.

[23] Cook TM, Woodall N, Harper J, Benger J on behalf of the Royal College of Anaesthetists fourth National Audit Project. Major complications of airway management in the UK: Results of the fourth National Audit Project of the Royal College of Anaesthetists and the difficult airway Society. Part 2: Intensive care and emergency departments. Bri J Anaesth 2011; 106: 632-642.

[24] Schälte G et al. The use of the Airtraq optical laryngoscope for routine tracheal intubation in high-risk cardiosurgical patients. BMC Research Notes 2011, 4:425.

[25] Nishikawa K , Hukuoka E, Kawagishi T, Shimodate Y. Efficacy of the Airtraq laryngoscope with a fiberoptic bronchoscope compared with that of Airtraq alone for tracheal intubation: A manikin study J Anesth 2011; 25:93-97.

[26] Agró F.E., Cataldo R., Mattei A. New devices and techniques for airway management. Minerva Anestesiology. 2009;75:141-149.

[27] Gordon YS Choi, Gavin M Joint; Chapter 29: Airway management and acute Airway obstruction; En: Andrew D. Bersten (director), OH'S Intensive Care Manual. Eight Edition. Elsevier. 2019. p 373-387.

[28] Pedro Tanaka, David Stolle Dueñas, Francisco Pérez-Cerdá Silvestre, Jesús Ruiz de las Heras, Jose Mª Calvo Vecino. Curso experto Universitario en el Manejo de la Vía aérea. Capítulo 6: Videolaringoscopios. Editorial Panamericana. P 30-32

[29] Sun F, Wang Y, Ma S, Zhu H, Yu X, Xu J; on behalf of Chinese Collaboration Group for Emergency Airway Management. Clinical consensus of emergency airway management. J Thorac Dis 2017;9(11):4599-4606. doi: 10.21037/jtd.2017.10.79 .

[30] Gerson DZ, Rosenblatt WH, Johansen MJ, et al. Use of the intubating LMA-Fastrach in 254 patients with difficult-to-manage airways. Anesthesiology 2001; 95: 1175.

[31] Irwin, R. S. Irwin and Rippe's Intensive Care Medicine, 8th Edition. Wolters Kluwer Health; 20171218. Retrieved from vbk://9781975102234201 71218.

[32] T.R. Craig, G.G. Lavery. Chapter 2: Airway Management in the Critically ill Adult. En: Joseph E. Parrillo (Director). Critical Care Medicine: Principles of diagnosis and management in the adult. Fifth edition. Elsevier. 2019 p 12-28.

[33] Francisco Pérez-Cerdá Silvestre, Ramón López Vicente, Jesús Ruiz de las Heras, Oscar Valencia Orgaz, Pedro Garrido Ortega, Sergio García Pérez. Curso Experto Universitario en el Manejo de la vía aérea. Capitulo 7: Fribrobroscoscopios y videofibroscopios. Editorial Médica Panamericana. P 22-29.

[34] M. Botana, A. Fernández-Villar, V. Leiro, C. Represas, A. Méndez, L. Piñeiro. Unidad de Técnicas Broncopleurales. Servicio de Neumología. Hospital Xeral de Vigo. Tracheal intubation guided by fibrobronchoscopy in patients with difficult airway. Predictive factors of the outcome. Scielo

[35] Alhomary M, Ramadan E, Curran E, Walsh SR. Videolaryngoscopy vs. fibreoptic bronchoscopy for awake tracheal intubation: A systematic review and meta-analysis. Anaesthesia 2018;73:1151-1161.

[36] Koga K, Asai T, Latto IP, Vaughan RS. Effect of the size of a tracheal tuve and the efficacy of the use of the laryngeal mask for fibrescope-aided tracheal intubation. Anaesthesia 1997; 52:512.

[37] Sidhu VS, Whitehead EM, Ainsworth QP, Smith M, CalderI. A technique of awake fibreoptic intubation. Experience in patients with cervical spine disease. Anaesthesia 1993;48:910-13. 95.

[38] Fuchs G, Schwarz G, Baumgartner A, Kaltenböck F, VoitAugustin H, Planinz W. Fiberoptic intubation in 327 neurosurgical patients with lesions of the cervical spine. J Neurosurg Anesth 1999;11:11-16.

[39] Badiger S, John M, Fearnley RA, Ahmad I, Asai T. Optimizing oxygenation and intubation conditions during awake fibreoptic intubation using a high-flow nasal oxygen-delivery system.Bri J Anaesth 2015;115:629-632.

[40] Ingrande J, Lemmens HJM. Dose adjustment of anaesthetics in the morbidly obese. Bri J Anaesth 2010; 105:i16–i23.

[41] Brookman CA, Teh HP, Morrison LM. Anticholinergics improve fibreoptic intubating conditions during general anaesthesia. Can J Anaesth 1997;44:165-167.

[42] Woodall NM, Harwood RJ, Barker GL, et al. Complications of awake fibreoptic intubation without sedation in 200 healthy anaesthetists attending a training course. Bri J Anaesth 2008;100:850-5. 60.

[43] Patil V, Barker GL, Harwood RJ, Woodall NM. Training course in local anaesthesia of the airway and fibreoptic intubation using course delegates as subjects. British J Anaesth 2002;89:586-593.

[44] Rosenstock CV, Thogersen B, Afshari A, Christensen AL, Eriksen C, Gíatke M. Awake fiberoptic or awake laryngoscopic tracheal intubation in patients with anticipated difficult airway management. Anesthesiology 2012;116(2): 1210-1216

[45] M. Haro Estarriol, M. Rubio Goday, MT. Casamitja Sot. Sección de Neumología. Hospital Universitario de Girona Doctor Josep Trueta. Avances en broncoscopia. Anales de Neumología 2013; 118 (3): 1641-1618

[46] Sørensen MK, Bretlau C, Gätke MR, Sørensen AM, Rasmussen LS. Rapid sequence induction and intubation with rocuronium–sugammadex compared with succinylcholine: A randomized trial. Br J Anaesth 2012; 108: 682-689.

[47] Collins JS, Lemmens HJM, Brodsky JB, Brock-Utne JG, Levitan RM. Laryngoscopy and morbid obesity: A comparison of the 'sniff' and 'ramped' positions. Obes Surg 2004; 14: 1171-1175.

[48] Murphy C, Wong DT. Airway management and oxygenation in obese patients. Can J Anaesth 2013; 60: 929-945.

[49] Rao SL, Kunselman AR, Schuler HG, Desharnais S. Laryngoscopy and tracheal intubation in the head-elevated position in obese patients: A randomized, controlled, equivalence trial. Anesth Analg 2008; 107: 1912-1918.

[50] Lu H Y, Jiang H, Zhu YS. Airtraq laryngoscope versus conventional Macintosh laryngoscope: A systematic review and meta-analysis. Anaesthesia 2011;66(12):1160-1167. doi: 10.1111/j.1365-2044.2011.06871.x.

[51] Maharaj CH et al. A comparison of tracheal intubation using the Airtraq or the Macintosh laryngoscope in routine airway management: A randomized, controlled clinical trial. Anaesthesia, 2006;61:1093-1099.

[52] Amathieu R et al. An algorithm for difficult airway management, modified for modern optical devices (Airtraq laryngoscope; LMA CTrach™): A 2-year prospective validation in patients for elective abdominal, gynecologic, and thyroid surgery. Anesthesiology 2011;114(1):25-33. doi: 10.1097/ALN.0b013e318201c44f.

[53] Koh KF, Hare JD, Calder I. Small tubes revisited. Anaesthesia 1998; 53: 46.

[54] Marfin AG, Iqbal R, Mihm F, Popat MT, Scott SH, Pandit JJ. Determination of the site of tracheal tube impingement during nasotracheal fibreoptic intubation. Anaesthesia 2006; 61: 646-650.